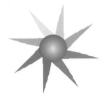

Perspective Press

THE

PHARMACY TECHNICIAN

FOURTH EDITION

MORTON PUBLISHING COMPANY
www.morton-pub.com

Morton Publishing

Fourth Edition
Copyright © 2010, 2007, 2004, 1999 by Morton Publishing Company

Printed in the United States of America.

Morton Publishing Company
925 West Kenyon Avenue, Unit 12
Englewood, CO 80110
phone: 1-303-761-4805
fax: 1-303-762-9923
www.morton-pub.com

International Standard Book Number

ISBN 10: 0-89582-828-6
ISBN 13: 978-0-89582-828-6

10 9 8 7 6 5 4 3 2

Library of Congress Control Number: 2009926153

Cover photo credit: ©iStockphoto.com/Steve Cole, christie and cole studio inc.

NOTICE

To the best of the Publisher's knowledge, the information presented in this book follows general practice as well as federal and state regulations and guidelines. However, please note that you are responsible for following your employer's and your state's policies and guidelines.

The job description for pharmacy technicians varies by institution and state. Your employer and state can provide you with the most recent regulations, guidelines, and practices that apply to your work.

The Publisher of this book disclaims any responsibility whatsoever for any injuries, damages, or other conditions that result from your practice of the skills described in this book for any reason whatsoever.

CONTENTS

Contents

PREFACE

The Pharmacy Technician and *The Pharmacy Technician Workbook & Certification Review* have successfully trained thousands of practicing pharmacy technicians and are officially endorsed by the American Pharmacists Association (APhA).

FEATURES

This book has been specially designed and developed to make learning easier and more productive.

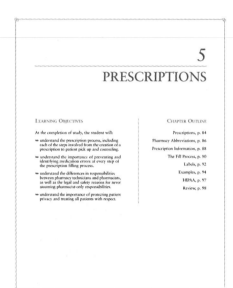

New: Each chapter opens with **Learning Objectives** and a **page-referenced Chapter Outline** to provide an overview of the chapter and allow for easy location of contents.

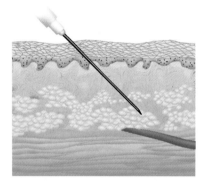

Illustrations are used extensively to provide information and reinforce text discussions.

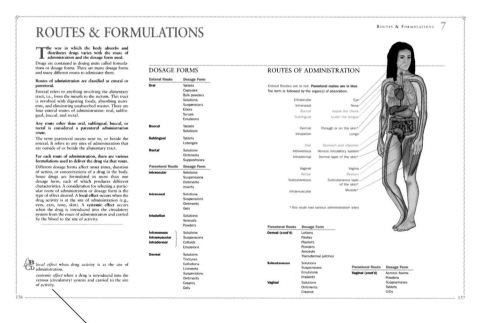

A distinctive **facing-page design** makes it easier to identify important points and to make connections between concepts. Illustrations are always on the same spread as corresponding text discussions. Topics are presented in perspective. Information is easy to find and understand.

A **running glossary,** represented by the symbol at left and shown in the page above, emphasizes important vocabulary throughout the text, making terms easy to locate and review.

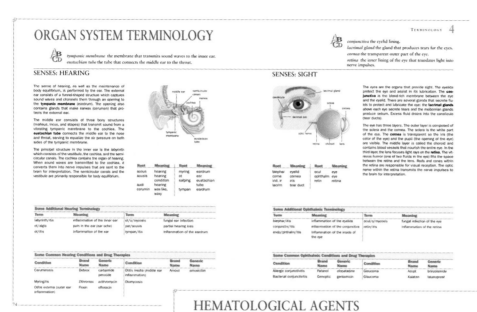

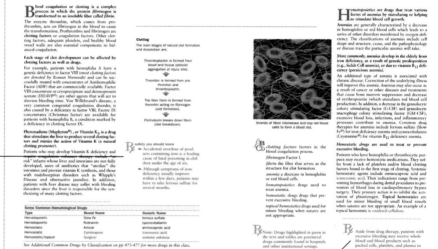

New: The *Fourth Edition* has more emphasis on **common disease conditions and corresponding drugs and drug therapies,** especially in the Organ Systems discussions in Chapter 4 (Terminology) and in Chapter 18, Common Drugs and Their Uses.

New: The *Fourth Edition* has more emphasis on quality and safety throughout the book, including new **Rx Safety You Should Know** features.

The **Rx symbol** indicates points of emphasis, useful tips, related content points, and information on additional resources that help provide a recipe for success.

End of chapter **Reviews** provide:

✔ a checklist of the **Key Concepts** in the chapter;

✔ **Match the Terms** exercise(s) that now include *all* ABCD key terms in the chapter (**new**);

✔ and **Multiple Choice** questions in the same sequence as the presentation of chapter topics.

KEY CHANGES IN THE FOURTH EDITION

This text has been carefully revised and updated throughout. Some of the more significant individual chapter changes are:

➡ Chapter 4 on *Terminology* now has two sets of tables for each organ system: an "Additional Terminology" table focusing on the terminology for common diseases, conditions, and/or treatments and a "Common Conditions and Drug Therapies" table that lists common conditions and the brand and generic names for corresponding drug therapies.

➡ In Chapter 5 on *Prescriptions*, the Common Abbreviations tables have been revised to clarify the categories of abbreviations and to provide prescription examples using the abbreviations. In addition, the sections on The Technician's Role and The Pharmacist's Role are revised and reorganized to put emphasis on the technician's role and the distinction between the technician and pharmacist roles.

➡ Chapter 6 on *Calculations* has new sections on Alligation and Powder Volume.

➡ Chapter 8 is now called *Parenterals: Sterile Compounding*. It has been significantly revised and re-organized with an expanded section on Administration Devices, a new section on Parenteral Incompatibilities, and a new section on Quality Assurance and Infection Control.

➡ Chapter 12 on *Information* has thoroughly updated information on all sources and the Common References section now emphasizes knowing when to use each source.

➡ Chapter 13 on *Inventory* has updated information on many topics including receiving and disposing of cytotoxic and other hazardous or non-returnable drugs, MSDS sheets, "fast movers and slow movers," seasonal drugs, preventing theft and drug diversion, hospital pharmacy inventory, automated systems, and durable and non-durable equipment supplies.

➡ Chapter15 on *Community Pharmacy* has updated and revised material on such topics as disease state management services and clinics, scanning original prescriptions, retrieving the correct drug when filling a prescription, the final check by the pharmacist, and filing hard copies of controlled substances prescriptions.

➡ Chapter 16 on *Hospital Pharmacy* has been carefully updated throughout with a new section on Technician Roles and an expanded section on Calculations.

➡ A new chapter 18 on *Common Drugs and Their Uses* integrates common drugs into each drug classification section and includes a list of Additional Common Drugs by Classification; has expanded discussions of many classification sections such as Antineoplastics; and highlights common hospital parenteral drugs in green where they appear throughout the chapter.

➡ The Appendices include Look-Alike / Sound-Alike Drugs, the Top 200 Brand Name Drugs, the Top 200 Generic Drugs, and a list of Commonly Refrigerated Drugs.

COMPANION WORKBOOK

The Pharmacy Technician Workbook and Certification Review, Fourth Edition offers hundreds of carefully explained key terms and concepts, over 1,000 exercises and problems for self-testing, *In the Workplace* sample documents and job-related information, and lists of the top 200 brand name drugs, top 200 generic drugs, and the top 200 drugs sorted by classification. This workbook can also be used in preparation for national certification exams such as the Pharmacy Technician Certification Exam (PTCE) and the Exam for Certification of Pharmacy Technicians (ExCPT). It provides two certification practice exams, one in the format of the PTCE and one in the format of the ExCPT. In addition, the *Workbook* contains a Calculations Practice Exam for practice in solving quantitative problems on the certification exams. ISBN: 978-0-89582-829-3.

ACKNOWLEDGMENTS

CONTRIBUTORS

We would like to thank the following people for their contributions to this book. Aside from developing and/or revising their specific chapter(s), they have been a great help with the whole book from making suggestions to providing general, and often frequent, assistance.

Robert P. Shrewsbury, Ph.D., R.Ph., Associate Professor of Pharmaceutics, University of North Carolina-Chapel Hill
> *Bob developed the material for Chapters 4, 7, 8, 9, 10, and 11, as well as the Appendix on Commonly Refrigerated Drugs. His involvement in this book has been invaluable.*

Brenda Vonderau, B.Sc. (Pharm.), Director, Medication Therapy Management Programs, Catalyst Rx
> *Brenda developed the Chapter on Prescriptions.*

Mary F. Powers, Ph.D., R.Ph., Associate Professor, University of Toledo College of Pharmacy
> *Mary developed the Financial Issues and Calculations chapters, revised what was the Classifications Appendix into a new Chapter 18 on Common Drugs and Their Uses, and prepared the lists of the top 200 brand name and generic drugs. In addition, Mary is the author of the Workbook accompanying this text. She has provided help and feedback throughout the development of the entire project, for which we are very grateful.*

Cindy B. Johnson, R.Ph., L.C.S.W., RxMentor Pharmacist, Humana
> *Cindy developed the Information chapter.*

Steve Johnson, BS., R.Ph., Meditech Lead Analyst, Catholic Health Initiatives
> *Steve revised the Inventory chapter. We are glad to have him on board.*

Ruth Duke, Pharm.D., Pharmacist, CVS Pharmacy
> *Ruth developed the material for the Community Pharmacy chapter and helped in getting valuable photography that has been transformed into art in this book.*

Pamela Nicoski, Pharm.D., Clinical Pharmacist, Loyola University Medical Center and Britta Penn, Pharm.D., Clinical Pharmacist, Children's Memorial Hospital
> *Pamela and Britta developed the Hospital Pharmacy chapter.*

Melanie V. Duhaine, R.N., B.S.N., M.Ed., Director of Nursing, Fairchild Manor, Senior-Associates of Western New York
> *Melanie developed what was the Classifications Appendix for the first three editions of the text.*

In addition we would like to thank the following reviewers who provided feedback on the previous editions which we used to help prepare the *Fourth Edition*: James Austin, R.N., B.S.N., CPhT, Program Chair, Pharmacy Technology Program, Weatherford College, Weatherford, Texas; CVS Pharmacy; Marisa Fetzer, Institute of Technology, Clovis, CA; Claudia Johnson, M.S.N., R.N.C., A.P.N., Allied Health Instructor, Pharmacy Technician Program, Polytech Adult Education; Mary Anna Marshall, CPhT, Instructor for PTCB Examination Review, CVS/Pharmacy Regional Intern Coordinator, Virginia Pharmacists Association, and Teacher in the Pharmacy Technician Program, Hanover High School, Richmond, VA; Tony David Ornelas, CPhT; Peter E. Vonderau, Sr., R.Ph., Pharmacy Manager, Scolari's Food & Drug, Inc.; and Walgreen Co.

Finally, we would like to thank Tammy Newnam for preparing all the in-text art and Hannah Hogan for designing and preparing the cover for the *Fourth Edition*. Patricia Billiot did a very thorough job proof-reading. And Dona Mendoza, Chrissy Morton, and Carter Fenton at Morton Publishers were always very helpful.

Perspective Press

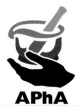

AMERICAN PHARMACISTS ASSOCIATION

BASIC PHARMACY AND PHARMACOLOGY SERIES

Dear Student or Instructor,

The American Pharmacists Association (APhA), the national professional society of pharmacists in the United States, and Morton Publishing Company, a publisher of educational texts and training materials in healthcare, are pleased to present this outstanding textbook, *The Pharmacy Technician, Fourth Edition*. It is one of a series of distinctive texts and training materials for basic pharmacy and pharmacology training published under this banner: *American Pharmacists Association Basic Pharmacy and Pharmacology Series*.

Each book in the series is oriented toward developing an understanding of fundamental concepts. In addition, each text presents applied and practical information on the skills necessary to function effectively in positions such as technicians and medical assistants who work with medications below the prescriber level and whose role in healthcare is increasingly important. Each of the books in the series uses a visual design to enhance understanding and ease of use and is accompanied by various instructional support materials. We think you will find them valuable training tools.

The American Pharmacists Association and Morton Publishing thank you for using this book and invite you to look at other titles in this series, which are listed below.

Thomas E. Menighan, BSPharm, MBA
Executive Vice President
Chief Executive Officer
American Pharmacists Association

Douglas N. Morton
President
Morton Publishing Company

TITLES IN THIS SERIES:

The Pharmacy Technician, Fourth Edition

The Pharmacy Technician Workbook and Certification Review, Fourth Edition

Medication Workbook for Pharmacy Technicians: A Pharmacology Primer (2012)

THE

PHARMACY TECHNICIAN

Fourth Edition

1

PHARMACY & HEALTH CARE

LEARNING OBJECTIVES

At the completion of study, the student will:

➡ be familiar with the overall history of pharmacy from ancient times through today.

➡ have an overall understanding of the pharmacy profession and the settings and economic environment in which it operates.

➡ have a general understanding of how computers are used in pharmacy.

ORIGINS

In earliest times, medicine was based in magic and religion.

Like many ancient peoples, Sumerians living between the Tigris and Euphrates rivers around 4,000 B.C. believed that demons were the cause of illness. They studied the stars and the intestines of animals for clues to the supernatural causes of man's condition and fate. In many cultures, physicians were priests, and sometimes considered gods or demi-gods. The Egyptian Imhotep, for example, born around 3,000 B.C., was a priest and adviser to pharaohs and was the first physician known by name. After his death, he was named a demi-god and eventually a god: the Egyptian god of medicine.

The supernatural approach to treating illness gradually gave way to a more scientific approach, based on observation and experimentation.

Around 400 B.C., the Greek physician Hippocrates developed a more scientific approach which has guided Western medicine for much of the time since. He promoted the idea of diagnosing illness based on careful observation of the patient's condition, not supernatural or other external elements. He also wrote the oath which physicians recited for centuries and still honor today: the Hippocratic Oath. From Hippocrates and others following in his footsteps, an approach to medicine in which natural causes were examined scientifically gradually grew to become the dominant approach to treating human illness.

 synthetic with chemicals, combining simpler chemicals into more complex compounds, creating a new chemical not found in nature as a result.

The Greek god of Medicine

The ancient Greek Aesculapius was said to have been such an extraordinary physician that he could keep his patients from dying and even raise the dead. This skill angered Pluto, the god of the underworld, because it reduced the number of his subjects. At Pluto's request, Zeus killed Aesculapius with a lightning bolt, then named him the god of medicine. Aesculapius' daughter, Panacea, became the goddess of medicinal herbs.

MEDICAL MYTH

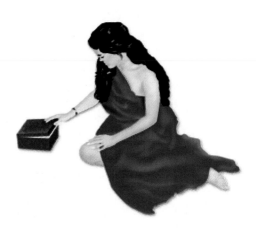

Pandora's Box

As punishment for Prometheus's theft of fire for mankind, the Greek god Zeus created Pandora and had her collect "gifts" for man from the gods. These gifts were really punishments that included disease and pestilence. They were released upon the world when Pandora opened her box.

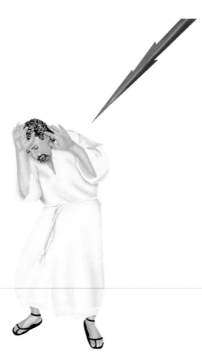

NATURE'S MEDICINE

A Treatment for Malaria

Malaria had long been one of the most deadly diseases in world history, until medicine made from the bark of a Peruvian tree, the Cinchona, was discovered. The medicine was quinine, popularly called "Jesuit's powder" for the Spanish priests that sent it to Europe from the New World. Its use along with preventive measures aimed at eradicating the cause of malaria brought the deadly disease under control.

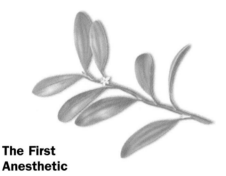

The First Anesthetic

Long before Spanish explorers noticed it, the Indians of the Andes chewed coca leaves for their medicinal effects, which included increased endurance. The active ingredient in the leaves was cocaine, which in 1884 was shown to be the first effective local anesthetic by Carl Koller, a Viennese surgeon. This discovery revolutionized surgery and dentistry, since previously anesthesia was administered on a general basis— that is, to the whole body. Eventually, because of its harmful properties when abused, a man-made substitute was developed, called procaine or Novocain®.

Besides looking to the supernatural, ancient man also looked to the natural world for medical answers.

Early man understood that plants and other natural materials had the power to treat or relieve illness. The ancient Sumerians used about 250 natural medicines derived from plants, many of which are still used today. Around 3000 B.C., the Chinese Emperor Shen Nung is said to have begun eating plants and other natural materials to determine which were poisonous and which were beneficial. One of the first known practitioners of "trial and error" drug testing, he is believed to have established 365 "herbs" that could be used in health treatments. Over the centuries, this number was gradually expanded by various Chinese physicians into the thousands. Herbal medicine remains a major component of Chinese medicine today.

Through the ages, people have used drugs to treat illnesses and other physical conditions.

Ancient cultures around the world used medicines made from natural sources, many of which contained drugs that we still use today. Over the past two centuries, however, science found ways to create **synthetic** drugs, which often have advantages in cost, effect, and availability. Some of these man-made drugs replaced natural drugs and others were for entirely new uses. Today, while we still rely on many drugs derived from natural sources, we use more than twice as many synthetically produced drugs as naturally produced ones. As a result, the number of illnesses and physical conditions that can be treated with drugs is constantly increasing.

Nature's Aspirin

The ancient Greek physicians Hippocrates and Dioscorides both wrote about the pain relieving ability of the bark of a white willow tree that grew in the Mediterranean. In the 1800's, more than 2,000 years after Hippocrates' time, the active ingredient in the willow bark, salicylic acid, was derived by chemists. However, because of difficulties in taking salicylic acid internally, acetylsalicylic acid, popularly known as aspirin, was developed and it eventually became the most widely used drug in the world.

MEDICINE THROUGH THE AGES

— A Timeline —

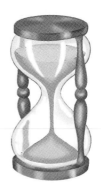

3000 B.C.

The **Egyptian Imhotep,** born around 3,000 B.C., was a priest and adviser to pharaohs and the first physician known by name. After his death, he was named a demi-god and eventually a god: the Egyptian god of medicine.

4000 B.C.

Ancient **Sumerians** studied the stars and animal intestines to divine man's fate and physical condition.

500 B.C.

The **Greek Alcmaeon,** a student of Pythagorus, saw diseases as a result of a loss of the body's natural equilibrium, rather than the work of the gods.

| 4000 B.C. | 3000 B.C. | 2000 B.C. | 1000 B.C. | 500 B.C. | 250 B.C. |

3000 B.C.

The **Chinese Emperor Shen Nung** is said to have begun tasting plants and other natural materials to determine which were poisonous and which were beneficial. One of the first known practitioners of "trial and error" drug testing, he is credited with establishing hundreds of herbal medicines.

1500 B.C.

The most complete record of ancient Egyptian medicine and pharmacology, called the **Papyrus Ebers,** dates back to 1500 B.C. This 1100 page scroll document includes about 800 prescriptions using 700 drugs, mostly derived from plants.

600 B.C.

A cult following **Aesculapius, the Greek god of Medicine,** established centers where medicine was practiced. These early clinics became training grounds for the great Greek physicians of later years.

400 B.C.

A number of medical documents are written by different Greek physicians under the name **Hippocrates.** The works avoid the supernatural and religious and represent an approach to medicine that is grounded in scientific reasoning and close observation of the patient. They contain writings about the conduct of physicians, including the famous Hippocratic oath.

 pharmacology the study of drugs—their properties, uses, application, and effects (from the Greek *pharmakon:* drug, and *logos:* word or thought).

pharmacognosy derived from the Greek words "pharmakon" or drug and "gnosis" or knowledge; the study of physical, chemical, biochemical and biological properties of drugs as well as the search for new drugs from natural sources.

100 B.C.

King Mithridates of Pontos practiced an early form of immunization by taking small amounts of poisons so that he could build his tolerance of them. It is said that he was so successful at this that when he eventually decided to kill himself through poisoning, he was unable to, and had to be killed by someone else. The potion Mithridates developed, Mithridaticum, was believed to be good at promoting health and was used for fifteen hundred years.

77 B.C.

Dioscorides, a Greek physician working in the Roman Legion, wrote the **De Materia Medica**, five books that described over 600 plants and their healing properties. His work was the main influence for Western pharmaceutics for over sixteen hundred years. One of the remedies he described was made from the bark of a type of willow tree, the active ingredient of which was salicylic acid, the natural drug on which acetylsalicylic acid (aspirin) is based. He also described how to get opium from poppies.

162 A.D.

The Greek physician **Galen** went to Rome and became the greatest name in Western medicine since Hippocrates both through his practice and extensive writings, nearly 100 of which survive. He believed there were four "humours" in man which needed to be in balance for good health, and he advocated "bleeding" to assist that balance. He also believed in the vigorous application of a scientific approach to medicine and his emphasis on education, observation, and logic formed the cornerstone for Western medicine.

| 200 B.C. | 100 B.C. | 1 A.D. | 100 A.D. | 200 A.D. |

---

200 B.C.

The first official Chinese "herbal," the **Shen Nung Pen Tsao**, listing 365 herbs for use in health treatments, is believed to have been published. This can be considered an early Chinese forerunner to the FDA approved drug list.

100 A.D.

The **Indian physician Charaka** wrote the **Charaka Samhita**, the first great book of Indian medicine, which among other things described over 500 herbal drugs that had been known and used in India for many centuries.

 Note: since the use of drugs goes so far back in history, we use many terms based on Greek or Latin words.

pharmacopeia an authoritative listing of drugs and issues related to their use.

pharmaceutical of or about drugs; also, a drug product.

panacea a cure-all (from the Greek *panakeia*, same meaning).

materia medica generally pharmacology, but also refers to the drugs in use (from the Latin materia, matter, and medica, medical).

MEDICINE THROUGH THE AGES

— A Timeline —

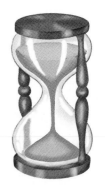

900 A.D.

The **Persian Rhazes** wrote one of the most popular textbooks of medicine in the Middle Ages, the **Book of Medicine Dedicated to Mansur**. A man of science, Rhazes was also an alchemist who believed he could turn lesser metal into gold. When he failed to do this, the Caliph ordered him beaten over the head with his own chemistry book until either his head or the book broke. Apparently, it was a tie. Rhazes lost sight in one eye but lived to continue his work.

1500 A.D.

When the Spanish found them, the **Indians of Mexico** had a well established pharmacology that included more than 1,200 drugs and was clearly the result of many hundreds of years of medical practice. One plant, the sarsaparilla, became very popular in Europe for its use on kidney and bladder ailments and can be found to this day in many medicinal teas.

1580 A.D.

In China, **Li Shi Zhen** completed the **Pen Tsao Kang Mu**, a compilation of nearly 2,000 drugs for use in treating illness and other conditions.

1630 A.D.

Jesuits sent **quinine** back to Europe in the early sixteen hundreds. Also called Jesuit's powder, it was the first drug to be used successfully in the treatment of the dreaded disease malaria.

Timeline: 750 | 1000 | 1250 | 1500 | 1750

1000 A.D.

Perhaps the greatest Islamic physician was **Avicenna**. His writings dominated medical thinking in Europe for centuries. He wrote a five volume encyclopedia, one of which was devoted to natural medications and another to compounding drugs from individual medications.

1500 A.D.

In the early fifteen hundreds, a Swiss alchemist who went by the name of **Paracelsus** rejected the "humoural" philosophy of Galen and all previous medical teaching other than Hippocrates. Though he had many critics, he is generally credited with firmly establishing the use of chemistry to create medicinal drugs. Included in his work is the first published recipe for the addictive drug laudanum, which became a popular though tragically abused drug for the next three hundred years.

1721 A.D.

Dr. Zabdiel Boylston becomes the first person in what is now the United States to administer a **smallpox vaccine**. Much of the Boston population was initially extremely suspicious. After several months, however, 249 people were eventually inoculated, six of whom died. This compared with 844 deaths among the 5,980 people who contracted the disease naturally.

1796

Edward Jenner successfully uses a vaccine from the milder cowpox disease to inoculate against smallpox.

antitoxin a substance that acts against a toxin in the body; also, a vaccine containing antitoxins, used to fight disease.

antibiotic a substance which harms or kills microorganisms like bacteria and fungi.

hormones chemicals produced by the body that regulate body functions and processes.

human genome the complete set of genetic material contained in a human cell.

1785 A.D.

The **British Physician, William Withering**, publishes his study of the **foxglove** plant and the drug it contained, **digitalis**, which became widely used in treating heart disease. Foxglove had been used since ancient times in various remedies but Withering described a process for creating the drug from the dried leaves of the plant and established a dosage approach.

1803

The German pharmacist **Frederich Serturner** extracts morphine from opium.

1846

In Boston, the first publicized operation using **general anesthesia** is performed. Ether is the anaesthetic.

1899

Acetylsalicylic acid, popularly known as **aspirin,** is developed because of difficulties in using salicylic acid, a drug contained in certain willow trees that had long been used in the external treatment of various conditions.

1921

In Toronto, Canada, **Frederick Banting** and **Charles Best** show that an extract of the hormone, **insulin,** will lower blood sugar in dogs and so may be useful in the treatment of the terrible disease diabetes. The biochemist James B. Collip then develops an extract of insulin pure enough to test on humans. The first human trial in January, 1922 proves successful and dramatically changes the prospects for all diabetics.

1957

Albert Sabin develops an **oral polio vaccine** using a weakened live virus that could be taken orally rather than by injection. However, because of risk of an associated disease from the live virus, only the injectable form of the vaccine is used to inoculate children after January 2000.

1960

The **birth control pill** is introduced.

1981

First documented cases of **AIDS.**

1987

AZT becomes the first drug approved by the FDA for AIDS treatment.

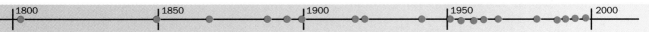

1864

Louis Pasteur's experiments show that microorganisms cause food spoilage, and that heat can be used to kill them and preserve the food. Though others had proposed principles of **"germ theory"** previously, Pasteur's work is instrumental in it becoming widely accepted.

1884

In 1884, **Carl Koller,** a Viennese surgeon, discovers that cocaine, the active ingredient in coca leaves, was useful as a local anesthetic in eye surgery, and cocaine is established as the **first local anesthetic**.

1890

Effective **antitoxins** are developed for diptheria and tetanus, giving a major boost to the development of medicines that fight infectious disease.

1928

In Britain, **Alexander Fleming** discovers a fungus which produces a chemical that kills bacteria. He names the chemical, **penicillin.** It is the first antibiotic drug.

1943

Russell Marker is able to create the **hormone progesterone,** the first reliable birth control drug, from a species of Mexican yam.

1951

James Watson and **Francis Crick** identify the structure of **DNA**, the basic component within the cell that contains the organism's genetic code.

1955

Dr. Jonas Salk succeeds in developing a refined **injectable polio vaccine** from killed polio virus. (In 1954 polio had killed more than 13,000 and crippled more than 18,000 Americans.)

1988

The **Human Genome Project** is begun with the goal of mapping the entire DNA sequence in the human genome, This information will provide a better understanding of hereditary diseases and allow the development of new treatments for them.

1989

Amgen, a **biotechnology** company that develops products based on advances in cellular and molecular biology, introduces its first product, Epogen, an anemia treatment for dialysis patients.

1996

HAART (Highly Active Anti-Retroviral Therapy) is introduced for AIDS treatment. Made up of a combination of one protease inhibitor and usually two antiretroviral drugs, it proves extremely effective in slowing HIV progress and is partially responsible for a 47% decrease in the AIDS death rate in 1997.

THE 20TH CENTURY

The average life span in the United States increased by over twenty years in the Twentieth Century.

In 1900, the average American lived only into their early fifties. By 2000, the average life expectancy at birth in the United States had risen to 77 years, and as of 2007 it was 77.9 years. Similar changes were seen throughout the industrialized world and to a lesser extent in developing countries. The growth of hospitals, advances in the treatment of disease, improved medical technology, better understanding of nutrition and health, and the rapid increase in the number of effective drugs and vaccines have all contributed to this profound change in improved life experience.

A major factor in the increased health and life expectancy seen in this century was the dramatic growth in pharmaceutical medicine.

Since the eighteenth century, there was a growing interest and success in creating man-made or synthetic medicines. The creation of aspirin in 1899 was followed by more pharmaceutical research and discoveries that spurred the growth of a worldwide industry committed to creating medicines for virtually every illness and condition. The discovery of the antibiotic penicillin was followed shortly by a World War in which its mass production was seen as critical to Allied success. This and other war-related drug needs stimulated the U.S. pharmaceutical industry to dramatically boost its capacity and production. Ever since, pharmaceutical research and development in the U.S. has grown substantially, making it the world's leading producer of medical pharmaceuticals.

LIVING LONGER

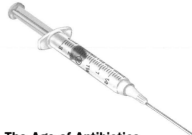

The Age of Antibiotics

In World War I, more soldiers died from infections than the wounds themselves. Although penicillin was discovered as an antibiotic in 1928, it was difficult to produce and for years not much was made of the discovery. With the start of World War II, however, British scientists looked again at penicillin and established that it was effective in fighting infections. Already under attack from Germany and unable to develop mass production methods for penicillin, the British sought help in the United States. In 1942, the Pfizer pharmaceutical company was able to develop a method for mass production of the drug, and by D-Day the Allied army was well stocked with it. Its use saved many thousands of lives during the war and revolutionized the pharmaceutical industry. A period of intense research and discovery in the field of antibiotics began, and many new antibiotics were developed which have dramatically contributed to improved health and increased life expectancy.

Living Longer

Improved pharmaceutical products have had a major effect on the life span of Americans and others in the twentieth century. In the U.S., the life span increased about 64% in the last century, with much of the increase due to the discovery and use of disease fighting drugs.

Source: National Center of Health Statistics

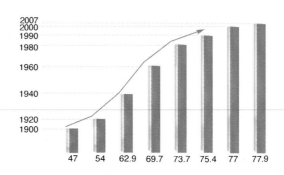

2007	2000	1990	1980	1960	1940	1920	1900
47	54	62.9	69.7	73.7	75.4	77	77.9

With the increasing availability of powerful drugs, their regulation became more important than ever.

Leaders and governments have long sought to regulate the use of medicinal drugs because of their effect on the population's health. The explosive growth of pharmaceuticals in the twentieth century made governments throughout the world keenly aware of the importance of setting and maintaining standards for their distribution and use.

In the United States, drug regulation is performed by the Food and Drug Administration.

FDA activity is a major factor in the nation's public health and safety. Before a drug can be marketed, it must be shown through testing that it is safe and effective for its intended use. Once marketed, the FDA monitors drugs to make sure they work as intended, and that there are no serious negative (adverse) effects from their use. If drugs that are marketed are found to have significant adverse effects, the FDA can recall them (take them off the market).

The discovery of new drugs requires a major investment of time, research, and development.

The pharmaceutical industry employs thousands of scientists and devotes about one-sixth of its income to research and development. Bringing a new drug to market is a long and difficult process in which the vast majority of research does not produce a successful drug. Thousands of chemical combinations must be tried in order to find one that might work as hoped. Once a potentially useful drug is created, it must undergo an extensive testing and approval process before it can be made available to the public. In the United States, the length of time from the beginning of development through testing and to ultimate FDA approval is often more than ten years.

THE DRUG INDUSTRY

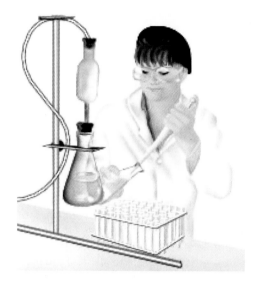

Patenting Discoveries

As with other scientific and technological areas, patenting new discoveries is an important part of the pharmaceutical development process since it protects against illegal copying of the discovery. The company holding the patent is then able to control the marketing of the product and use this as a way to recover their original investment. Since patenting generally occurs long before a drug is approved, however, a company generally has only about ten years of patent protection left in which to market their product without competition from direct copies called "generic" versions. For more information, see the section on New Drug Approval and Marketed Drugs in Chapter 3.

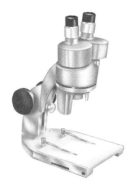

It's in the Genes

One of the most exciting areas of pharmaceutical research is performed by molecular biologists studying human genes. While antibiotics are the answer for many infectious diseases, many other diseases which seemed based on heredity are effectively untreatable. The study of the human genome has shown that many diseases are related to genetic defects. This has led to the creation of new drugs that can successfully treat many diseases previously considered untreatable. As a result, the field of biotechnology has become the most dynamic area of pharmaceutical research and development.

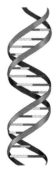

PHARMACY TODAY

A "prescription" drug is one that has been ordered or "prescribed" by a physician or other licensed prescriber to treat a patient. Though physicians occasionally give patients the actual medication, in most cases the individual who dispenses the prescribed medication to the patient is a pharmacist. Pharmacists at the more than 50,000 community pharmacies account for approximately half of the distribution of prescription drugs in the United States. The rest reach consumers primarily through hospitals, mass merchandisers, food stores, mail order pharmacies, clinics, and nursing home— all of which employ pharmacists for the dispensing of medications.

The pharmacist has consistently been rated as one of the most highly trusted professionals in the U.S.

The sheer number of available drugs, their different names and costs, multiple prescriptions from different physicians, and the involvement of third-party insurers are among the many factors which make using prescription drugs a complex area for consumers. As a result, they rely on pharmacists to provide information and advice on prescription and over-the-counter medications in easy to understand language. They also routinely ask the pharmacist to make recommendations about less expensive generic substitutes for a prescribed drug.

In 1990, the U.S. Congress required pharmacists to provide counseling services to Medicaid patients in the Omnibus Budget Reconciliation Act (OBRA).

Since then, a number of states have begun requiring this for all patients, and it is generally considered a fundamental service for pharmacists to provide.

Between 1997 and 2007 the number of prescriptions filled in the United States increased by 72% while the number of pharmacists employed increased by approximately 15%.

To help with this increasingly complex environment, pharmacists use powerful computerized tools and specially-trained assistants. Computers put customer profiles, product, inventory, pricing, and other essential information within easy access. Pharmacy technicians perform many tasks that pharmacists once performed.

THE PHARMACIST

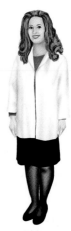

A Trusted Profession

Pharmacists consistently rank as one of the mostly highly trusted and ethical professions in the United States, according to Gallup Polls. In 2008, the top five professions were:

1. Nurses
2. Pharmacists
3. Medical Doctors
4. Police Officers
5. Clergy

Education

To become a pharmacist, an individual must have earned a Doctor of Pharmacy degree from an accredited college of pharmacy (of which there are about 93 in the U.S.), pass a state licensing exam (in some states), and perform experiential training under a licensed pharmacist. Once licensed, the pharmacist must receive continuing education to maintain their license. Pharmacists seeking to teach, do research, or work in hospitals often must have postdoctoral training in the form of residency and fellowship training. Three out of five pharmacists work in community pharmacies; one out of four in hospitals.

PHARMACY SETTINGS

Most pharmacists and pharmacy technicians work in either a community pharmacy or hospital setting, with community pharmacy being the area of greatest employment (about half of all pharmacists and technicians). However, there are a number of other environments where significant employment can be found. The primary environments for pharmacist and technician employment are:

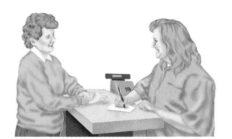

- **community pharmacies:** the area of greatest employment.
- **hospitals:** the next greatest area of employment.
- **mail order operations:** pharmacy businesses that provide drugs by mail to patients—a fast growing area.
- **long-term care:** residence facilities that provide care on a long-term rather than acute or short-term basis.
- **managed care:** care that is managed by an insurer, such as Kaiser Permanente.
- **home care:** care provided to patients in their home, often by a hospital or by a home care agency working with a home care pharmacy.

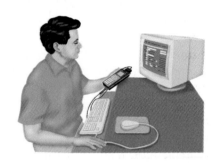

ECONOMIC TRENDS

Between 1970 and 2000, total health care costs in the United States increased by over 1,500 percent to $1.353 trillion dollars. By 2010 costs are projected to increase to $2.726 trillion.

As a result of these escalating costs, there have been increasing efforts by government, industry, and consumers to find ways to control the costs of care. Though drugs represent only a small fraction of overall health care expenses, they have also been included in these efforts.

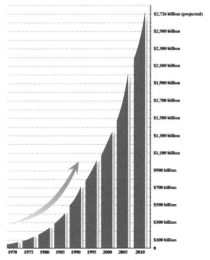

- A result of the managed care movement is that the majority of prescriptions are now paid by private third parties such as HMO's and other insurance companies, instead of directly by consumers.
- Along with this is a trend toward the use of closed "formularies," lists of drugs which are approved for use. These lists rely substantially on substituting generic drugs in place of more expensive brands that may be prescribed by the physician.
- Another cost-cutting trend is the increasing use of "therapeutic substitution" in which a chemically different drug that performs a similar function is substituted, usually because it is less expensive.

Source for illustration and data: U.S. Statistical Abstract

COMPUTERS IN PHARMACY

Pharmacies use powerful computerized tools that help productivity.

Computerized pharmacy management systems put customer profiles, product, inventory, pricing, and other essential information within easy access. They also automate elements like label printing, inventory management, stock reordering, and billing. As a result, pharmacies and pharmacists dispense more prescriptions and information than ever before.

Pharmacy computer systems may be developed by the user to meet specific needs, purchased ready-made, or provided by a drug wholesaler.

Wholesalers provide inventory management systems to their customers as part of their service. The wholesaler actually owns the system. It is primarily designed for placing orders with the wholesaler, though it may also contain various other elements. Large pharmacy chains have the business volume to justify the expense of developing comprehensive systems that are tailored to their needs. Smaller operations usually buy a commercially available system. Whatever the operation, a computerized pharmacy management system is an indispensable productivity tool.

Although each pharmacy computer system has its own specific features, many general principles of computer usage apply to all systems.

The most important element is stated in the classic computer axiom: garbage in, garbage out. That is, the information produced by the computer is only as good as the information that is entered into it. This means special care has to be taken when entering information (generally called data) to make sure it is correct. A simple mistake in data entry can result in the wrong medication being given to the wrong patient or any number of other serious problems.

℞ Keyboard skills: Considering how much data entry is required, being able to type at least forty-five words per minute is an important skill.

Computer knowledge: Many systems use personal computers or similar custom hardware, so familiarity with using computers is important.

A SAMPLE COMPUTER SYSTEM

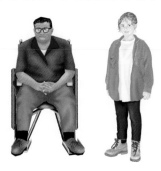

Patient Profile

Allows complete information about patients, including prescribers, insurer, and medication history, and medical history, including allergies; identifies drug interactions for patients taking multiple medications.

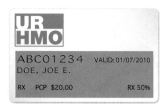

UR HMO

ABC01234   VALID: 01/07/2010
DOE, JOE E.
RX   PCP $20.00   RX 50%

Billing

Checks policies of third parties such as HMOs and insurers; authorizes third party transactions and credit cards electronically.

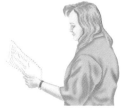

Management Reporting

Forecasting, financial analysis.

data information that is entered into and stored in a computer system.

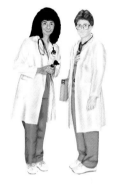

Prescriber Profile

Includes state identification numbers and affiliations with facilities and insurers.

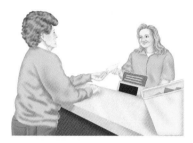

Education/Counseling

Patient information about drugs, usage, interactions, allergies, etc.

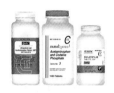

Product Selection

Locates items by various means (brand name, generic name, product code, category, supplier, etc.). Gives updates of prices and other product information.

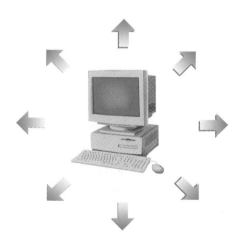

Pharmacy computer systems generally offer most or all of these features, as well as a number of others.

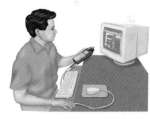

Inventory

Adjusts inventory as prescriptions are filled; analyzes turnover; produces status reports; automatically re-orders based on inventory levels, generates purchase orders.

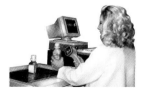

Pricing

Provides prices for medications and possible substitutes; automatically updates prices; scans prices from bar codes.

Security

Password protection restricts access to authorized users for different features.

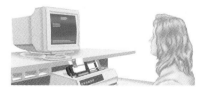

Labeling

Creates label, receipt, customer information, and usage instructions.

REVIEW

KEY CONCEPTS

ORIGINS

- ✔ People have used drugs derived from plants to treat illnesses and other physical conditions for thousands of years.

- ✔ The ancient Greeks used the bark of a white willow tree to relieve pain. The bark contained salicylic acid, the natural forerunner of the active ingredient in aspirin.

- ✔ Cocaine was the first effective local anesthetic.

MEDICINE THROUGH THE AGES

- ✔ The foxglove plant contains the drug digitalis, which has been widely used in treating heart disease.

- ✔ Louis Pasteur's experiments show that microorganisms cause food spoilage, and that heat can be used to kill them and preserve the food.

- ✔ Frederick Banting and Charles Best showed that an extract of the hormone, insulin, lowered blood sugar in dogs and might be useful in the treatment of diabetes.

- ✔ Alexander Fleming discovered the antibiotic chemical, penicillin.

- ✔ The Human Genome Project is an attempt to map the entire DNA sequence in the human genome. This information will provide a better understanding of hereditary diseases and how to treat them.

THE 20TH CENTURY

- ✔ The average life span in the United States increased by over twenty years in the Twentieth Century.

- ✔ In World War I, more soldiers died from infections than the wounds themselves; in World War II, the mass production of antibiotic penicillin saved thousands of lives and was seen as a critical factor in the success of the Allied forces.

PHARMACY TODAY

- ✔ To become a pharmacist in the United States, an individual must graduate from an accredited college of pharmacy, pass a state licensing exam, and perform an internship working under a licensed pharmacist.

- ✔ Once licensed, the pharmacist must receive continuing education to maintain their license.

- ✔ The cost of health care in the United States from 1970 to 2000 rose by over 1,500 percent; costs are estimated to increase an additional 100% between 2000 and 2010 to $2.726 trillion.

- ✔ Increasing costs of health care have brought increased efforts to control the cost of prescription drugs, one aspect of which is the use of closed "formularies" that rely substantially on substituting generic drugs in place of more expensive brands.

COMPUTERS IN PHARMACY

- ✔ Computerized pharmacy management systems put customer profiles, product, inventory, pricing, and other essential information within easy access. One result has been that pharmacies and pharmacists dispense more prescriptions and information than ever before.

SELF TEST

MATCH THE TERMS   *the answer key begins on page 511*

1. antibiotic ____

2. antitoxin ____

3. data ____

4. hormones ____

5. human genome ____

6. materia medica ____

7. panacea ____

8. pharmaceutical ____

9. pharmacognosy ____

10. pharmacology ____

11. pharmacopeia ____

12. synthetic ____

a. combining simpler chemicals into more complex ones, creating a new chemical not found in nature.

b. an authoritative listing of drugs and issues related to their use.

c. of or about drugs; also, a drug product.

d. a cure-all.

e. the study of drug properties, uses, application, and effects.

f. generally pharmacology, but also refers to the drugs in use.

g. a substance that acts against a toxin in the body.

h. a substance which harms or kills microorganisms like bacteria and fungi.

i. chemicals produced by the body that regulate body functions and processes.

j. the complete set of genetic material contained in a human cell.

k. the study of physical, chemical, biochemical and biological properties of drugs as well as the search for new drugs from natural sources.

l. information that is entered into and stored in a computer system.

CHOOSE THE BEST ANSWER   *the answer key begins on page 511*

1. The first physician known by name was
   a. Prometheus.
   b. Hippocrates.
   c. Imhotep.
   d. Aesculapius.

2. Hippocrates approach to medicine was based on
   a. superstition.
   b. careful observation.
   c. astrology.
   d. animal behavior.

3. The ancient Greek goddess of Medicinal Herbs was
   a. Pandora.
   b. Panacea.
   c. Hippocrates.
   d. Euphrates.

4. Derived from the bark of the Peruvian tree, "Jesuit's powder," used along with preventive measures, helps keep this disease under control.
   a. smallpox
   b. malaria
   c. polio
   d. tuberculosis

REVIEW

5. Aspirin is made from salicylic acid from the bark of the _____ tree.
   a. willow
   b. cinchona
   c. tea
   d. fig

6. _____ was the first effective local anesthetic.
   a. Quinine
   b. Cocaine
   c. Heroin
   d. Morphine

7. Around 3,000 B.C. _____ established, by trial and error, about 365 herbs that could be used as health treatments.
   a. Imhotep
   b. Hippocrates
   c. Aesculapius
   d. the Chinese Emperor Shen Nung

8. The _____ from _____ is an 1100 page scroll document containing about 800 prescriptions using 700 drugs mostly derived from plants.
   a. pharmacopeia, 2005
   b. "herbal, 200 B.C.
   c. Papyrus Ebers, 1500 B.C.
   d. De Materia Medica, 77 B.C.

9. The first great book of Indian medicine describing over 500 herbal drugs that had been used for centuries was written in
   a. 500 B.C.
   b. 500 A.D.
   c. 100 A.D.
   d. 1,000 A.D.

10. The Persian Rhazes who wrote one of the most popular textbooks of medicine in the middle ages was a man of science and
    a. an alchemist.
    b. a sorcerer.
    c. a politician.
    d. a god.

11. _____ was a(n) _____ physician who wrote a five volume encyclopedia in _____, one of which was devoted to natural medicines and another compounding drugs from individual medications.
    a. Li Shi Zen, Chinese, 1580 A.D.
    b. Zabdiel Boylston, colonial, 1721 A.D.
    c. William Withering, British, 1785 A.D.
    d. Avicenna, Islamic, 1000 A.D.

12. An authoritative listing of drugs and issues related to their use is a(an)
    a. pharmaceutical.
    b. pharmacology.
    c. pharmacopeia.
    d. panacea.

13. _____ showed that heat can be used to kill microorganisms associated with food spoilage.
    a. Pasteur
    b. Banting and Best
    c. Watson and Crick
    d. Fleming

14. _____ discovered penicillin could kill some bacteria.
    a. Banting and Best
    b. Watson and Crick
    c. Fleming
    d. Marker

15. _____ are substances produced by the body to regulate body functions and processes.
   a. Hormones
   b. Antitoxins
   c. Antibiotics
   d. Genomes

16. _____ identified the structure of DNA.
   a. Watson and Crick
   b. Banting and Best
   c. Serturner
   d. Koller

17. The pharmaceutical manufacturing industry devotes about _____ of its income to research and development.
   a. 1/10
   b. 1/6
   c. 1/3
   d. 1/2

18. _____ protect(s) against illegal copying of new discoveries.
   a. Generics
   b. Brand names
   c. Patenting
   d. The FDA

19. The FDA is required to
   a. ensure that a drug is safe and effective for its intended use.
   b. to monitor a drug after it is marketed to ensure it works as intended.
   c. to monitor a drug for any adverse effects.
   d. all of the above.

20. The length of time from the beginning of development of a new drug to FDA approval is often more than _____ years.
   a. two
   b. five
   c. ten
   d. twenty

21. In most cases the individual who dispenses the prescribed medication to the patient is the
   a. prescribing physician.
   b. nurse.
   c. medical office assistant.
   d. pharmacist.

22. The Omnibus Budget Reconciliation Act (OBRA) requires that pharmacists provide
   a. counseling services to all patients.
   b. mail order medication to Medicaid patients.
   c. counseling services to Medicaid patients.
   d. HMO coverage to all patients.

23. To become a pharmacist in the United States:
   a. an individual must graduate from an accredited college of pharmacy, pass a state licensing exam, and perform experiential training working under a licensed pharmacist.
   b. an individual must graduate from a non-accredited college of pharmacy and pass a state licensing exam.
   c. no internship experience is required unless the pharmacist intends to practice in community pharmacy.
   d. an individual must graduate from an accredited college of pharmacy, and perform an internship working under a licensed pharmacist, however, no examination is required.

REVIEW

24. The area of greatest employment for pharmacists is
    a. hospitals.
    b. mail order operations.
    c. community pharmacies.
    d. managed care.

25. The pharmacy technician may find the greatest employment opportunities in
    a. the hospital setting.
    b. the community setting.
    c. home health care.
    d. mail order operations.

26. In managed care, care is managed by a(an)
    a. patient.
    b. physician.
    c. pharmacist.
    d. insurer.

27. Lists of drugs approved for use by managed care organizations are called
    a. OBRA.
    b. mail order operations.
    c. HMOs.
    d. formularies.

28. Information that is entered and stored into a computer, such as a patient's name, is called
    a. product.
    b. inventory.
    c. data.
    d. billing.

2

THE PHARMACY TECHNICIAN

LEARNING OBJECTIVES

At the completion of study, the student will:

➡ be familiar with the overall aspects of the pharmacy technician job and the general role of the pharmacy technician in relation to the pharmacist.

➡ know what personal standards are expected of the pharmacy technician.

➡ understand the overall scope of HIPAA regulations as they relate to interactions between health care providers and patients as well as the patient's health information.

➡ understand the range of training programs and what agencies establish training and certification regulations, and what organization accredits training programs.

➡ know what technicians must do in order to receive certification and how often it must be renewed.

PHARMACY TECHNICIAN

In health care, "technicians" are individuals who are given a basic level of training designed to help them perform specific tasks.

This training often is provided at community and technical colleges or even on the job. By comparison, health care "professionals" such as physicians and pharmacists receive more extensive and advanced levels of education.

To perform their duties, pharmacists today rely upon the assistance of trained support staff called pharmacy technicians.

Technicians perform essential tasks that do not require the pharmacist's skill or expertise. They work under the direct supervision of a licensed pharmacist who is legally responsible for their performance.

Pharmacy technicians perform such tasks as filling prescriptions, packaging doses, performing inventory control, and keeping records.

Having technicians perform these tasks gives the pharmacist more time for activities which require a greater level of expertise, such as counseling patients. As the job of the pharmacist has become more complex, the need for pharmacy technicians has increased. As a result, pharmacy technician is a rapidly growing occupation offering many opportunities. As of 2008, there were about 326,300 pharmacy technicians employed in the United States and it is estimated this number will grow by at least 31% through 2018.

Like pharmacists, most pharmacy technicians are employed in community pharmacies and hospitals.

However, they are also employed by or in clinics, home care, long term care, mail order prescription pharmacies, nuclear pharmacies, internet pharmacies, pharmaceutical wholesalers, the Federal Government, and various other settings. Depending upon the specific setting and job, they may perform at different levels of specialization and skill. An introductory level technician job at a pharmacy requires general skills. In various hospital and other environments, there are specialized technician jobs which require more advanced skills developed from additional education, training and experience. Compensation for these specialized positions is greater than it is for entry level positions.

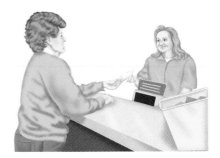

receiving prescriptions

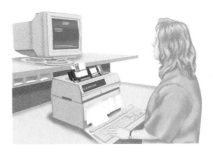

using computers

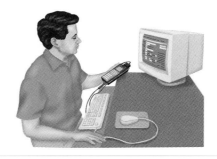

inventory control

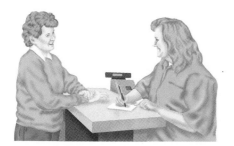

taking patient information

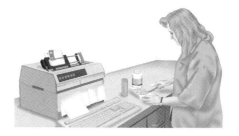

filling prescriptions

The Pharmacy Technician

The activities on these pages may be part of a pharmacy technician's job responsibilities. However, **specific responsibilities and tasks for pharmacy technicians differ by setting and are described in writing by each employer** through job descriptions, policy and procedure manuals, and other documents. What individuals may and may not do in their jobs is often referred to as their "scope of practice." The pharmacist's scope of practice is of course much greater than the technician's. As part of their job requirement, all technicians are required to know specifically what tasks they may and may not perform, as well as which tasks must be performed by the pharmacist.

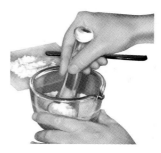

compounding

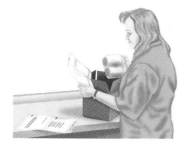

ordering

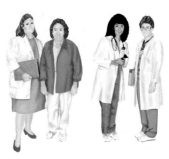

working with a team of health care professionals

PERSONAL STANDARDS

There are personal standards for pharmacy technicians.

Employers may specify these standards as part of the job requirement. Many, though not all, are outlined on these pages. There are standards for behavior, skill, health, hygiene, and appearance. Anyone seeking to become a pharmacy technician should consider how they compare in each of these areas and what they must do to excel in them.

The pharmacy technician is a member of a team, the patient's health care team.

For this team to succeed, all its members, including the technician, must work together for the welfare of the patient. If a member of the team fails to perform as required, including the technician, there can be serious consequences for the patient. Anyone wishing to become a pharmacy technician must be able to work cooperatively with others, communicate effectively, perform as expected, and act responsibly. The patient's welfare depends upon it.

Respect for the Patient

The patient's welfare is the most important consideration in health care. To ensure this, various government laws and professional standards guarantee basic patient rights and require health care providers to explain them to patients.

The 1996 **Health Insurance Portability and Accountability Act** made health care providers responsible for the privacy and security of all identifiable patient health information (also called Protected Health Information or PHI), in any form, whether it is electronic, on paper or orally communicated. Among other things, this means that computer files must be protected; any electronic transmission of health information, including claims and billing, must be done via HIPAA-compliant electronic data interchange (EDI); there can be no discussion of patient information within earshot of others; no casual discussion with anyone, including a patient's family members or friends, of a patient or patient information; directing patients to a private area when discussing medications or other personal health issues; making sure files and documents are securely stored where no unauthorized person can access them.

THE TECHNICIAN: A PERSONAL INVENTORY

Technicians should have these personal qualities:

✔ **Dependable**
The patient, the pharmacist, and the patient's health care team will depend upon you performing your job as required, including showing up on time for scheduled work hours. You must do what you are required to do, whether anyone is observing you or not.

✔ **Detail Oriented**
Patients must receive medications exactly as they have been prescribed. Drugs, whether prescription or over the counter, can be dangerous if misused, and mistakes by pharmacy technicians can be life-threatening.

✔ **Trustworthy**
You will be entrusted with confidential patient information, dangerous substances, and perishable products. In addition, many drugs are very expensive and you will be trusted to handle them appropriately.

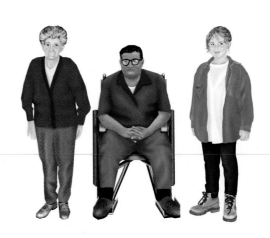

inventory to make an accounting of items on hand; also, with people, to assess characteristics, skills, qualities, etc.

confidentiality the requirement of health care providers to keep all patient information private among the patient, the patient's insurer, and the providers directly involved in the patient's care.

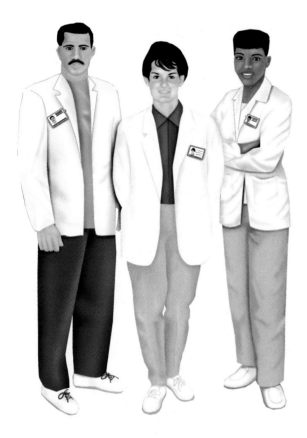

Technicians must follow these personal guidelines:

✔ Health

You must maintain good physical and mental health. If you become physically or mentally run-down, you increase the chance of making serious mistakes.

✔ Hygiene

Practice good hygiene. You will interact closely with others. Poor hygiene may hurt your ability to be effective. You will also be expected to perform in infection free conditions and poor hygiene can violate this requirement.

✔ Appearance

Your uniform and personal clothing should be neat, clean, and functional. Shoes should be comfortable. Clothes should allow the freedom of movement necessary to perform your duties. Hair should be well-groomed and pulled back if long. Fingernails should be neat and trim.

Technicians must be capable and competent in the following skill areas:

✔ Mathematics and Problem Solving

You will routinely perform mathematical calculations in filling prescriptions and other activities.

✔ Language and Terminology

You must learn the specific pharmaceutical terminology and medical abbreviations (e.g., QID, QS) that will be used on your job.

✔ Computer Skills

You will regularly use computers for entering patient information, maintaining inventory, filling prescriptions, and so on.

✔ Interpersonal Skills

You will interact with patients/customers, your supervisor, co-workers, physicians, and others. You must be able to communicate, cooperate, and work effectively.

℞ There are legal aspects to many of these standards. Failing to follow them can hurt your job performance and result in legal violations.

TRAINING & COMPETENCY

Training and *competency* requirements for pharmacy technicians differ from setting to setting.

Technician training is generally based on job requirements for the specific workplace, particular skills involved, any applicable professional standards, and state regulations. Specific training and certification requirements are set by each state's board of pharmacy. Regulations vary considerably but almost all states require some form of technician training.

An example of a model curriculum for technician training is that of The American Society of Health-System Pharmacists (ASHP).

The ASHP is the leading association for pharmacists practicing in hospitals, and other health care systems. Their curriculum provides a national standard for developing technician competency. It can be adapted to different pharmacy settings and the specific needs of an individual training program. Training programs that meet ASHP standards can receive accreditation from it in recognition of having done so. The ASHP curriculum is also endorsed by the Pharmacy Technician Educator's Council (PTEC).

Your training program will prepare you to do your job.

The ASHP maintains a directory of over 250 schools and training institutions that offer technician training programs; most of these programs have been accredited by the ASHP and the remainder have applied for accreditation. These programs are found in community, technical, and career colleges, as well in on-the-job settings such as community pharmacies, hospitals and other institutional settings.

Your employer will monitor and document your competency.

Your employer is legally responsible for your performance and therefore your competency. In addition to monitoring this on a daily basis, you will receive regularly scheduled performance reviews. The frequency of performance reviews will vary by employer and be indicated in your job description or other employee information. Through these reviews and other means, your employer will document your competency to perform your job.

TRAINING

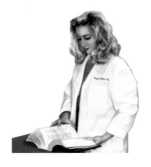

Training Program

Depending upon your setting, you will receive training in some or all of the following areas:

- drug laws
- terminology
- prescriptions
- calculations
- drug routes and forms
- drug dosage and activity
- infection control
- compounding
- preparing IV admixtures
- biopharmaceutics
- drug classifications
- inventory management
- pharmacy literature

An important part of training is exposure to actual workplace settings. Many technicians receive this in the form of on-the-job training from their employer or as internships through community colleges or other training programs.

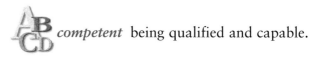

competent being qualified and capable.

COMPETENCY

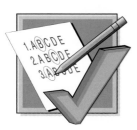
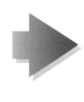

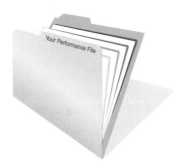

Testing

Demonstration of competency during training will generally be through written tests and practical demonstrations. In on-the-job training or internships, your performance will be directly judged by the supervising pharmacist.

Continuing Education

Pharmacy is a dynamic field that changes constantly. There are always new drugs, treatments, methods and other developments. As a result, continuing education is a critical element in maintaining competency for pharmacy technicians. In order to perform your job as required, you must continually learn new information. Ultimately, this will make your job more interesting and you more effective.

Performance

After you have qualified as competent, your employer will continue to monitor and document your performance and competency throughout your employment. These files may include:

➡ performance reviews,
➡ complaints,
➡ comments by your supervisor and and other appropriate personnel.

Most jobs also have a probation period during which time the pharmacy technician is expected to learn certain skill sets. If competency is not met, the technician may receive an extended probation period or be dismissed from the job.

 For information regarding ASHP accredited programs, contact:

The American Society of Health-System
  Pharmacists
7272 Wisconsin Ave.
Bethesda, MD 20814
301-657-3000
http://www.ashp.org

CERTIFICATION

Since there is no federal standard for training or competency, a valuable career step for pharmacy technicians is getting national *certification.*

To receive certification in most states, technicians must pass a standardized national examination, such as the Pharmacy Technician Certification Exam (PTCE) offered by the Pharmacy Technician Certification Board (PTCB), the Exam for the Certification of Pharmacy Technicians (ExCPT) given by the Institute for the Certification of Pharmacy Technicians (ICPT), or another exam approved by their state board. These exams test the technician's knowledge and competency in basic pharmacy functions and activity areas. While certification is mainly voluntary, as of January, 2010 the PTCB had certified over 363,000 pharmacy technicians.

Certification is a mark of achievement that employers, colleagues, and others will recognize.

If you pass a national certification examination, you will be able to use the CPhT designation after your name. This designation stands for Certified Pharmacy Technician. Beyond verifying your competence as a technician, this indicates that you have a high level of knowledge and skill and can be given greater responsibilities. This in turn means that you may earn more, and will probably cost your employer less time and money for training. Studies have also shown that certified technicians have lower turnover, higher morale, greater productivity, and make fewer errors. Some employers may pay for the cost of a certification exam (if successfully completed) and/or provide training assistance for a certification exam.

Certification must be renewed every two years.

Because pharmacy is a constantly changing field, maintaining skills and competence requires continuing education. In order to renew their certification every two years, CPhTs must meet requirements of 20 contact hours of pharmacy-related continuing education, including at least one hour in pharmacy law. Up to ten contact hours of continuing education can occur at the CPhT's practice site under the supervision of a registered pharmacist, and these hours can be customized to fit the specific needs of the CPhT.

PTCE AND ExCPT

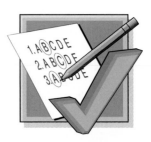

Both exams are certified by the National Commission for Certifying Agencies (NCCA), last two hours, and are administered in a computerized testing environment. To take either exam, candidates must have completed high school or have a GED, and have never been convicted of a felony.

The Pharmacy Technician Certification Exam (PTCE) contains 90 multiple choice questions and tests these areas:

- ➡ assisting the pharmacist in serving patients (66% of the exam);
- ➡ maintaining medication and inventory control systems (22% of the exam);
- ➡ participating in the administration and management of pharmacy practice (12% of the exam).

In addition to the requirements stated above, candidates for the PTCE must have never been convicted of a pharmacy or drug-related misdemeanor . To pass the exam, candidates must score at least 650 out of a possible 900.

The Exam for the Certification of Pharmacy Technicians (ExCPT) contains 110 multiple choice questions and tests these areas:

- ➡ regulations and technician duties (~25% of the exam);
- ➡ drugs and drug products (~23% of the exam);
- ➡ dispensing process (~52% of the exam).

In addition to the requirements stated above for both tests, candidates for the ExCPT must be at least 18 years old.

---

 certification a legal proof or document that an individual meets certain objective standards, usually provided by a neutral professional organization.

In accordance with the Americans with Disabilities Act (ADA), special accommodations will be provided for persons with documented disabilities taking a national certification exam.

Sample PTCE Questions

The sample questions below reflect the "choose the best answer" format of the PTCE. This type of question requires careful reading and judgment. In some cases, there may be more than one answer that is at least partially correct. However, there will only be one correct answer that is the best and most complete answer.

answers:
1. 4
2. 1
3. 1
4. 2
5. 4
6. 4

1. Pharmacies located in hospitals are required to follow regulations of this organization:

1. ASHP
2. USP
3. ASCP
4. JCAHO

2. Of the following schedules of drugs, which is for drugs with no accepted medical use in the United States?

1. Schedule I
2. Schedule II
3. Schedule III
4. Schedule IV

3. Of the following needles, which size is the most likely to cause coring?

1. 13 G
2. 16 G
3. 20 G
4. 23 G

4. A solution of Halperidol (Haldol®) contains 2 mg/ml of active ingredient. How many grams would be in 473 ml of this solution?

1. 9.46 gm
2. 0.946 gm
3. 0.0946 gm
4. 0.00946 gm

5. You have a 70% solution of Dextrose 1000 ml. How many Kg of Dextrose is in 400 ml of this solution?

1. 280 Kg
2. 28 Kg
3. 2.8 Kg
4. 0.28 Kg

6. Which is the largest capsule size?

1. size 5
2. size 3
3. size 1
4. size 0

More sample exam questions and practice exams can be found in the workbook accompanying this text, *The Pharmacy Technician Workbook and Certification Review, Fourth Edition.*

For information regarding the PTCE contact the Pharmacy Technician Certification Board by mail at 2215 Constitution Avenue, NW, Washington, DC 20037-2985, by phone at (800) 363-8012, by fax at (202) 429-7596, or by visiting their website at www.ptcb.org.

For information regarding ExCPT, contact Exam for the Certification of Pharmacy Technicians by mail at 2536 S Old Hwy 94, Suite 224, St. Charles, Mo 63303, by phone at (314) 442-6775, by fax at (866) 203-9213 or by e-mail at info@icptmail.org.

REVIEW

KEY CONCEPTS

PHARMACY TECHNICIAN

- ✔ Pharmacy technicians perform essential tasks that do not require the pharmacist's skill or expertise.

- ✔ Pharmacy technicians work under the direct supervision of a licensed pharmacist who is legally responsible for their performance.

- ✔ The specific responsibilities and tasks for pharmacy technicians differ by setting and are described in writing by each employer through job descriptions, policy and procedure manuals, and other documents.

- ✔ Having technicians perform these tasks gives the pharmacist more time for activities which require a greater level of expertise, such as consulting with patients.

- ✔ What individuals may and may not do in their jobs is often referred to as their "scope of practice."

- ✔ Like pharmacists, most pharmacy technicians are employed in community pharmacies and hospitals.

- ✔ However, they are also employed in clinics, home care, long term care, mail order prescription pharmacies, and various other settings.

- ✔ In various hospital and other environments, there are specialized technician jobs which require more advanced skills developed from additional education, training and experience.

PERSONAL STANDARDS

- ✔ Pharmacy technicians are entrusted with confidential patient information, dangerous substances, and perishable products.

- ✔ Drugs, whether prescription or over the counter, can be dangerous if misused, and mistakes by pharmacy technicians can be life-threatening.

- ✔ Pharmacy technicians routinely perform mathematical calculations in filling prescriptions and other activities.

- ✔ Pharmacy technicians must learn the specific pharmaceutical terminology that will be used on the job.

- ✔ Pharmacy technicians must be able to communicate, cooperate, and work effectively with others.

TRAINING AND COMPETENCY

- ✔ Standards for pharmacy technician training or competency are established by the state boards of pharmacy; regulations vary considerably but most states require some form of technician training.

CERTIFICATION

- ✔ Although certification is mainly voluntary, many states recognize PTCB certification and some require pharmacy technicians to take the PTCE or other exam approved by their state board.

- ✔ The CPhT designation, Certified Pharmacy Technician, is good for two years. It verifies an individual's competence as a technician, and indicates a high level of knowledge and skill.

SELF TEST

MATCH THE TERMS *the answer key begins on page 511*

1. certification _____

2. competent _____

3. confidentiality _____

4. inventory _____

5. personal inventory _____

6. professionals _____

7. scope of practice _____

8. technicians _____

a. what individuals may and may not do in their jobs.

b. to assess one's personal characteristics, skills, qualities, etc.

c. the requirement of health care providers to keep all patient information private among the patient, the patient's insurer, and the providers directly involved in the patient's care.

d. being qualified and capable to perform a task or job.

e. a legal proof or document that an individual meets certain objective standards, usually provided by a neutral professional organization.

f. individuals who are given a basic level of training designed to help them perform specific tasks.

g. individuals who receive extensive and advanced levels of education before being allowed to practice, such as physicians and pharmacists.

h. to make an accounting of items on hand.

CHOOSE THE BEST ANSWER *the answer key begins on page 511*

1. _____ are individuals who are given a basic level of training designed to help them perform specific tasks.
   a. LPNs
   b. DOs
   c. Professionals
   d. Technicians

2. In pharmacy, technicians perform essential tasks that do not require _____ skill or expertise.
   a. the clerk's
   b. the pharmacist's
   c. scientific
   d. mathematical

3. Specialized technician jobs in hospitals have _____ compensation than entry level positions.
   a. less
   b. about the same
   c. greater

4. Specific responsibilities and tasks for pharmacy technicians differ by setting and are described in writing by each
   a. technician.
   b. local police department.
   c. employer.
   d. state board of pharmacy.

5. The pharmacy technician can do the following functions except
   a. take patient information.
   b. fill prescription orders.
   c. compound prescription orders.
   d. advise patients on medications.

6. What individuals may and may not do on their jobs is referred to as their
   a. job responsibilities.
   b. scope of practice.
   c. opinion.
   d. employee guidelines.

REVIEW

7. The term that describes making an accounting of items on hand is a/an
   a. policy.
   b. inventory.
   c. ordering.
   d. re-ordering.

8. The Health Insurance Portability and Accountability Act of 1996
   a. governs how often insurance companies can merge with each other.
   b. makes insurers accountable to patients for reimbursement of approved medical costs.
   c. is a set of general rather than legal guidelines regarding the privacy of patient health information.
   d. requires health care providers to be responsible for the privacy and security of a patient's protected health information.

9. Under HIPAA, PHI stands for
   a. Personal Health Information.
   b. Protected Health Information.
   c. Professional Health Information.
   d. Programmed Health Information.

10. Pharmacy technicians should be detail oriented. This means
   a. patients must receive medications exactly as they have been prescribed.
   b. an incorrect strength will always be detected by the pharmacist.
   c. technicians do not need to be careful because the pharmacist is supposed to find and correct all technician errors.

11. Good hygiene is important for pharmacy technicians because of the interactions with other persons and the expectation of performing in _____ conditions.
   a. warm
   b. cold
   c. infection free
   d. sunny

12. Pharmacy technicians must be capable and competent in mathematics and problem solving because
   a. all medications that are available on prescription cannot lead to overdose death.
   b. pharmacists always check their work.
   c. all medications come pre-mixed and pre-packaged.
   d. mathematical calculations are routinely used.

13. Pharmacy technicians must be capable and competent with computer skills because
   a. pharmacists will check their data entry.
   b. pharmacists do all of the computer work.
   c. pharmacists should operate the computer.
   d. technicians regularly use computers.

14. Pharmacy technicians must be capable and competent in the area of interpersonal skills. This means
   a. they must be able to communicate, cooperate, and work effectively.
   b. they must socialize with their co-workers.
   c. the pharmacist should obtain all confidential information from the patient.
   d. they must make friends with every patient.

15. Training and certification requirements for pharmacy technicians are set by
   a. each state's board of pharmacy.
   b. the ASHP
   c. the PTCB.
   d. the federal government.

16. The _____ is the leading association for pharmacists practicing in hospitals and other health care systems.
   a. ASHP
   b. PTCB
   c. PTEC
   d. APhA

17._____ typically monitor and document competency of pharmacy technicians.
a. Employers
b. Technicians
c. Pharmacists
d. PTCB

18. Any complaints received regarding an employee's employment
a. are discarded after two weeks.
b. are discarded after one year.
c. are discarded within one week after the complaint was received.
d. may be kept in the employee's performance/personnel file.

19. Training that occurs in actual workplace settings is called
a. performance-based training.
b. on-the-job training.
c. community college training.
d. certified training.

20._____ is another term for being qualified and capable.
a. Realistic
b. Competent
c. Professional
d. Technical

21. In the United States, two organizations that performs pharmacy technician certification are the
a. APhA and ASHP.
b. PTCB and ICPT.
c. ASHP and PTEC.
d. PTEC and APhA.

22. The Pharmacy Technician Certification Exam (PTCE) tests:
a. 66% on assisting the pharmacist in serving patients, 22% on maintaining medications and inventory control systems, and 12% on participating in pharmacy administration and management.
b. 22% on assisting the pharmacist in serving patients, 66% on maintaining medications and inventory control systems, and 12% on participating in pharmacy administration and management.
c. 12% on assisting the pharmacist in serving patients, 66% on maintaining medications and inventory control systems, and 22% on participating in pharmacy administration and management.
d. 12% on assisting the pharmacist in serving patients, 22% on maintaining medications and inventory control systems, and 66% on participating in pharmacy administration and management.

23. To take the PTCE exam, candidates
a. need only submit an application form.
b. must be working at a pharmacy.
c. need to have completed an ASHP accredited training program.
d. must have a high school diploma or GED by the application deadline and have never been convicted of a felony or a pharmacy or drug-related misdemeanor.

24. Certification must be renewed every
a. three years.
b. year.
c. two years.
d. four years.

REVIEW

25. After passing a pharmacy technician national certification exam, pharmacy technicians may use the following designation after their name:
    a. PT
    b. RPhT
    c. CPhT
    d. none of the above

26. CPhTs need _____ of continuing education every _____ years to renew certification.
    a. 30 hours, 2
    b. 10 hours, 1
    c. 30 hours, 3
    d. 20 hours, 2

27. Continuing education for CPhTs must contain _____ in pharmacy law every _____ years.
    a. one hour, one
    b. two hours, one
    c. one hour, two
    d. two hours, two

DRUG REGULATION & CONTROL

LEARNING OBJECTIVES

At the completion of study, the student will:

➥ know the key legislative acts governing pharmacy practice.

➥ understand the FDA process for new drug approval.

➥ understand the process by which patents expire making a drug eligible for release under a pharmaceutical or generic name, and what approval procedures manufacturers must go through.

➥ know the different requirements for labels and product labeling for stock medications, prescription containers, controlled substances, and over-the-counter drugs.

➥ know the restrictions for the different categories of over-the-counter drugs.

➥ know the five groups of controlled substances and restrictions for each.

➥ know when a DEA number is required and how to check it.

➥ know when and how to fill out and process DEA Form 222.

➥ be aware of other key DEA forms and when they are required.

➥ know the process for FDA drug recalls.

DRUG REGULATION

— A TIMELINE —

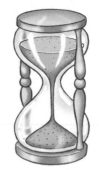

There are many laws in the United States concerning the safety and effectiveness of food, drugs, medical devices, and cosmetics. Regardless of whether a product is produced in the United States or is imported, it must meet the requirements of these laws. The leading enforcement agency at the federal level for these regulations is the Food and Drug Administration. On these pages are brief descriptions of U.S. federal laws and their significance.

Food and Drug Act of 1906

Prohibited interstate commerce in adulterated or misbranded food, drinks, and drugs. Government pre-approval of drugs is required.

1927 Food, Drug and Insecticide Administration

The law enforcement agency is formed that would be renamed in 1930 as the Food and Drug Administration.

1950 Alberty Food Products v. U.S.

The United States Court of Appeals rules that the purpose for which a drug is to be used must be included on the label.

| 1900 | 1910 | 1920 | 1930 | 1940 | 1950 |

1914 Harrison Tax Act

In response to growing addiction to opiates and cocaine-containing medicines, the Harrison Tax Act established that manufacturers, pharmacists, importers, and physicians prescribing narcotics should be licensed and required to pay a tax.

1938 Food, Drug and Cosmetic (FDC) Act

In response to the fatal poisoning of 107 people, primarily children, by an untested sulfanilamide concoction, this comprehensive law requires new drugs be shown to be safe before marketing.

1951 Durham-Humphrey Amendment

This law defines what drugs require a prescription by a licensed practitioner and requires them to include this **legend** on the label: "Caution: Federal Law prohibits dispensing without a prescription" or the more recent "Rx Only."

The Thalidomide Lesson

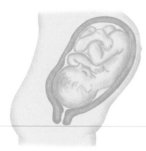

In 1962, a new sleeping pill containing the drug, thalidomide, was found to cause severe birth defects when used by pregnant women. This included lost limbs and other major deformities that affected thousands of children in Europe, where the drug had been widely used. In the United States, the drug was not yet approved for marketing and was only being used in tests, so it affected a small number of children. However, the nature of the defects and the number of children affected created a public demand in the U.S. for tighter drug regulation that resulted in the Kefauver-Harris Amendment. From then on, drugs would have to be shown to be both safe and effective before they could be marketed in the United States.

Later studies found thalidomide to be safe and effective in treating multiple myeloma and it is now approved for that use. However, an FDA Alert remains on the drug stating that both men and women must agree in writing to their understanding of the risks of thalidomide and actions they must take while being treated with it.

legend drug any drug which requires a prescription and either of these "legends" on the label: "Caution: Federal law prohibits dispensing without a prescription," or "Rx only."

1962 Kefauver-Harris Amendment

Requires drug manufacturers to provide proof of both safety and effectiveness before marketing the drug.

1966 Fair Packaging and Labeling Act

This requires all consumer products in interstate commerce to be honestly and informatively labeled.

1970 Controlled Substances Act (CSA)

The CSA classifies five levels of drugs (controlled substances) that have potential for abuse and therefore restricts their distribution. The Drug Enforcement Administration (DEA) as a division of the Justice Department was established by the CSA and enforces its regulations.

1976 Medical Device Amendment

Requires pre-market approval for safety and effectiveness of life-sustaining and life-supporting medical devices.

1987 Prescription Drug Marketing Act

Restricts distribution of prescription drugs to legitimate commercial channels and requires drug wholesalers to be licensed by the states.

1990 Omnibus Budget Reconciliation Act (OBRA)

Among other things, this act requires pharmacists to offer counseling to Medicaid patients regarding medications.

1990 Anabolic Steroid Control Act

This act was passed to "address the abuse of steroids by athletes, and, especially, youngsters and teenagers."

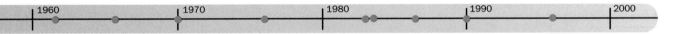

1960   1970   1980   1990   2000

1970 Poison Prevention Packaging Act

Requires child-proof packaging on all controlled and most prescription drugs dispensed by pharmacies. Non-child-proof containers may only be used if the prescriber or patient requests one.

1983 Orphan Drug Act

Provides incentives to promote research, approval, and marketing of drugs needed for the treatment of rare diseases.

1984 Drug Price Competition and Patent Term Restoration Act (Hatch-Waxman)

This act allowed for both the extension of drug patent terms and quicker introduction of lower-cost generic drugs.

1996 Health Insurance Portability and Accountability Act

Among other things this act defined the scope of health information that may and may not be shared among health care providers without patient consent and provided for broad and stringent regulations to protect patients' right to privacy. All "covered entities," meaning any health care provider using electronic claims transmissions, billing or other electronic transfer of patient information are required to be compliant with HIPAA privacy and security regulations. These regulations govern the transfer of patient health information whether it is communicated electronically, on paper, or orally.

℞ **safety you should know**
The FDA's Center for Drug Evaluation and Research provides an Index to Drug-Specific Information (www.fda.gov/cder/drug/DrugSafety/DrugIndex.htm) with patient, consumer and healthcare professional information sheets, including FDA Alerts. The Center also works with drug manufacturers to develop risk management programs for drugs with FDA Alerts, such as the iPLEDGE program for Accutane. Health care professionals, wholesalers, pharmacies and patients must register in the iPLEDGE program to prescribe, distribute, fill prescriptions for, or use Accutane.

NEW DRUG APPROVAL

All new drugs, whether made domestically or imported, require FDA approval before they can be marketed in the United States.

A new drug is any drug proposed for marketing after 1938 that was not already recognized as safe and effective. This represents the vast majority of drugs on the market.

Before it will be approved, a new drug must be shown to be both safe and effective and that its benefits substantially outweigh its risks.

It is the responsibility of the drug manufacturer (not the FDA) to provide proof of this to the FDA's Center for Drug Evaluation and Research (CDER). The proof is based on extensive testing which begins in the laboratory, where chemical analysis is performed, and moves on to animal testing and then clinical trials with people. The FDA estimates that the testing process currently takes 8.5 years.

"Clinical trials" involve testing the drug on people.

Clinical tests begin with small numbers of participants over a short period of time and eventually expand into large groups of participants over long periods. Trial participants must give their informed consent. Among other things, it means the person must be told of the risks of the treatment along with other treatment options in language they can understand. Participants are also free to leave the trial at any time they wish.

placebo an inactive substance given in place of a medication.

pediatric having to do with the treatment of children.

Testing Children

Children are not included in trials until a drug has been fully tested on adults. Drugs which have not been tested on children generally state on the label that their safety and effectiveness has not been established for children. Some drugs, however, may carry label information for **pediatric** use that is based on studies of adults and other pediatric treatment information. The Pediatric Labeling Rule mandates that all drugs have pediatric dosing and safety information on their labels if the drug has potential use for pediatric patients.

TESTING

Animal Testing

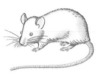

Once laboratory testing of a proposed new drug is finished, the drug is tested on animals before it will be tested on humans. Drug companies try to use as few animals and to treat them as humanely as possible. Since different species often react differently, more than one species is usually tested. Drug absorption into the bloodstream is monitored carefully. Only a fraction of a percent of drugs tested on animals are ever tested on humans.

Placebos

Placebos are inactive substances, not real medications, that are administered to give the patient the impression he or she is receiving a potentially effective medication. This provides a valuable comparison against patients who receive a test drug. Patients in trials must freely agree to the possibility that they may be given a placebo. They must also be informed of an effective treatment if one is available.

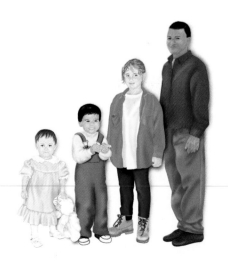

Testing Phases in Humans

There are three phases of testing a new drug in humans. Testing begins with a small number of participants for a short time and this gradually increases to a large number of participants over long periods of time. The goals of each phase also change from indicating a minimal level of safety to ultimately verifying the safety, effectiveness and dosage for widespread use. Only about 25% of drugs tested in phase 1 successfully complete phase 3 and are approved for marketing. Once a drug becomes available to the public, additional information is collected about safety, efficacy, and uses, and this additional post-marketing surveillance is sometimes called phase 4.

phase 1

➡ **20–100 patients**
➡ **time: several months**
➡ **purpose: mainly safety**

phase 2

➡ **up to several hundred patients**
➡ **time: several months to two years**
➡ **purpose: short-term safety but mainly effectiveness**

phase 3

➡ **several hundred to several thousand patients**
➡ **time: one to four years**
➡ **purpose: safety, dosage, and effectiveness**

D uring the trial phase, a proposed new drug is called an investigational new drug (IND).

It is available for use only within the trial groups unless granted a special "treatment" status which is sometimes given to provide relief to critically ill patients outside of clinical trials. An example of this is AZT, which was used on thousands of AIDS patients who were not part of a clinical trial prior to the drug receiving FDA approval. It is worth noting, however, that such drugs are extremely expensive and are excluded from coverage by most insurers and HMOs.

Tests are "controlled" by comparing the effect of a proposed drug on one group of patients with the effect of a different treatment on other patients.

Patients have the same condition and similar characteristics and are placed in either treatment groups or control groups at random to make sure the groups have essentially the same characteristics. The control group may receive no drug at all, a placebo, a drug known to be effective, or a different dose of the same drug.

The patients in a trial are always "blind" to the treatment.

They are not told which group (controlled or treatment) they are in. In a "double-blind" test, neither the patients nor the physicians know whether the patient is receiving the active drug or a placebo. This prevents patients and/or their physicians from imagining effects one way or the other. Medical results alone determine the drug's effectiveness and its safety.

Medical Products Other Than Drugs

Medical devices and biological products such as insulin and vaccines must also meet FDA testing and approval requirements. The *Center for Devices and Radiological Health (CDRH)* is responsible for devices. The *Center for Biologics Evaluation and Research (CBER)* is responsible for biological products made from living organisms.

Source: Food and Drug Administration

MARKETED DRUGS

A patent for a new drug gives its manufacturer an exclusive right to market the drug for a specific period of time under a brand name. During this time, the manufacturer attempts to recover the costs of the drug's research and development. A drug patent is in effect for 17 years from the date of the drug's discovery. Since the testing and approval process takes years to complete, for many years drugs reached the market with only half their patent time left. To compensate for this, the Hatch-Waxman Act of 1984 provided for up to five year extensions of patent protection to the patent holders to make up for time lost while products went through the FDA approval process.

Once a patent for a brand drug expires, other manufacturers may copy the drug and release it under its pharmaceutical or "generic" name.

Manufacturers of generic drugs do not need to perform the safety and effectiveness testing required of new drugs. However, they need to demonstrate that the drug is **pharmaceutically equivalent** to the proprietary (patented brand) drug—that it has same active ingredients, same dosage form, same route of administration, and same strength, and that it is **therapeutically equivalent**—that the body's use of the drug is the same. This is measured by the rate and extent to which the active ingredients are absorbed into the bloodstream. Evaluations of generic drug products can be found in the FDA "Orange Book."

Over-The-Counter (OTC) drugs are drugs which do not require a prescription.

They can be used upon the judgment of the consumer. There are over 100,000 OTC drugs in 80 therapeutic categories marketed. The FDA publishes acceptable ingredients for OTC drugs in "Drug Monographs." The manufacturer of an OTC drug must follow monograph requirements to be able to market their drug without undergoing the FDA new drug approval process. Though some OTC drugs were available before FDA approval was required, the FDA has been reviewing them under the "OTC Drug Review Program," and all new OTC drugs require FDA approval.

LABELS AND PRODUCT LABELING

While all drugs are required to have clear and accurate information for all labels, inserts, packaging, and so on, there are different information requirements for various categories of drugs. Information requirements for OTC drugs are designed to enable consumers to use them without medical advice. Manufacturers of prescription drugs do not have to include directions for use on their labels since such directions must be supplied by the prescriber and dispenser. In many cases, important associated information may not fit on the label itself, and it will be provided in the form of an insert, brochure, or other document that is referred to as **product labeling.** We'll look at labels and label information requirements on these next few pages.

Look-Alike, Sound-Alike

Federal laws require that a drug and/or its container not be imitative of another drug so that the consumer will be misled. Nevertheless, there are many drugs with similar sounding names in similar looking packages. It is therefore essential for pharmacy technicians to pay close attention to the details of drug names and packaging. Using the wrong drug can have very serious consequences. A list of some Look-Alike and Sound-Alike drugs is in the Appendix A.

 For more information on pharmaceutical and therapeutic equivalents and the Orange Book, see Chapter 10 of this text and Chapter 3 of *The Pharmacy Technician Workbook and Certification Review, Fourth Edition.*

 pharmaceutical equivalent drug products that contain identical amounts of the same active ingredients in the same dosage form.

therapeutic equivalent pharmaceutical equivalents that produce the same effects in patients.

product labeling important associated information that is not on the label of a drug product itself, but is provided with the product in the form of an insert, brochure, or other document.

OTC LABELS

Active Ingredient (In Each Tablet)	Purpose
Chlorpheniramine Maleate 4 mg...Antihistamine	

Uses: for the temporary relief of these symptoms of hay fever
- ► sneezing   ► runny nose   ► itchy, watery eyes

Warnings

Ask a Doctor Before Use
If You Have:

- ► glaucoma
- ► a breathing problem such as emphysema or chronic bronchitis
- ► difficulty in urination due to enlargement of the prostate gland

If You Are:

- ► taking sedatives or tranquilizers

When Using This Product:

- ► marked drowsiness may occur
- ► alcohol, sedatives, and tranquilizers may increase the drowsiness effect
- ► avoid alcoholic beverages
- ► use caution when driving a motor vehicle or operating machinery
- ► excitability may occur, especially in children

If pregnant or breast-feeding, ask a health professional before use.
Keep out of reach of children. In case of overdose, get medical help right away.

Directions:

Adults and children over 12 years:	Take 1 tablet every 4 to 6 hours as needed. Do not take more than 6 tablets in 24 hours.
Children 6 to under 12 years:	Take 1/2 tablet every 4 to 6 hours as needed. Do not take more than 3 tablets in 24 hours.
Children under 6 years:	Ask a doctor.

FDA label format for OTC medications

Many over-the-counter products have labels that are difficult to read, understand, or both. To the left is a label format adopted by the FDA to make it easier to read and understand the information currently contained on over-the-counter medication labels.

Over-the-counter medications do not require a prescription but sometimes prescriptions are written for them for insurance or other reasons. In addition, patients often seek counseling regarding the use of over-the-counter medications. As a result, the pharmacy technician will deal with OTC medications regularly and should be familiar both with their label information and how to handle inquiries about them.

Since OTC medications are not without risks, all patients requesting information on them should be referred to the pharmacist. OTC medications may have significant drug interactions with prescription drugs the patient may be taking which could lead to serious adverse effects, including death.

The following information should be contained on the labels of over-the-counter medications.

- ➥ product name
- ➥ name and address of manufacturer or distributor
- ➥ list of all active and other ingredients
- ➥ amount of contents
- ➥ adequate warnings
- ➥ adequate directions for use

BEHIND-THE-COUNTER OTC MEDICATIONS

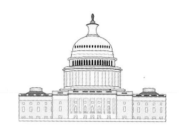

While most OTC medications are not kept behind the pharmacy counter, some are, even if a prescription is not required. These medications may at times be sold without a prescription, but with restrictions on their sale.

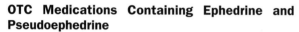

OTC Medications Containing Ephedrine and Pseudoephedrine

The Combat Methamphetamine Epidemic Act requires that some OTC cold and allergy medications must be kept behind the counter. OTC medications containing ephedrine, pseudoephedrine or phenylpropanolamine are affected by this law, although phenylpropanolamine is no longer available in OTC medications.

The **Combat Methamphetamine Epidemic Act** sets daily and monthly restrictions (3.6 grams per day and 7.5 grams per month) on the amount of ephedrine or pseudoephedrine that can be sold to an individual. The law also requires purchasers to present photo identification, and requires retailers to keep personal information about the purchasers for at least two years after each purchase. It is important to note that some state or local laws may call for additional restrictions on the sale of ephedrine and pseudoephedrine-containing OTCs.

As part of the Combat Methamphetamine Epidemic Act appropriately trained pharmacy technicians may be allowed to sell OTC medications containing ephedrine or pseudoephedrine. The following rules must be followed:

✔ The pharmacy or store cannot exceed the established daily and monthly limits for the OTC sale of ephedrine or pseudoephedrine to any one customer.

✔ The pharmacy or store must maintain written or electronic records for a period of two years that contain the following elements:

➡ Product name
➡ Quantity sold
➡ Name and address of purchaser
➡ Date and time of the sale
➡ Proof of identification
➡ Signature of the purchaser

Ingredient	Number of Tablets
30 mg Pseudoephedrine HCl	146
60 mg Pseudoephedrine HCl	73
120 mg Pseudoephedrine HCl	36
240 mg Pseudoephedrine HCl	18

Ingredient	Number of Milliliters
15 mg/1.6 ml Pseudoephedrine HCl	468
7.5 mg/5 ml Pseudoephedrine HCl	2929
15 mg/5 ml Pseudoephedrine HCl	1464
30 mg/5 ml Pseudoephedrine HCl	732
60 mg/5 ml Pseudoephedrine HCl	366

The daily sales limit of pseudoephedrine base is 3.6 grams per purchaser, regardless of number of transactions.

 Combat Methamphetamine Epidemic Act (CMEA) Federal law that sets daily and monthly limits on OTC sale of pseudoephedrine and ephedrine.

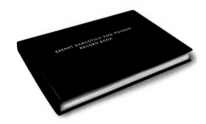

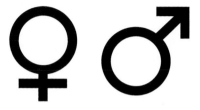

Exempt Narcotics

Exempt narcotics are medications that contain habit-forming ingredients but can be sold by a pharmacist without a prescription to persons at least eighteen years of age. For example, there are some cough syrups that contain a small amount of codeine and do not require a prescription according to federal, state, or local law.

Certain rules apply to the sale of exempt narcotics:

✔ Dispensing of exempt narcotics is made only by a pharmacist, although the actual cash register transaction may be completed by a pharmacy technician after a pharmacist has approved and documented the dispensing.

✔ Limits for how many dosage units can be sold in any given 48-hour period are followed.

✔ Purchasers of exempt narcotics are at least 18 years old, and purchasers not known by the pharmacist must provide suitable identification.

✔ A bound record book containing the name and address of the purchaser, the name and quantity of exempt narcotic purchased, the date of each purchase, and the name or initials of the pharmacist who dispensed the substance to the purchaser is maintained.

Emergency Contraceptives

Plan B® is a drug indicated for emergency contraception (EC). Plan B® has **dual marketing** status and that means that it has both prescription drug status and OTC drug status.

While a prescription is required to dispense EC to patients under 17 years old, pharmacists may sell Plan B® without a prescription to individuals 17 years and older. A special program called CARE, which stands for Convenient Access, Responsible Education, provides that Plan B® is available only through pharmacies and other health care facilities licensed to dispense prescription drugs. Packages of Plan B® that can be sold OTC bear the statement "Rx only for women younger than age 17." Pharmacies that stock Plan B® as an OTC must keep the product behind the counter and confirm the patient's age by requesting to see government-issued identification.

Additionally, pharmacists in some states have authority to prescribe and dispense EC under protocol to patients under 17 years old. Alaska, California, Hawaii, Maine, Massachusetts, New Hampshire, New Mexico, Vermont, and Washington law provides pharmacists with authority to prescribe and dispense EC under protocol.

Exempt narcotics Medications with habit-forming ingredients that could be dispensed by a pharmacist without a prescription to persons at least eighteen years of age.

Dual marketing Status of medications like Plan B® that are classified as both prescription drugs and OTC drugs.

SAMPLE LABELS

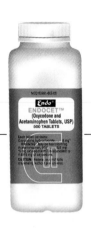

MANUFACTURER STOCK LABEL

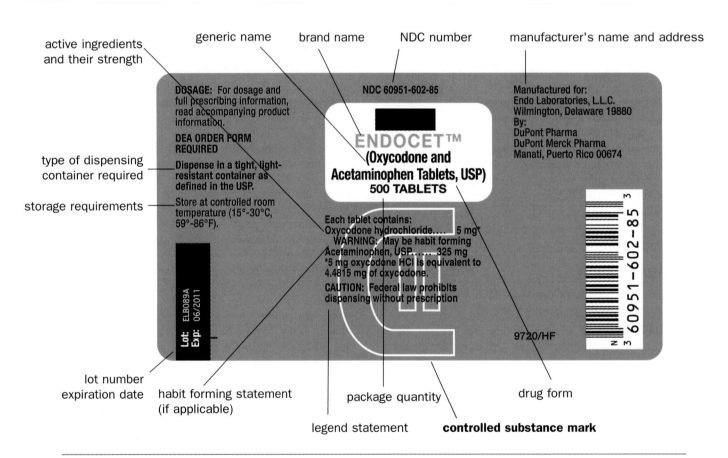

active ingredients and their strength

generic name

brand name

NDC number

manufacturer's name and address

type of dispensing container required

storage requirements

lot number expiration date

habit forming statement (if applicable)

package quantity

legend statement

drug form

controlled substance mark

DOSAGE: For dosage and full prescribing information, read accompanying product information.

DEA ORDER FORM REQUIRED

Dispense in a tight, light-resistant container as defined in the USP.

Store at controlled room temperature (15°-30°C, 59°-86°F).

Lot: ELB089A
Exp: 06/2011

NDC 60951-602-85

ENDOCET™
(Oxycodone and Acetaminophen Tablets, USP)
500 TABLETS

Each tablet contains:
Oxycodone hydrochloride.... 5 mg*
WARNING: May be habit forming
Acetaminophen, USP...... 325 mg
*5 mg oxycodone HCl is equivalent to 4.4815 mg of oxycodone.

CAUTION: Federal law prohibits dispensing without prescription

Manufactured for:
Endo Laboratories, L.L.C.
Wilmington, Delaware 19880
By:
DuPont Pharma
DuPont Merck Pharma
Manati, Puerto Rico 00674

3 60951-602-85

9720/HF

Product Labeling

In addition to a container label, manufacturer prescription drugs must also be accompanied by product labeling, sometimes called the "package insert" or "prescribing information," which includes information on the following: clinical pharmacology, indications and usage, contraindications, warnings, precautions, adverse reactions, drug abuse and dependence, dosage, and packaging. This information is designed to inform both the prescriber and the dispenser regarding the drug.

NDC (National Drug Code) Numbers

An NDC number is an identification number assigned by the manufacturer to a drug product. Each NDC number has 3 sets of numbers: the first set indicates the manufacturer; the second set indicates the medication, its strength, and dosage form; and the third set indicates the package size. Note that depending on whether it is an older or newer drug product, the first set of numbers could have four or five digits and the second set of numbers could have three or four digits. The last set of numbers always has two digits.

controlled substance mark the mark (CII–CV) which indicates the control category of a drug with a potential for abuse.

DISPENSED PRESCRIPTION DRUG LABEL

Minimum requirements on prescription labels for most drugs generally are as follows:

- ✔ name and address of dispenser
- ✔ prescription serial number
- ✔ date of prescription or filling
- ✔ expiration date
- ✔ name of prescriber

And any of the following that are stated in the prescription:

- ✔ name of patient
- ✔ directions for use
- ✔ cautionary statements

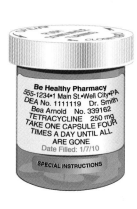

Certain drugs have greater requirements, and many states impose greater requirements.

Typical elements on a prescription label:

name and address of dispenser

date filled

prescription number

patient name

directions for use

name, quantity, strength, manu-facturer and dosage form

expiration date

prescriber

initials of the dispensing pharmacist

refills available

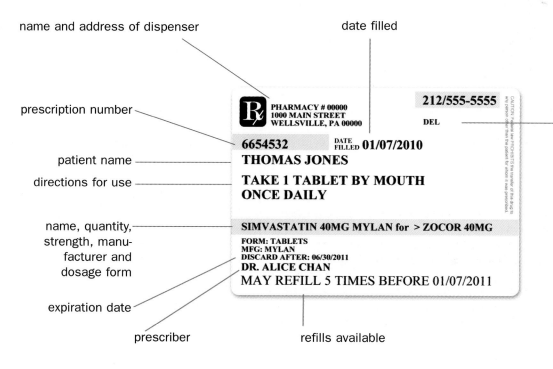

CONTROLLED SUBSTANCES

The government tightly controls the use of drugs that can be easily abused.

The U.S. Congress established the Controlled Substances Act of 1970 (CSA). It identified five groups or schedules of drugs as **controlled substances** and put strict guidelines on their distribution. This act also requires manufacturers, distributors, or dispensers of controlled substances to register with the Drug Enforcement Administration (DEA) of the Justice Department. This created a "closed system" in which only registered parties can distribute these drugs.

The five control schedules are as follows*:

Schedule I:

➥ Each drug has a high potential for abuse and no accepted medical use in the United States. It may not be prescribed. Heroin, various opium derivatives, and hallucinogenic substances are included on this schedule.

Schedule II:

➥ Each drug has a high potential for abuse and may lead to physical or psychological dependence, but also has a currently accepted medical use in the United States. Amphetamines, opium, cocaine, methadone, and various opiates are included on this schedule.

Schedule III:

➥ Each drug's potential for abuse is less than those in Schedules I and II and there is a currently accepted medical use in the U.S., but abuse may lead to moderate or low physical dependence or high psychological dependence. Anabolic steroids and various compounds containing limited quantities of narcotic substances such as codeine are included on this schedule.

Schedule IV:

➥ Each drug has a low potential for abuse relative to Schedule III drugs and there is a current accepted medical use in the U.S., but abuse may lead to limited physical dependence or psychological dependence. Phenobarbital, the sedative chloral hydrate, and the anesthetic methohexital are included in this group.

Schedule V:

➥ Each drug has a low potential for abuse relative to Schedule IV drugs and there is a current accepted medical use in the U.S., but abuse may lead to limited physical dependence or psychological dependence. Compounds containing limited amounts of a narcotic such as codeine are included in this group.

*21 USC (United States Code) Sec. 812 as of 1/96. Note: these schedules are revised periodically. It is important to refer to the most current schedule.

REGULATIONS

Labels

Manufacturers must clearly label controlled drugs with their control classification.

Record Keeping

Distributors are required to maintain accurate records of all controlled substance activity, including accurate records of inventory and drugs dispensed. Schedule II records must be kept for seven years and all other records for two years, unless the state requirement is different. Schedule II prescription records must also be kept separate from non-controlled drug records, though in some cases they may be kept with other controlled drug records.

Security for Controlled Drugs

Schedule II drugs are generally stored in a locked, tamper-proof narcotics cabinet that is usually secured to the floor or wall. Schedule III, IV, and V drugs may be kept openly on storage shelves in retail and hospital settings.

Joint Responsibility

By law, both the prescriber and the dispenser of the prescription have joint responsibility for the legitimate medical purpose of the prescription. This is primarily intended to ensure that controlled substances not be prescribed for inappropriate reasons.

DEA Number

All prescribers of controlled substances must be authorized by the DEA. They are assigned a DEA number which must be used on all controlled drug prescriptions.

controlled substances five groups of drugs identified by the 1970 Controlled Substances Act (CSA) as having the potential for abuse and whose distribution is therefore strictly controlled by five control schedules set forth in the CSA.

Additional DEA Forms are discussed on pages 46-47.

SAMPLE LABELS AND DEA 222 ORDER FORM

Manufacturer containers and labels for C-II, C-III, and C-IV controlled drug products. Note that the control substance marks are prominent.

DEA Form 222 (at right) is used to order C-I and C-II substances. It must be filled out in pen, typewriter, or indelible pencil and be signed by an authorized person, in triplicate. Copy 1 is retained by the supplier, Copy 2 is forwarded to the DEA, and Copy 3 is retained by the purchaser (for example, the pharmacy). The purchaser must record on Copy 3 the number of containers received and the dates the drugs were received. Each form has its own unique serial number issued when the form is requested and all forms must be kept on-hand for two years, even if they are filled out incorrectly. This form can be requested on-line from www.deadiversion.usdoj.gov/drugreg/index.html. Note that C-III–C-V don't require federal order forms because of their lower potential for abuse.

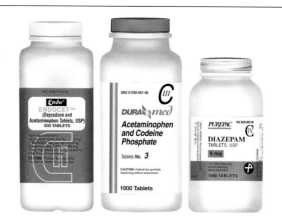

CONTROLLED SUBSTANCE PRESCRIPTIONS

Controlled-substance prescriptions have greater requirements at both federal and state levels than other prescriptions, particularly Schedule II drugs. On controlled substance prescriptions, the DEA number must appear on the form and the patient's full street address must be entered.

On Schedule II prescriptions, the form must be signed by the prescriber. In many states, there are specific time limits that require Schedule II prescriptions be promptly filled. Quantities are limited and generally refills are not allowed.

Federal requirements for Schedules III–V are less stringent than for Schedule II. For example, faxed prescriptions are allowed and they may be refilled up to five times within a six month period. However, state and other regulations may be stricter than federal requirements, so it is necessary to know the requirements for your specific job setting.

Working the DEA Formula: An Example

DEA numbers are required by federal law. They have two letters followed by seven single-digit numbers, e.g., AB1234563. **To check a DEA number on a prescription, use the following formula:** Add the sum of the first, third and fifth digits to twice the sum of the second, fourth, and sixth digits; the total should be a number whose last digit is the same as the last digit of the DEA number on the prescription. For example, using the number AB1234563, since $(1 + 3 + 5) + 2 \times (2 + 4 + 6) = 33$, the DEA number is consistent with the formula.

ADDITIONAL DEA FORMS

Although DEA Form 222 (see page 45) is the most frequently used DEA form, manufacturers, distributors, and dispensers of controlled substances are also required to use specific DEA forms to register with the DEA and otherwise monitor inventory.

Below is a list of all DEA forms and some samples of more commonly used forms. They are available online at www.deadiversion.usdoj.gov/drugreg/index.html.

DEA Forms

- ➡ DEA Form-224 (Application for New Registration)
- ➡ DEA Form-224a (Renewal Application for Registration)
- ➡ DEA Form-224b (Retail Pharmacy Registration Affidavit for Chain Renewal)
- ➡ DEA Form-222 (U.S. Official Order Forms—Schedule ! & II)
- ➡ DEA Form-41 (Registrants Inventory of Drugs Surrendered)
- ➡ DEA Form-106 (Report of Theft or Loss of Controlled Substances)
- ➡ DEA Form-363 (New Application Registration)—Narcotic Treatment Program
- ➡ DEA Form-363a (Application for DEA Registration)—NTP renewal registration
- ➡ DEA Form-510 (Application for Registration)—for Chemical Registration

This is an example of **Application for New Registration (DEA Form-224)** for retail pharmacies, hospitals/clinics, practitioners, teaching institutions and mid-level practitioners. The form requests information such as the business activity, drug schedules, state license number and state controlled substance number (if required).

Source: www.deadiversion.usdoj.gov/drugreg/index.html and Pharmacist's Manual, U.S. Department of Justice, Drug Enforcement Administration, Office of Diversion Control.

This is an example of a **Registrants Inventory of Drugs Surrendered (DEA Form-41).** The form requests information such as the mailing address, DEA number, name of drug or preparation, number of containers, contents (number of grams, tablets, ounces or other units per container), and controlled substance content in each unit.

This is an example of a **Report of Theft or Loss of Controlled Substances (DEA Form 106)**. The form requests information such as the name and address of the registrant, phone number, name of the police department contacted, type of theft or loss, purchase value to registrant and name of carrier.

PUBLIC SAFETY

Though the FDA approval process is quite thorough, it is impossible to fully prove that a drug is safe for use.

No matter how many people participate in the clinical trials, the number is always just a fraction of how many will use a drug once it is approved. So there is always the risk that the drug may produce adverse side effects when used on a larger population. To monitor this, the FDA maintains a reporting program called MedWatch which encourages health care professionals to report **adverse effects** that occur from the use of an approved drug or other medical product. MedWatch does not monitor vaccines. That is performed by the Vaccine Adverse Event Reporting System (VAERS).

The FDA has several options if it determines that a marketed drug presents a risk of illness, injury, or gross consumer deception.

It may seek an **injunction** that prevents the manufacturer from distributing the drug; it may seize the drug; or it may issue a **recall** of the drug or certain lots of the drug. Of these, recalls are considered the most effective, largely because they involve the cooperation of the manufacturer, which after all is the only party that knows where the drugs have been distributed. As a result, recalls are the FDA's preferred means of removing dangerous drugs from the market.

adverse effect an unintended side effect of a medication that is negative or in some way injurious to a patient's health.

injunction a court order preventing a specific action, such as the distribution of a potentially dangerous drug.

recall the action taken to remove a drug from the market and have it returned to the manufacturer.

A Manufacturer Recall

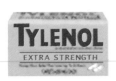

When someone tampered with a small number of Tylenol capsule packages and fatally poisoned seven people, Johnson & Johnson immediately recalled the capsules from the market. This swift and responsible action resulted in a highly favorable public response and increased popularity for Tylenol—and Johnson & Johnson.

RECALLS

Recalls are, with a few exceptions, voluntary on the part of the manufacturer. However, once the FDA requests a manufacturer recall a product, the pressure to do so is substantial. The negative publicity from not recalling would significantly damage a company's reputation, and the FDA would probably take the manufacturer to court, where criminal penalties could be imposed. The FDA can also require recalls in certain instances with infant formulas, biological products, and devices that pose a serious health hazard. Manufacturers may of course recall drugs on their own and do so from time to time for any number of reasons.

Recall Classifications

There are three classes of recalls:

Class I

Where there is a strong likelihood that the product will cause serious adverse effects or death.

Class II

Where a product may cause temporary but reversible adverse effects, or in which there is little likelihood of serious adverse effects.

Class III

Where a product is not likely to cause adverse effects.

safety you should know

Voluntary MedWatch reports for adverse reactions to drugs may be submitted online at https://www.accessdata.fda.gov/scripts/medwatch/, by telephone (1-800-FDA-1088), fax, or mail. Forms can be downloaded from http://www.fda.gov/medwatch/getforms.htm. Adverse reactions to vaccines are reported through the Vaccine Adverse Event Reporting System (VAERS) maintained by the Centers for Disease Control (CDC) and the FDA. The VAERS phone number is 1-800-822-7967; web submissions and downloadable forms are available at http://vaers.hhs/gov.

How an FDA requested recall works:

Reports of adverse effects

The FDA receives enough reports of adverse effects or misbranding that it decides the product is a threat to the public health. It contacts the manufacturer and recommends a recall.

Manufacturer agrees to recall

If the manufacturer agrees to a recall, they must establish a recall strategy with the FDA that addresses the depth of the recall, the extent of public warnings, and a means for checking the effectiveness of the recall. The depth of the recall is identified by wholesale, retail, or consumer levels. The effectiveness may require anything from no follow-up to a complete follow-up check of everyone who should have been notified of the recall. Checks can be made by personal visit, phone calls, or letters.

Customers contacted

Once the strategy is finalized, the manufacturer contacts its customers by telegram, mailgram, or first-class letters with the following information:

✔ the product name, size, lot number, code or serial number, and any other important identifying information.

✔ reason for the recall and the hazard involved.

✔ instructions on what to do with the product, beginning with ceasing distribution.

Recalls listed publicly

Recalls are listed in the weekly FDA Enforcement Report.

LAW AND THE TECHNICIAN

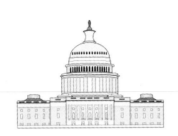

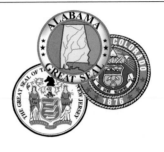

FEDERAL LAW

Federal laws provide a foundation for the state laws which govern pharmacy practice. In addition to the specific drug laws enforced by the FDA and DEA, there are federal laws regulating the treatment of patients (especially in nursing homes) that apply to various aspects of pharmacy practice. These laws guarantee certain patient rights including privacy and confidentiality, right to file complaints, information necessary for informed consent, and the right to refuse treatment.

A major piece of legislation affecting patients' privacy rights and how health care providers may or may not use patient health information is the Health Insurance Portability and Accountability Act of 1996. In an effort to streamline health care costs, this act encourages providers to use electronic transactions and allows a minimum amount of patient health information to be transferred among providers, without patient consent, for purposes of treatment, payment or administrative operations. At the same time, to protect patients' rights, HIPAA makes the health care provider responsible for maintaining the privacy and security of patient information, informing the patient of their privacy policies and procedures, and allowing the patient to both review and correct any records.

STATE LAW

In each state, the State Department of Professional Regulation is responsible for licensing all prescribers and dispensers. There are also state boards of pharmacy that administer state regulations for the practice of pharmacy in the state. In many cases, state regulations are stricter than federal, and the stricter state regulation must be followed. By definition, this means that the lesser Federal requirements are also being met. Following both state and federal regulations is mandatory.

Each state has specific regulations which may or may not be different from other states. For example, a few states allow pharmacists to prescribe under limited conditions. Many allow nurse practitioners and physician assistants to prescribe. When states allow non-physicians to prescribe, they limit their scope of authority. That is, a non-physician prescriber may only prescribe for certain conditions and must follow a strict set of rules (called a **protocol**) that determines the prescription. Non-physician prescribers include dentists, veterinarians, pharmacists, nurse practitioners, and physician assistants. Since states differ on many aspects of pharmacy practice, including who may and may not prescribe, it is necessary to know your own state's regulations, a copy of which can be obtained from your state's Board of Pharmacy.

States regulate the work of pharmacy technicians largely by holding the pharmacist supervising a technician responsible for the technician's performance. If a technician fails to observe any relevant law, the supervising pharmacist is subject to a penalty by the state board. As a result, the supervising pharmacist must explain all the regulations (federal, state, and local) that apply to the technician as part of the job description, and must work with the technician to assure **compliance** with those regulations.

protocol specific guideline for practice.

compliance doing what is required.

negligence failing to do something that should or must be done.

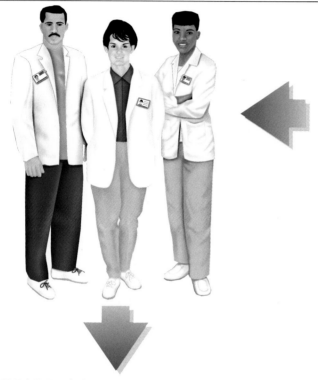

LIABILITY

Legal liability means you can be prosecuted for misconduct. This is true even if you are directed to do it by a supervisor, physician, patient, or customer. Misconduct doesn't necessarily mean you intended to do something, or even that you actively did it. You can be guilty of misconduct by simply failing to do something you should have done. This is called **negligence**, and is the most common form of misconduct. Here are some ways the pharmacy technician can be negligent:

➡ incorrectly labeling the prescription;
➡ failing to maintain patient confidentiality;
➡ failing to recognize expired drugs;
➡ calculation errors;
➡ dispensing the wrong medication;
➡ incorrect handling of controlled substance;
➡ inaccurate record keeping.

For information about a pharmacy technician liability insurance policy, see Chapter 12.

OTHER STANDARDS

Besides the FDA, DEA, and the State Board of Pharmacy, there are various professional bodies and associations which set and maintain pharmacy standards. These include:

➡ **American Society of Health-System Pharmacists:** The ASHP is a 30,000 member association for pharmacists practicing in hospitals, HMOs, long-term care facilities, home care agencies, and other health care systems. It is an accrediting organization for pharmacy residency and pharmacy technician training programs.

➡ **United States Pharmacopeia:** The USP is a voluntary not-for-profit organization that sets standards for the manufacture and distribution of drugs and related products in the United States. These standards are directly referred to by federal and state laws and are published in the "United States Pharmacopeia and the National Formulary."

➡ **Joint Commission on Accreditation of Health Care Organizations:** JCAHO is an independent non-profit organization that establishes standards and monitors compliance for nearly twenty thousand health care programs in the United States. JCAHO-accredited programs include hospitals, health care networks, HMOs, and nursing homes, among others.

➡ **The American Society for Consultant Pharmacists:** The ASCP sets standards for practice for pharmacists who provide medication distribution and consultant services to nursing homes.

Basic criminal and civil laws also apply to pharmacy technicians, which means that crimes like theft, discrimination, sexual harassment, fraud, etc., are punishable just as they would be outside of your job.

REVIEW

KEY CONCEPTS

DRUG REGULATION

✔ In the United States, the leading federal enforcement agency for regulations concerning drug products is the Food and Drug Administration.

✔ The distribution of drugs that may be easily abused is controlled by the Drug Enforcement Administration (DEA) within the Justice Department.

✔ Manufacturers' containers for prescription drugs must have this legend on the label: "Rx only."

✔ Pharmacists must offer counseling to patients regarding medications.

NEW DRUG APPROVAL

✔ Before it is approved for marketing, a new drug must be shown to be both safe and effective and that its benefits substantially outweigh its risks.

✔ Placebos are inactive substances, not real medications, that are used to test the effectiveness of drugs.

MARKETED DRUGS

✔ Once a patent for a brand drug expires, other manufacturers may copy the drug and release it under its generic name.

BEHIND-THE-COUNTER OTC MEDICATIONS

✔ Some OTC medications are kept behind the counter even if they do not require a prescription. These include OTC medications containing ephedrine and pseudoephedrine; exempt narcotics; and emergency contraceptives.

SAMPLE LABELS

✔ The minimum requirements on prescription labels for most drugs are as follows: name and address of dispenser, prescription serial number, date of prescription or filling, name of prescriber, name of patient, directions for use, and cautionary statements.

CONTROLLED SUBSTANCES

✔ Manufacturers must clearly label controlled drugs with their control classification.

✔ All prescribers of controlled substances must be registered with the DEA and are assigned a DEA number which must be used on all controlled drug prescriptions.

ADDITIONAL DEA FORMS

✔ Although DEA Form 222 is the most frequently used DEA form, manufacturers, distributors and dispensers of controlled substances are also required to use specific DEA forms to register with the DEA and otherwise monitor inventory.

PUBLIC SAFETY

✔ Recalls are, with a few exceptions, voluntary on the part of the manufacturer.

LAW AND THE TECHNICIAN

✔ Federal laws provide a foundation for the state laws which govern pharmacy practice.

✔ State boards of pharmacy are responsible for licensing all prescribers and dispensers and administering regulations for the practice of pharmacy in the state.

✔ Legal liability means you can be prosecuted for misconduct, including negligence.

SELF TEST

MATCH THE TERMS   *he answer key begins on page 511*

1. adverse effect ____

2. Combat Methamphetamine Epidemic Act (CMEA) ____

3. compliance ____

4. controlled substance mark ____

5. controlled substances ____

6. dual marketing ____

7. exempt narcotics ____

8. injunction ____

9. legend drug ____

10. liability ____

11. NDC (National Drug Code) ____

12. negligence ____

13. pediatric ____

14. pharmaceutical equivalent ____

15. placebo ____

16. product labeling ____

17. protocol ____

18. recall ____

19. therapeutic equivalent ____

a. medications with habit-forming ingredients that can be dispensed by a pharmacist without a prescription to persons at least 18 years of age.

b. any drug which requires a prescription and this "legend" on the label: Rx only.

c. failing to do something you should have done.

d. important associated information that is not on the label of a drug product itself.

e. legal responsibility for costs or damages arising from misconduct or negligence.

f. status of medications like Plan B® that are classified as both prescription and OTC drugs.

g. the action taken to remove a drug from the market and have it returned to the manufacturer.

h. the mark (CII–CV) which indicates the control category of a drug with a potential for abuse.

i. the number on a manufacturer's label indicating the manufacturer and product information.

j. Federal law that sets daily and monthly limits on OTC sale of pseudoephedrine and ephedrine.

k. an inactive substance given in place of a medication.

l. having to do with the treatment of children.

m. drug products that contain identical amounts of the same active ingredients in the same dosage form.

n. pharmaceutical equivalents that produce the same effects in patients.

o. five groups of drugs identified by the 1970 Controlled Substances Act (CSA) as having the potential for abuse and whose distribution is therefore strictly controlled by five control schedules set forth in the CSA.

p. an unintended side effect of a medication that is negative or in some way injurious to a patient's health.

q. a court order preventing a specific action, such as the distribution of a potentially dangerous drug.

r. specific guideline for practice.

s. doing what is required.

REVIEW

CHOOSE THE BEST ANSWER

the answer key begins on page 511

1. Both domestic and imported drugs require approval by (a/the) _____ before they can be marketed in the United States.
   a. FDA
   b. US Marshal
   c. DEA
   d. US Customs

2. The _____ prohibited interstate commerce in adulterated or mis-branded food, drinks, and drugs.
   a. 1938 Food, Drug and Cosmetic (FDC) Act
   b. Food and Drug Act of 1906
   c. Harrison Act
   d. 1990 Omnibus Budget Reconciliation Act (OBRA)

3. In response to growing addiction to opiates and cocaine-containing medicines, the Harrison Narcotic Act of 1914 required that all manufacturers, importers and physicians prescribing narcotics be
   a. licensed.
   b. taxed.
   c. licensed and taxed.
   d. fined.

4. The Food and Drug Administration was initially named the
   a. Food, Drug, and Alcohol Commission.
   b. Food, Drug, and Weapons Administration.
   c. Food, Drug, and Hazardous Substance Regulatory Agency.
   d. Food, Drug, and Insecticide Administration.

5. Because of fatal poisoning from liquid sulfanilamide, the _____ required new drugs be shown to be safe before marketing.
   a. Food and Drug Act of 1906
   b. 1938 Food, Drug and Cosmetic Act
   c. 1951 Durham Humphrey Amendment
   d. 1990 Omnibus Budget Reconciliation Act (OBRA)

6. The _____ required child-proof packaging for most prescription drugs.
   a. Food, Drug and Cosmetic Act
   b. Poison Prevention Packaging Act
   c. Durham-Humphrey Amendment
   d. Kefauver-Harris Amendment

7. The 1984 Hatch-Watchman Act allowed for
   a. quicker introduction of generic drugs only.
   b. extension of drug patent terms only.
   c. quicker introduction of drugs and extension of drug patent terms.
   d. introduction of generic versions of trade drugs regardless of patent terms.

8. Pharmacists were required to offer counseling to Medicaid patients by the
   a. Durham-Humphrey Amendment.
   b. 1990 Omnibus Budget Reconciliation Act (OBRA).
   c. Kefauver-Harris Amendment.
   d. Harrison Act.

9. Drugs that require prescriptions are _____ drugs.
   a. Durham
   b. Humphrey
   c. legend
   d. Kefauver

10. An inactive substance given in place of a medication during clinical trials is a
    a. pediatric.
    b. phase 2.
    c. phase 3.
    d. placebo.

11. The FDA requires _____ phases of testing in humans.
    a. two
    b. three
    c. four
    d. five

12. The main purpose of phase 2 clinical trials is
    a. dosage.
    b. economics.
    c. animals.
    d. effectiveness.

13. Phase 3 clinical trials generally have _____ participants.
    a. several hundred to several thousand
    b. 20–100 patients
    c. less than 10
    d. up to several hundred patients

14. The Pediatric Labeling Rule of 1994 mandated that
    a. all drug trials include children after a drug has been fully tested on adults.
    b. all drugs carry label information for pediatric use based on studies of adults and other pediatric treatment information.
    c. all drugs have pediatric dosing and safety information on their labels if the drug has potential use for pediatric patients.
    d. all drug labels indicated whether they have been tested on children.

15. After a patent has expired for a medication, other manufacturers may copy the drug and release it under the _____ name.
    a. generic
    b. trade
    c. brand
    d. patent

16. Manufacturers of generic drugs
    a. need to perform the same safety and effectiveness testing required for new drugs.
    b. do not need to perform the same safety and effectiveness testing but do need to demonstrate that a drug is pharmaceutically equivalent to the corresponding proprietary drug.
    c. do not need to perform the same safety and effectiveness testing but do need to demonstrate that a drug is therapeutically equivalent to the corresponding proprietary drug.
    d. do not need to perform the same safety and effectiveness testing but do need to demonstrate that a drug is both pharmaceutically and therapeutically equivalent to the corresponding proprietary drug.

17. Drugs that do not require a prescription are _____ drugs.
    a. FDA
    b. OTC
    c. Durham-Humphrey
    d. legend

18. The Combat Methamphetamine Epidemic Act requires that OTC cold and allergy medications that contain which of the following drugs be kept behind the counter?
    a. antihistamine
    b. methamphetamine
    c. ephedrine and pseudoephedrine
    d. antitussive

REVIEW

19. Pharmacy technicians may sell exempt narcotics
    a. without approval from the pharmacist if they record the sale in a record book.
    b. only with approval from the pharmacist.
    c. after the pharmacist has approved and documented the sale in a record book.
    d. without approval or documentation of the sale.

20. A prescription to dispense Plan B®
    a. is not required.
    b. is required for patients under 17.
    c. is required for patients 17 years of age and under.
    d. is required for patients 17 years of age and under unless otherwise allowed by state law.

21. Of the following Schedule of drugs, which one deals with drugs that have no accepted medical use in the United States?
    a. Schedule I
    b. Schedule II
    c. Schedule III
    d. Schedule IV

22. Amphetamines, opium, cocaine, and methadone are in DEA Schedule _____ because they have accepted medical use, but have a high potential for abuse and may lead to physical or psychological dependence.
    a. II
    b. III
    c. IV
    d. V

23. The FDA reporting system for adverse effects that occur from use of approved drugs is called
    a. Class I.
    b. MedWatch.
    c. VAERS.
    d. Class II.

24. _____ drug recalls are issued by manufacturers when there is a strong likelihood that the product will cause serious adverse effects or death.
    a. Class I
    b. Class II
    c. Class III
    d. Class IV

25. A technician could be prosecuted for misconduct called _____ if s/he incorrectly labeled a prescription.
    a. liability
    b. insubordination
    c. negligence
    d. compliance

26. Basic criminal and civil laws, like theft, discrimination, sexual harassment, and fraud, apply to pharmacy technicians.
    a. True
    b. False

27. Pharmacies located in the health care institutions (hospitals, etc.) are required to follow regulations of this organization:
    a. ASHP
    b. USP
    c. ASCP
    d. JCAHO

TERMINOLOGY

LEARNING OBJECTIVES

At the completion of study, the student will:

➡ explain the common nomenclature system used in medical science terminology.

➡ be familiar with the medical science terminology associated with major body organ systems.

➡ be familiar with common organ disease states and drugs used to treat the disease states.

➡ recognize how the common nomenclature system is used in naming drug classes.

➡ appreciate the complexity of medical abbreviations utilized to shorten terminology used in medical communications.

TERMINOLOGY

Medical dictionaries contain thousands of words that are used in medicine and pharmacy.

Many of the words don't look like words commonly used in literature or speech, and at first glance they can be quite intimidating. But the secret to learning medical science terminology is to learn that there is a system, or order, to it. The purpose of this chapter is to explain this system.

Medical science terminology is made up of a small number of *root words*.

Most of these root words originate from either Greek or Latin words. Words developed from the Greek language are most often used to refer to diagnosis and surgery. Words from the Latin language generally refer to the anatomy of the body.

Numerous *suffixes* and *prefixes* are attached to the root word.

The suffixes and prefixes give specifics to the meaning of the root word. The suffix is a modifier attached to the end of the root word, and the prefix is attached to the front of the root word. So each medical science term will have at least one root word and then a suffix or prefix to complete the meaning. It is not required that every root word have both a suffix and a prefix. Each root word could have just one. In general, prefixes are used less frequently than suffixes.

***Combining vowels* are used to connect the prefix, root word, or suffix parts of the term.**

In some cases the combining vowel can be used to combine the various parts of the word. And there are some cases where the combining vowel is not used at all. Sometimes a combining vowel is added to make the word easier to pronounce. The most common combining vowel is the letter "o."

root word the base component of a term which gives it a meaning that may be modified by other components.

suffix a modifying component of a term located at the end of the term.

prefix a modifying component of a term located at the beginning of the term.

combining vowel a vowel used to connect the prefix, root word, or suffix parts of a term.

Root	Prefix
Suffix	C.V.

ROOT WORDS

The root word is the foundation of medical science terminology. Root words can immediately identify what part of the body a term relates to. For example, consider this list of common root words and the parts of the body to which they refer:

Root	Part of Body
card	heart
cyst	bladder
gastr	stomach
hemat	blood
hepat	liver
my	muscle
pector	chest
neur	nerve
pneum	lung
ocul	eye
derma	skin
ven	vein
mast	breast
oste	bone
nephr	kidney
ot	ear

If a phrase contains the word "cardiac," it is referring to the heart, since "card" is the root word of the word cardiac. The word "ocular" would refer to the eye since "ocul" is the root word of the word ocular.

 Learning the most popular roots, suffixes, and prefixes will help you to understand a large amount of pharmaceutical terminology.

Medical Term

Medical and pharmaceutical nomenclature is a system made up of these four elements:

➡ **root words** ➡ **prefixes**
➡ **suffixes** ➡ **combining vowels**

PREFIXES

A prefix is added to the beginning of a root word to clarify its meaning. For example, *"derma"* is the root word for skin, or things related to the skin, and *"xero"* is a prefix used to describe things that are dry. So:

xero + derma = xeroderma

➡ *meaning:* a "dry skin" condition

Consider another example. The root word for vision is *"opia,"* and the prefix for double is *"dipl."* So:

dipl + opia = diplopia

➡ *meaning:* double vision

For a final example, consider the prefix *"sub"* and the root *"lingu."* "Sub" means under or beneath, and "lingu" is the root word for tongue. So:

sub + lingu = sublingu

➡ *meaning:* under the tongue

However, there are few English words ending in "u," and so this combination is further modified with the typical suffix *"al"* which means "pertaining to," as in:

sub + lingu + al = sublingual

➡ *meaning:* pertaining to under the tongue

SUFFIXES

The suffix is added to the end of a root word to clarify the meaning. Sometimes the connection is made without the aid of a connecting vowel.

Root	Suffix
gastr (stomach)	**itis** (inflammation)

➡ **gastritis**: inflammation of the stomach

Root	Suffix
neur (nerve)	**algia** (pain)

➡ **neuralgia**: pain in the nerve

Sometimes a combining vowel (CV) is used to complete the connection of the different word parts.

1st Root	2nd Root	Suffix	CV
pneum (lung)	**thorax** (chest)		**o**

➡ **pneumothorax**: area of the chest containing the lungs

1st Root	2nd Root	Suffix	CV
card (heart)	**my** (muscle)	**pathy** (disease)	**i, o**

➡ **cardiomyopathy**: disease in the heart muscle tissue

COMBINING THE ELEMENTS

The last combination possibility is to have a prefix and a suffix attached to a root word.

Prefix	Root	Suffix
hypo (low)	**glyc** (sugar)	**emia** (blood)

➡ **hypoglycemia**: low blood sugar

Prefix	Root	Suffix
hyper (high)	**thyroid** (thyroid)	**ism** (state of)

➡ **hyperthyroidism**: too much thyroid activity

And then there is always the possibility that a combining vowel (CV) will be used within a word.

Prefix	Root	Suffix	CV
peri (around)	**dont** (teeth)	**ic** (pertaining to)	**o**

➡ **periodontic**: around the teeth

PREFIXES

Root	Prefix
Suffix	C.V.

Below are common prefixes used in medical and pharmaceutical science terminology.

Prefix	Meaning	Prefix	Meaning
a	without	medi	middle
ambi	both	melan	black
an	without	meso	middle
ante	before	meta	beyond, after, changing
anti	against	micro	small
bi	two or both	mid	middle
brady	slow	mono	one
chlor	green	multi	many
circum	around	neo	new
cirrh	yellow	pan	all
con	with	para	alongside of or abnormal
contra	against	peri	around
cyan	blue	polio	gray
dia	across or through	poly	many
dis	separate from or apart	post	after
dys	painful, difficult	pre	before
ec	away or out	pro	before
ecto	outside	pseudo	false
endo	within	purpur	purple
epi	upon	quadri	four
erythr	red	re	again or back
eu	good or normal	retro	after
exo	outside	rube	red
hemi	half	semi	half
heter	different	sub	below or under
hyper	above or excessive	super	above or excessive
hypo	below or deficient	supra	above or excessive
im	not	sym	with
immun	safe, protected	syn	with
in	not	tachy	fast
infra	below or under	trans	across, through
inter	between	tri	three
intra	within	ultra	beyond or excessive
iso	equal	uni	one
leuk	white	xanth	yellow
macro	large	xer	dry

SUFFIXES

Root	Prefix
Suffix	C.V.

Below are common suffixes used in medical and pharmaceutical science terminology.

Suffix	Meaning	Suffix	Meaning
ac	pertaining to	oid	resembling
al	pertaining to	ole	small
algia	pain	oma	tumor
ar	pertaining to	opia	vision
ary	pertaining to	opsia	vision
asthenia	without strength	osis	abnormal condition, increase
cele	pouching or hernia	osmia	smell
cyesis	pregnancy	ous	pertaining to
cynia	pain	paresis	partial paralysis
eal	pertaining to	pathy	disease
ectasis	expansion or dilation	penia	decrease
ectomy	removal	phagia	swallowing
emia	blood condition	phasia	speech
genic	origin or production	philia	attraction for
gram	record	phobia	fear
graph	recording instrument	plasia	formation
graphy	recording process	plasty	surgical repair or reconstruction
ia	condition of	plegia	paralysis, stroke
iasis	condition, formation of	rrhage	to burst forth
iatry	treatment	rrhea	discharge
ic	pertaining to	sclerosis	narrowing, constriction
icle	small	scope	examination instrument
ism	condition of	scopy	examination
itis	inflammation	spasm	involuntary contraction
ium	tissue or structure	stasis	stop or stand
lith	stone, calculus	tic	pertaining to
logy	study of	tocia	childbirth, labor
lysis	breaking down or dissolution	tomy	incision
malacia	softening	toxic	poison
megaly	enlargement	tropic	stimulate
meter	measuring instrument	ula	small
metry	measuring process	ule	small
mycosis	fungal infection	y	condition, process of

ORGAN SYSTEM TERMINOLOGY

A good way to learn medical science terminology is to learn it based on the different organ systems in the body.

There are names for structures and parts of organ systems that form the root words used in medical science terminology. These names have to be learned. Then they can be applied to understand or to construct words.

The cardiovascular system distributes blood throughout the body using blood vessels called arteries, capillaries, and veins. Blood transports nutrients to the body's cells and carries waste products away from them. Blood is made up of red blood cells, white blood cells, platelets, and plasma. Erythrocytes (red blood cells) transport oxygen from the lungs to the body and carbon dioxide from the cells to the lungs. Leukocytes (white blood cells) fight bacterial infections by producing antibodies.

Blood is pumped through the cardiovascular system by the heart. Valves within the heart maintain the flow of blood in only one direction. Conductive tissue which is unique to the heart muscle is responsible for the heartbeat.

When blood is forced out of the heart, the increased pressure on the system is called the **systolic phase**. When blood pressure is monitored, this pressure is reported (in mm Hg) as the first number of a two number sequence. The **diastolic phase**, or relaxation phase, is the second number reported in blood pressure monitoring. Blood pressures are reported as systole/diastole, i.e., 120/80. A sphygmomanometer is used to measure blood pressure.

CARDIOVASCULAR SYSTEM

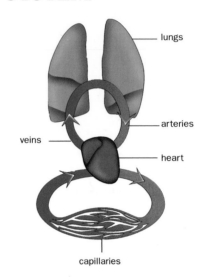

Root	Meaning	Root	Meaning
angi	vessel	phleb	vein
aort	aorta	stenosis	narrowing
card	heart	thromb	clot
oxy	oxygen	vas(cu)	blood vessel
pector	chest	ven	vein

Some Additional Cardiovascular System Terminology

Term	Meaning	Term	Meaning
ather/o/scler/osis	hardening of the artery	thromb/osis	blood clots in the vascular system
card/io/my/o/pathy	disease of the heart muscle	ven/ous	pertaining to the veins
hyper/tension	high blood pressure		

Some Common Cardiovascular Conditions and Drug Therapies

Condition	Brand Name	Generic Name	Condition	Brand Name	Generic Name
Atrial fibrillation	Coumadin	warfarin	Coronary artery disease	Norvasc	amlodipine
Atrial fibrillation	Lopressor	metroprolol	Coronary artery disease	Plavix	clopidogrel
Congestive heart failure	Coreg	carvedilol	Hypertension	Diovan	valsartan
Congestive heart failure	Vasotec	enalapril	Hypertension	Lasix	furosemide

systolic phase the blood pressure as the heart is pumping blood into the cardiovascular system.

diastolic phase the blood pressure after the heart has completed a pumping stroke.

endocrine system a system of glands that secrete hormones into the bloodstream.

ENDOCRINE SYSTEM

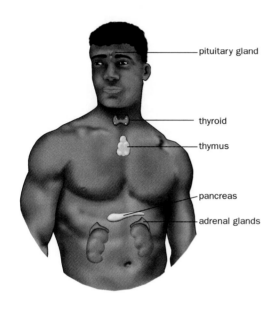

- pituitary gland
- thyroid
- thymus
- pancreas
- adrenal glands

The **endocrine system** consists of the glands that secrete hormones, chemicals that assist in regulating body functions.

Several organs act as endocrine glands as well as members of other organ systems. For example, the liver, stomach, pancreas, and kidneys are members of the endocrine system as well as other organ systems. Organs that belong primarily to the endocrine system include the pituitary gland, the adrenal glands, the thyroid gland, and the gonads (ovaries and testes).

The pituitary gland produces multiple hormones and is located at the base of the brain. It controls the body's growth and releases hormones into the bloodstream that control much of the activity of the other glands. The thyroid gland is located just below the larynx and releases hormones important for regulating body metabolism. There are four smaller parathyroid glands located on the thyroid gland. The thymus gland is located beneath the sternum. The pancreas is best known for its production of insulin and glucagon. The small adrenal glands are located on top of the kidneys. They produce such hormones as aldosterone, cortisol (hydrocortisone), androgens, and estrogens. The medulla region of the adrenal glands produce the catecholamines adrenaline (epinephrine) and noradrenaline (norepinephrine).

Root	Meaning	Root	Meaning
adrena	adrenal	pancreat	pancreas
glyc	sugar	somat	body
lipid	fat	thym	thymus
nephr	kidney	thyr	thyroid

Some Additional Endocrine System Terminology

Term	Meaning	Term	Meaning
endo/crine	pertaining to glands that secrete hormones into the bloodstream	hyper/lipid/emia	increase of lipids in the blood
		hypo/thyroid/ism	a deficiency of thyroid secretion
hyper/glyc/emia	high blood sugar	somat/ic	pertaining to the body

Some Common Endocrine System Conditions and Drug Therapies

Condition	Brand Name	Generic Name	Condition	Brand Name	Generic Name
Diabetes insipidus	Pitressin	vasopressin	Hyperthyroidism	Tapazole	methimazole
Diabetes mellitus	Humalog	insulin lispro	Hypoaldosteronism	Florinef	fludrocortisone
Diabetes mellitus	Novolin R	insulin regular	Hypothyroidism	Levoxyl	levothyroxine
Diabetes mellitus	Orinase	tolbutamide			

ORGAN SYSTEM TERMINOLOGY

GASTROINTESTINAL TRACT

The gastrointestinal (GI) tract is located in the abdomen, and is surrounded by the peritoneal lining. The GI tract contains the organs that are involved in the digestion of foods and the absorption of nutrients. These organs include the stomach, small and large intestine, gallbladder, liver, and pancreas.

The GI tract is sometimes inappropriately referred to as the **alimentary tract.** The alimentary tract refers to the system that goes from the mouth to the anus. The alimentary tract contains organs such as lips, tongue, teeth, salivary glands, pharynx, esophagus, rectum, and anus, in addition to the GI tract.

Several organs contribute to the digestion of foods by secreting enzymes into the small intestine when food is present. Ducts carry bile from the liver (hepatic duct) and the gallbladder (cystic duct) to the duodenum. The pancreas is located behind the stomach and also contributes enzymes to the digestive process.

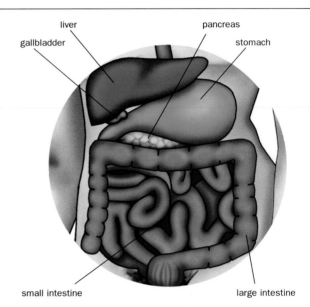

Root	Meaning	Root	Meaning
chol	bile	gastr	stomach
col	colon	hepat	liver
duoden	duodenum	lapar	abdomen
enter	intestine	orexia	appetite
esophag	esophagus	pancreat	pancreas

Some Additional Gastrointestinal Tract Terminology

Term	Meaning	Term	Meaning
an/orexia	loss of appetite	gastr/itis	inflammation of the stomach
col/itis	inflamed or irritable colon	hepat/oma	liver tumor
hepat/itis	inflammation of the liver		

Some Common Gastrointestinal Conditions and Drug Therapies

Condition	Brand Name	Generic Name	Condition	Brand Name	Generic Name
Constipation	Colace	docusate	Nausea, Vomiting	Compazine	prochlorperazine
Diarrhea	Lomotil	diphenoxylate w/ atropine	Ulcers	Nexium	esomeprazole
			Ulcers	Tagamet	cimetidine
GERD (Gastrointestinal reflux disease)	Prilosec	omeprazole			

alimentary tract the organs from the mouth to the anus. The GI tract is a portion of the alimentary tract.

integumentary system the body covering, i.e., skin, hair, and nails.

INTEGUMENTARY SYSTEM

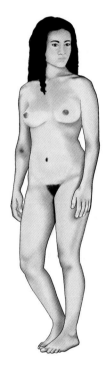

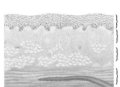

epidermis
dermis
subcutaneous
muscle

The covering of the body is referred to as the **integumentary system**. It is the body's first line of defense, acting as a barrier against disease and physical hazards. It also helps control body temperature by releasing heat through sweat or by constricting blood vessels to act as insulation. It includes the skin, hair, and nails.

Hair is made of keratinized cells. Finger nails and toenails are also composed of keratin. The mammary glands, or breasts, are also considered part of the integumentary system.

The skin is composed of the epidermis and dermis. The epidermis has no blood or nerves and is constantly discarding dead cells. The dermis, which is made of living cells, contains capillaries, nerves, and lymphatics. The dermis also contains the sebaceous glands, sweat glands, and hair.

The subcutaneous layer of tissue is beneath the dermis but is closely interconnected to it. It separates the skin from the other organs (for example, the muscular system, as in the illustration).

Root	Meaning	Root	Meaning
adip	fat	kerat	hard
cutane	skin	mast	breast
derma(t)	skin	necr	death (of cells, etc.)
hist	tissue	onych	nail

Some Additional Integumentary System Terminology

Term	Meaning	Term	Meaning
dermat/itis	skin inflammation	sub/cutane/ous	beneath the skin
kerat/osis	area of increased hardness	trans/derm/al	through the skin
onych/mycosis	fungal infection of the nails		

Some Common Integumentary System Conditions and Drug Therapies

Condition	Brand Name	Generic Name	Condition	Brand Name	Generic Name
Acne	Accutane	isotretinoin	Herpes labialis (cold sores)	Abreva	docosanol
Acne vulgaris	Retin-A	retinoic acid, tretinoin	Impetigo	Keflex	cephalexin
			Impetigo	Zithromax	azithromycin
Atopic dermatitis	Elidel	pimecrolimus	Psoriasis	Dovonex	calcipotriene
Atopic dermatitis	Protopic	tacrolimus			

ORGAN SYSTEM TERMINOLOGY

 lymphocytes a type of white blood cells (leukocytes) that helps the body defend itself against bacteria and diseased cells.

LYMPH AND BLOOD SYSTEMS

The lymphatic system is responsible for collecting plasma water that leaves the blood vessels, filtering it for impurities through its lymph nodes, and returning the lymph fluid back to the general circulation. The lymphatic system is the center of the body's immune system.

The largest organ in the system is the spleen. It is responsible for removing old red blood cells from the circulation. It is also a storage organ for **lymphocytes,** a type of white blood cell that attacks bacteria and disease cells. Lymphocytes release antibodies that destroy disease cells and provide immunity against them.

The thymus, tonsils, spleen, and adenoids are lymphoid organs outside the network of the lymphatic system.

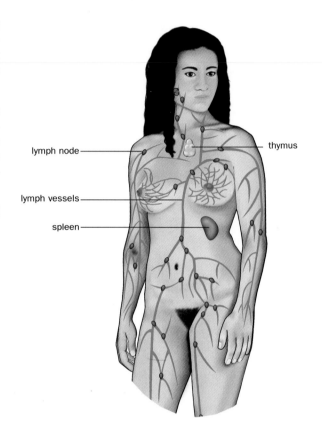

Root	Meaning	Root	Meaning
aden	gland	lymph	lymph
cyt	cell	splen	spleen
hemat	blood	thromb	clot
hemo	blood	thym	thymus
leuk	white		

Some Additional Lymph and Blood Systems Terminology

Term	Meaning	Term	Meaning
an/emia	decrease in red blood cells	leuk/emia	increase in white blood cells
hemat/oma	a collection of blood, often clotted	splen/ectomy	removal of the spleen
		thym/oma	tumor of the thymus
hemo/philia	a disease in which the blood does not clot normally		

Some Common Lymph and Blood Systems Conditions and Drug Therapies

Condition	Brand Name	Generic Name	Condition	Brand Name	Generic Name
Anemia	Procrit	epoetin alfa	Lymphoma, Multiple myeloma	Cytoxan	cyclophosphamide
Hemophilia	Kogenate-FS	antihemophilic factor	Non-Hodgkin's lymphoma	Rituxan	rituximab
Leukemia	Gleevec	imatinib			

flexor movement an expansion or outward movement by muscles.

MUSCULAR SYSTEM

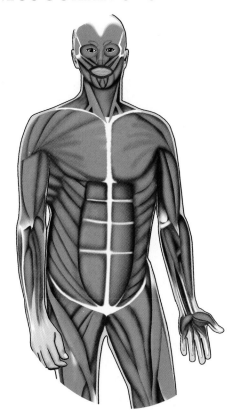

The word muscle comes from the Latin *mus* (mouse) and *cle* (little) because muscle movements resemble a mouse moving under a cover.

The body contains more than 600 muscles which give shape and movement to it. The skeletal muscles are attached to the bones by tendons. The muscles themselves are striated, i.e., made up of fibers.

The action of most muscles is called voluntary, because it is controlled consciously. Involuntary muscles operate automatically and are found in the heart, the stomach, or in the walls of blood vessels.

Some muscles produce an outward or **flexor movement** and these are called agonist muscles. Antagonist muscles are the ones that contract or bring the limb back to the original position.

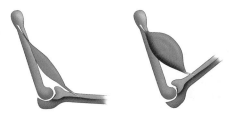

expansion and contraction of muscles

Root	Meaning	Root	Meaning
chondr	cartilage	fibr	fiber
my	muscle	tendin	tendon

Some Additional Muscular System Terminology

Term	Meaning	Term	Meaning
chondr/o/malacia	softening of cartilage	my/o/plasty	plastic surgery of muscle tissue
fibr/o/my/algia	chronic pain in the muscles	tendin/itis	inflammation of a tendon
my/o/necr/o/sis	increase in muscle death		

Some Common Muscular System Conditions and Drug Therapies

Condition	Brand Name	Generic Name	Condition	Brand Name	Generic Name
Fibromyalgia	Cymbalta	duloxetine	Muscle spasm	Valium	diazepam
Fibromyalgia	Lyrica	pregabalin	Rheumatoid arthritis	Mobic	meloxicam
Gout	Indocin	indomethacin	Spasticity	Lioresal	baclofen
Gout	Zyloprim	allopurinol	Tendinitis	Naprosyn	naproxen
Multiple sclerosis	Copaxone	glatiramer			

ORGAN SYSTEM TERMINOLOGY

NERVOUS SYSTEM

The most complex of the body organ systems is the nervous system, the body's system of communication. The **neuron** (nerve cell) is the basic functional unit in this system. There are over 100 billion neurons in the brain alone. Neurons also transmit information from the brain to the entire body.

The primary parts of this system are the brain and the spinal cord, called the central nervous system (CNS). The peripheral nervous system is composed of nerves that branch out from the spinal cord.

There are subdivisions of the peripheral nervous system called the autonomic nervous system and the somatic nervous system. The autonomic nervous system controls the automatic functions of the body, e.g., breathing, digestion, etc. The somatic nervous system controls the voluntary actions of the body, e.g., muscle movements.

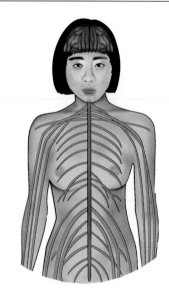

central and peripheral nervous systems

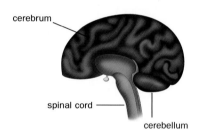

brain and spinal cord

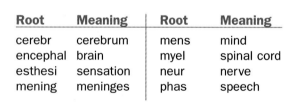

Root	Meaning	Root	Meaning
cerebr	cerebrum	mens	mind
encephal	brain	myel	spinal cord
esthesi	sensation	neur	nerve
mening	meninges	phas	speech

Some Additional Nervous System Terminology

Term	Meaning	Term	Meaning
de/men/tia	disorientation, confusion, loss of memory	encephal/itis	inflammation of the brain
		mening/itis	inflammation of the meninges
dys/phasia	difficulty in speaking	neur/algia	severe pain along a nerve

Some Common Nervous System Conditions and Drug Therapies

Condition	Brand Name	Generic Name	Condition	Brand Name	Generic Name
Depression	Elavil	amitriptyline	Parkinson's disease	Requip	ropinirole
Epilepsy	Depakote	divalproex sodium	Parkinson's disease	Sinemet	carbidopa and levodopa
Epilepsy	Klonopin	clonazepam	Psychosis	Seroquel	quetiapine
HSV encephalitis	Zovirax	acyclovir	Psychosis	Zyprexa	olanzapine

neuron the functional unit of the nervous system.
osseous tissue the rigid portion of the bone tissue.

SKELETAL SYSTEM

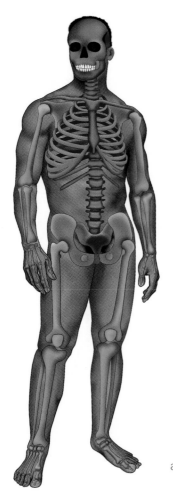

The skeletal system protects soft organs and provides structure and support for the body's organ systems. Made up largely of hard **osseous tissue**, it is a living system that undergoes dynamic changes throughout life.

The system's 206 bones are called axial (the skull and the vertebra surrounding the spinal column) or appendicular (arms, legs, and connecting bones). They are held together at joints by connective tissue called ligaments and cartilage. Joints range from rigid to those allowing full motion (e.g., the ball and socket joints of the hips and shoulders).

Root	Meaning	Root	Meaning
arthr	joint	oste	bone
carp	wrist	patell	knee cap
crani	skull	ped, pod	foot
dactyl	finger or toe	pelv	pelvis
femor	thigh bone	phalang	bones of fingers and toes
fibul	small, lower leg bone	rachi	vertebrae
		spondyl	vertebrae
humer	upper arm bone	stern	sternum, breastbone
		tibi	large lower leg bone

axial **and** appendicular **skeleton**

Some Additional Skeletal System Terminology

Term	Meaning	Term	Meaning
arthr/itis	inflammation of the joint	oste/o/carcin/oma	cancerous bone tumor
carp/al	pertaining to the wrist	rach/itis	inflammation of the spine
oste/o/arthr/itis	chronic bone and joint disease		

Some Common Skeletal System Conditions and Drug Therapies

Condition	Brand Name	Generic Name	Condition	Brand Name	Generic Name
Arthritis	Celebrex	celecoxib	Osteoporosis	Fosamax	alendronate
Arthritis, Spondylitis	Enbrel	etanercept	Paget's disease	Didronel	etidronate
Osteoporosis	Actonel	risedronate	Rheumatoid arthritis	Mobic	meloxicam

ORGAN SYSTEM TERMINOLOGY

FEMALE REPRODUCTIVE SYSTEM

The female reproductive system produces hormones (e.g., estrogen, progesterone), controls menstruation, and provides for childbearing. The system contains the vagina, uterus, fallopian tubes, ovaries, and the external genitalia.

The mammary glands (located in breast tissue) are also associated with the female reproductive system. The mammary glands produce and secrete milk at childbirth.

The vagina is a muscular tube that leads from an external opening to the cervix and uterus. The uterus is a hollow, pear-shaped organ. The fallopian tubes transport eggs from the ovary to the uterus. The ovaries are located on each side of the uterus. In sexually mature females, the uterus is prepared for the possibility of fertilization and pregnancy each month during the menstrual cycle.

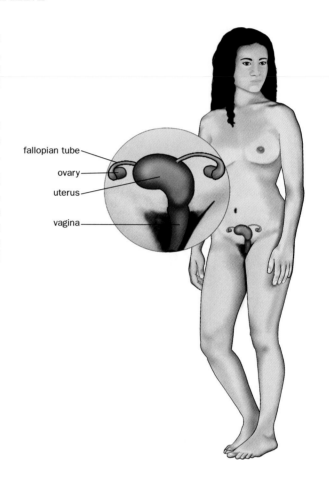

Root	Meaning	Root	Meaning
gynec	woman	metr	uterus
hyster	uterus	ovari	ovary
lact	milk	salping	fallopian tube
mamm	breast	toc	birth
mast	breast	uter	uterine
men	menstrua-tion		

Some Additional Female Reproductive System Terminology

Term	Meaning	Term	Meaning
a/men/o/rrhea	absence of menstruation	endo/metr/i/osis	abnormal growth of uteral tissue
dys/men/o/rrhea	menstrual pain	mast/itis	inflammation of the breast
dys/toc/ia	difficult childbirth	vagin/itis	inflammation of the vagina

Some Common Female Reproductive System Conditions and Drug Therapies

Condition	Brand Name	Generic Name	Condition	Brand Name	Generic Name
Breast cancer	Ellence	epirubicin	Menopausal symptoms	Premarin	conjugated estrogens
Chlamydia	Zithromax	azithromycin			
Dysmenorrhea	Cataflam	diclofenac	Ovulation induction	Clomid	clomiphene
Endometriosis	Synarel	nafarelin			

MALE REPRODUCTIVE SYSTEM

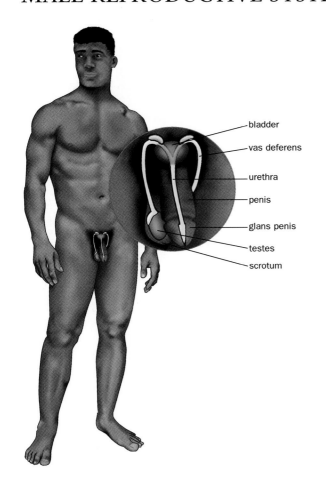

bladder
vas deferens
urethra
penis
glans penis
testes
scrotum

The male reproductive system produces sperm and secretes the hormone testosterone. The primary male sex organs are the testes (also called testicles). They are the oval-shaped organs enclosed in the scrotum.

The seminal glands, located at the base of the bladder, produce part of the seminal fluid. They have ducts that lead into the vas deferens which carry the sperm from the testes. The prostate gland is located at the upper end of the urethra. The penis (glans penis) is the external organ for urination and sexual intercourse. The tip of the penis is covered by the prepuce (foreskin). The urethra, by which urine and semen leave the body, is inside the penis.

Root	Meaning	Root	Meaning
andr	male	sperm	sperm
balan	glans penis	vas	vessel, duct
prostat	prostate gland	test	testis, testicle
semin	semen		

Some Additional Male Reproductive System Terminology

Term	Meaning	Term	Meaning
a/sperm/ia	inability to secrete sperm	semin/oma	tumor of the testes
balan/itis	inflammation of the glans penis	vas/ectomy	removal of a segment of the vas deferens
prostat/itis	inflammation of the prostate		

Some Common Male Reproductive System Conditions and Drug Therapies

Condition	Brand Name	Generic Name	Condition	Brand Name	Generic Name
Benign prostatic hyperplasia	Flomax	tamsulosin	Erectile dysfunction	Levitra	vardenafil
			Erectile dysfunction	Cialis	tadalafil
Benign prostatic hyperplasia	Proscar	finasteride	Genital HSV infection	Valtrex	valacyclovir
			Prostate cancer	Casodex	bicalutamide

ORGAN SYSTEM TERMINOLOGY

RESPIRATORY SYSTEM

The respiratory system brings oxygen into the body through inhalation and expels carbon dioxide gas through exhalation. It produces sound for speaking and helps cool the body.

Respiratory muscles (especially the diaphragm) expand the lungs automatically, causing air to be inhaled into the upper respiratory tract. The pleural cavity surrounds the lungs and provides lubrication for respiration. The pharynx directs food into the esophagus and air into the trachea. The larynx contains the vocal cords. The trachea, or windpipe, connects to the two bronchi (bronchial tubes) that enter the lungs.

As air enters through the nose, it is warmed, moistened, and filtered. Inside the lungs, the bronchial tubes branch out and lead to the alveolar sacs that are the site of gas exchange within the lungs. The lungs have specialized tissues called **alveoli** that are responsible for the exchange of gases between the blood and inhaled air.

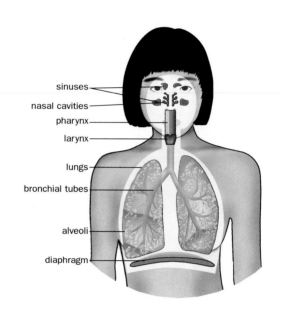

Root	Meaning	Root	Meaning
aer	air	ox	oxygen
aero	gas	pector	chest
bronch	bronchus	pneum	lung, air
capn	carbon dioxide	pulmon	lung
		rhin	nose
laryng	larynx	sinus	sinus
nas	nose		

Some Additional Respiratory System Terminology

Term	Meaning	Term	Meaning
bronch/itis	inflammation of the bronchial membranes	pector/algia	chest pain
		pneum/o/nia	bacterial infection of the lungs
hyper/capn/ia	excessive carbon dioxide in the blood	rhin/itis	inflammation of the nose
		sinus/itis	inflammation of the sinuses

Some Common Respiratory System Conditions and Drug Therapies

Condition	Brand Name	Generic Name	Condition	Brand Name	Generic Name
Allergic rhinitis	Zyrtec	cetirizine	Chronic obstructive pulmonary disease (COPD)	Combivent	albuterol and ipratropium
Asthma	Theo-24	theophylline			
Bronchospasms, COPD	Spiriva	tiotropium	Mucolytic therapy	Mucomyst	N-acetylcysteine
Bronchospasms, COPD	Ventolin	albuterol			

alveoli a part of the lungs where gases are exchanged between blood and the air.

nephron the functional unit of the kidney responsible for removing wastes from the blood and producing urine.

URINARY TRACT

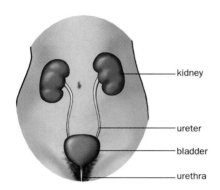

The urinary tract is responsible for removing waste materials from the blood. The urinary tract includes the kidneys, ureters, urinary bladder, and urethra.

The primary organ of the urinary tract is the kidney. The **nephron** is the functional unit of the kidney. There are several million nephrons in the kidneys. Urine is produced as plasma water is filtered through the glomerulus and the filtrate is collected in the tubule. Waste materials from the blood may also be filtered into the tubule or may be secreted into the tubule at sites other than the glomerulus. The filtrate that moves along the tubule is called urine.

Urine leaves the kidney through the ureters and collects in the bladder. It is excreted from the bladder through the urethra.

Root	Meaning	Root	Meaning
albumin	protein	ur	kidney
cyst	bladder	uria	urine, urination
lith	stone	ureter	ureter
nephr	kidney	urethr	urethra
ren	kidney	vesic	bladder

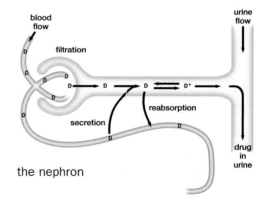

the nephron

Some Additional Urinary Tract Terminology			
Term	**Meaning**	**Term**	**Meaning**
an/uria	inability to produce urine	keto/uria	ketone bodies in the urine
cyst/itis	inflammation of the bladder	nephr/itis	inflammation of the kidney
dys/uria	painful urination	poly/uria	excessive urination
lith/iasis	formation of any stone		

Some Common Urinary Tract Conditions and Drug Therapies					
Condition	**Brand Name**	**Generic Name**	**Condition**	**Brand Name**	**Generic Name**
Cystinuria	Capoten	captopril	Urinary tract infection (UTI)	Macrobid	nitrofurantoin
Cystitis	Cipro	ciprofloxacin	Urinary tract infection (UTI)	Raniclor	cefaclor
Glomerulonephritis	Solu-medrol	methylprednisolone	Urolithiasis (kidney stones) pain management	Voltaren	diclofenac
Urinary incontinence	Detrol	tolterodine			

ORGAN SYSTEM TERMINOLOGY

 tympanic membrane the membrane that transmits sound waves to the inner ear.
eustachian tube the tube that connects the middle ear to the throat.

SENSES: HEARING

The sense of hearing, as well as the maintenance of body equilibrium, is performed by the ear. The external ear consists of a funnel-shaped structure which captures sound waves and channels them through an opening to the **tympanic membrane** (eardrum). The opening also contains glands that make earwax (cerumen) that protects the external ear.

The middle ear consists of three bony structures (malleus, incus, and stapes) that transmit sound from a vibrating tympanic membrane to the cochlea. The **eustachian tube** connects the middle ear to the nose and throat, serving to equalize the air pressure on both sides of the tympanic membrane.

The principal structure in the inner ear is the labyrinth which consists of the vestibule, the cochlea, and the semicircular canals. The cochlea contains the organ of hearing. When sound waves are transmitted to the cochlea, it converts them into nerve impulses that are sent to the brain for interpretation. The semicircular canals and the vestibule are primarily responsible for body equilibrium.

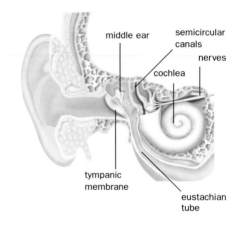

Root	Meaning	Root	Meaning
acous	hearing	myring	eardrum
acusis	hearing condition	ot	ear
		salping	eustachian tube
audi	hearing		
cerumin	wax-like, waxy	tympan	eardrum

Some Additional Hearing Terminology

Term	Meaning	Term	Meaning
labyrinth/itis	inflammation of the inner ear	ot/o/mycosis	fungal ear infection
ot/algia	pain in the ear (ear ache)	par/acusis	partial hearing loss
ot/itis	inflammation of the ear	tympan/itis	inflammation of the eardrum

Some Common Hearing Conditions and Drug Therapies

Condition	Brand Name	Generic Name	Condition	Brand Name	Generic Name
Ceruminosis	Debrox	carbamide peroxide	Otitis media (middle ear inflammation)	Amoxil	amoxicillin
Myringitis	Zithromax	azithromycin	Otomycosis	Nizoral	ketoconazole
Otitis externa (outer ear inflammation)	Floxin	ofloxacin			

conjunctiva the eyelid lining.

lacrimal gland the gland that produces tears for the eyes.

cornea the transparent outer part of the eye.

retina the inner lining of the eye that translates light into nerve impulses.

SENSES: SIGHT

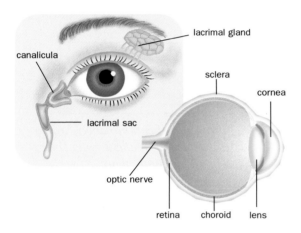

The eyes are the organs that provide sight. The eyelids protect the eye and assist in its lubrication. The **conjunctiva** is the blood-rich membrane between the eye and the eyelid. There are several glands that secrete fluids to protect and lubricate the eye: the **lacrimal glands** above each eye secrete tears and the meibomian glands produce sebum. Excess fluid drains into the canalicula (tear ducts).

The eye has three layers. The outer layer is composed of the sclera and the cornea. The sclera is the white part of the eye. The **cornea** is transparent so the iris (the color of the eye) and the pupil (the opening of the eye) are visible. The middle layer is called the choroid and contains blood vessels that nourish the entire eye. In the third layer, the lens focuses light rays on the **retina.** The vitreous humor (one of two fluids in the eye) fills the space between the retina and the lens. Rods and cones within the retina are responsible for visual reception. The optic nerve within the retina transmits the nerve impulses to the brain for interpretation.

Root	Meaning	Root	Meaning
blephar	eyelid	ocul	eye
corne	cornea	ophthalm	eye
irid, ir	iris	retin	retina
lacrim	tear duct		

Some Additional Ophthalmic Terminology

Term	Meaning	Term	Meaning
blephar/itis	inflammation of the eyelids	ocul/o/mycosis	fungal infection of the eye
conjunctiv/itis	inflammation of the conjunctiva	retin/itis	inflammation of the retina
endo/phthalm/itis	inflammation of the inside of the eye		

Some Common Ophthalmic Conditions and Drug Therapies

Condition	Brand Name	Generic Name	Condition	Brand Name	Generic Name
Allergic conjunctivitis	Patanol	olopatadine	Glaucoma	Azopt	brinzolamide
Bacterial conjunctivitis	Genoptic	gentamicin	Glaucoma	Xalatan	latanoprost
Blepharitis (eyelid infection)	Polytrim	polymyxin, trimethoprim	Superficial ocular infection	Maxitrol	neomycin/ polymyxin
Chronic dry eye	Restasis	cyclosporine			

DRUG CLASSIFICATIONS

The same system used to interpret medical science terminology can be used to interpret drug classification names.

A classification is a grouping of drugs that have some properties in common.

For example, penicillin, cefoxitine, and ciprofloxacin are used to treat bacterial infections, so they are grouped in a class called anti-infectives.

Each of the drugs mentioned above has unique properties, but they all share the property of being effective against bacterial infections. So the classification name "anti-infective" is created by combining "anti" and "infective" into anti-infective, meaning "against infection." Since much of drug therapy is based on opposing some physiological process in the body, many drug classes begin with the prefix "anti" or "ant."

Root	Prefix
Suffix	C.V.

Drug classification names can be understood by identifying their components.

THE "AGAINST" CLASSES

Some examples of the "anti" classes of drugs

antacid	relieves gastritis, ulcer pain, indigestion and heartburn
antianginal	relieves heart pain
anticoagulant	dissolves or prevents blood clots
anticonvulsant	prevents seizures
antidepressant	prevents depression
antidiarrheal	stops diarrhea
antiemetic	prevents nausea and vomiting
antihistamine	blocks the effects of histamine
antihyperlipidemic	lowers high cholesterol levels
antihypertensive	reduces high blood pressure
anti-inflammatory	reduces inflammation
antipruritic	prevents or relieves itching
antispasmodic	relieves intestinal cramping
antitussive	relieves coughing by inhibiting cough reflex

OTHER CLASSES

Here are examples of other classification names which can be understood by breaking down the term into its medical terminology components.

de + conges + tant	**decongestant:**	reduces nasal congestion
an + alges + ic	**analgesic:**	without pain, kills pain
hypo + glyc + emic	**hypoglycemic:**	reduces blood sugar levels
hypo + lipid + emic	**hypolipidemic:**	reduces blood lipid (cholesterol) levels
kerat + o + lytic	**keratolytic:**	destroys hard skin layers such as warts
contra + cep + tive	**contraceptive:**	prevents pregnancy
psych + o + tropic	**pyschotropic:**	changes mental states
sperm + i + cide	**spermicide:**	destroys sperm

MEDICAL ABBREVIATIONS

Many medical and pharmaceutical terms are abbreviated for ease of communication and record notation.

It has been estimated that about 10,000 abbreviations are used in the medical sciences. Many abbreviations are specific for one institution or one area of the country. It is also possible that one abbreviation may have more than one meaning. When in doubt, the pharmacy technician should verify the meaning of an abbreviation.

Common Medical Abbreviations

ADD	Attention deficit disorder		IO, I/O	Fluid intake and output
ADR	Adverse drug reaction		IOP	Intraocular pressure
AIDS	Acquired immunodeficiency syndrome		IV	Intravenous
AV	Atrial-ventricular		KVO	Keep veins open
AMI	Acute myocardial infarction		LBW	Low birth weight
ANS	Autonomic nervous system		LDL	Low density lipoprotein
AWP	Average wholesale price		LOC	Loss of consciousness
BM	Bowel movement		MI	Myocardial infarction
BP	Blood pressure		MICU	Medical intensive care unit
BPH	Benign prostatic hyperplasia		MRI	Magnetic resonance imaging
BS	Blood sugar		NKA	No known allergies
BSA	Body surface area		NPO	Nothing by mouth
CA	Cancer		NS	Normal saline
CAD	Coronary artery disease		NVD	Nausea, vomiting, diarrhea
CF	Cardiac failure		OR	Operating room
CHF	Congestive heart failure		PMH	Past medical history
CMV	Cytomegalovirus		PUD	Peptic ulcer disease
CNS	Central nervous system		PVD	Peripheral vascular disease
COPD	Chronic obstructive pulmonary disease		RA	Rheumatoid arthritis
CVA	Cerebrovascular accident (stroke)		RBC	Red blood count or red blood cell
DAW	Dispense as written		s	Without
D/C	Discontinue		SBP	Systolic blood pressure
DM	Diabetes melitus		SOB	Short of breath
DOB	Date of birth		STD	Sexually transmitted diseases
DUR	Drug utilization review		T	Temperature
Dx	Diagnosis		T&C	Type and cross-match
EC	Enteric coated		TB	Tuberculosis
ECG, EKG	Electrocardiogram		TEDS	Thrombo-embolic disease stockings
ENT	Ears, nose, throat		TPN	Total parenteral nutrition
ER	Emergency room		Tx	Treatment
FH	Family history		U	Units
GERD	Gastroesophageal reflux disease		U/A	Urinalysis
GI	Gastrointestinal		UCHD	Usual childhood diseases
Gtt	Drop		URD	Upper respiratory diseases
HA	Headache		UTI	Urinary tract infection
HBP	High blood pressure		VD	Venereal disease
HDL	High density lipoprotein		VS	Vital signs
HIV	Human immunodeficiency virus		WBC	White blood count or white blood cell
HR	Heart rate		WT	Weight

REVIEW

KEY CONCEPTS

TERMINOLOGY

✔ Much of medical science terminology is made up of a combination of root words, suffixes, and prefixes that originated from either Greek or Latin words.

✔ A prefix is added to the beginning of a root word and a suffix is added to the end of a root word to clarify the meaning.

✔ Combining vowels are used to connect the prefix, root word, or suffix parts of the term.

✔ It is not necessary that a root word have a prefix, suffix, and combining vowel.

ORGAN SYSTEM TERMINOLOGY

✔ The cardiovascular system circulates blood throughout the body in blood vessels called arteries, capillaries, and veins.

✔ The endocrine system consists of the glands that secrete hormones (chemicals that assist in regulating body functions).

✔ The GI tract contains the organs that are involved in the digestion of foods and the absorption of nutrients.

✔ The integumentary system (i.e., the body's covering) is the first line of defense against disease and physical hazards.

✔ The lymph and blood systems are the center of the body's immune system.

✔ The body contains more than 600 muscles which give it shape and produce movement.

✔ The nervous system is the body's system of communication. The neuron (nerve cell) is its basic functional unit.

✔ The skeletal system protects soft organs and provides structure and support for the body's organ systems.

✔ The female reproductive system produces hormones (estrogens, progesterone), controls menstruation, and provides for childbearing.

✔ The male reproductive system produces sperm and secretes the hormone testosterone.

✔ The respiratory system brings oxygen into the body through inhalation and expels carbon dioxide gas through exhalation.

✔ The primary organ of the urinary tract is the kidney; each kidney has millions of nephrons that help remove waste materials from the blood.

✔ The sense of hearing, as well as maintenance of the body's equilibrium, is the function of the ear.

✔ The eye is the sensitive organ involved in sight. Several body mechanisms are involved in protecting this organ (e.g., tear production, blinking).

DRUG CLASSIFICATIONS/MEDICAL ABBREVIATIONS

✔ The same system used in medical science terminology can be applied to the names given to various drug classes.

✔ There are an estimated 10,000 medical abbreviations used in medical science. Many abbreviations are specific to an institution or area of the country.

SELF TEST

MATCH THE TERMS: I   *the answer key begins on page 511*

1. through the skin _____
2. blood tumor _____
3. ven _____
4. ot _____
5. gastr _____
6. hardening of artery _____
7. muscle repair _____
8. otalgia _____
9. liver tumor _____
10. card _____
11. cyst _____
12. derma _____
13. loss of appetite _____

a. athersclerosis
b. kidney
c. chest
d. transdermal
e. eye
f. heart
g. hematoma
h. myoplasty
i. encephalitis
j. bladder
k. blood
l. bone
m. breast

14. hemat _____
15. hepat _____
16. mast _____
17. increase in white blood cells _____
18. nephr _____
19. neur _____
20. ocul _____
21. oste _____
22. brain inflammation _____
23. pector _____
24. pneum _____
25. my _____

n. ear
o. earache
p. vein
q. liver
r. anorexia
s. lung
t. muscle
u. nerve
v. skin
w. stomach
x. leukemia
y. hepatoma

MATCH THE TERMS: II   *the answer key begins on page 511*

1. alimentary tract _____
2. alveoli _____
3. combining vowel _____
4. conjunctiva _____
5. cornea _____
6. diastolic phase _____
7. endocrine system _____
8. eustachian tube _____
9. flexor movement _____

a. the organs from the mouth to the anus.
b. an expansion or outward movement by muscles.
c. a part of the lungs where gases are exchanged between blood and the air.
d. the eyelid lining.
e. a vowel used to connect the prefix, root word, or suffix parts of a term.
f. the blood pressure after the heart has completed a pumping stroke.
g. a system of glands that secrete hormones into the blood stream.
h. the transparent outer part of the eye.
i. the tube that connects the middle ear to the throat.

REVIEW

MATCH THE TERMS: III   *the answer key begins on page 511*

1. integumentary system ____

   a. the inner lining of the eye that translates light into nerve impulses.

2. lacrimal gland ____

   b. the body covering, i.e., skin, hair, and nails.

3. lymphocytes ____

   c. a type of white blood cells (leukocytes) that helps the body defend itself against bacteria and diseased cells.

4. nephron ____

   d. the functional unit of the kidney responsible for removing wastes from the blood and producing urine.

5. neuron ____

   e. the gland that produces tears for the eyes.

6. osseous tissue ____

   f. the base component of a term which gives it a meaning that may be modified by other components.

7. prefix ____

   g. a modifying component of a term located at the end of the term.

8. retina ____

   h. a modifying component of a term located at the beginning of the term.

9. root word ____

   i. the blood pressure as the heart is pumping blood into the cardiovascular system.

10. suffix ____

   j. the functional unit of the nervous system.

11. systolic phase ____

   k. the rigid portion of the bone tissue.

12. tympanic membrane ____

   l. the membrane that transmits sound waves to the inner ear.

CHOOSE THE BEST ANSWER   *the answer key begins on page 511*

1. Medical science terminology has a _____ ____ in every word.
   a. root word
   b. suffix
   c. combining vowel
   d. all of the above

2. The _____ is a modifier attached to the end of the root word and the _____ is a modifier attached to the front of the root word.
   a. prefix, suffix
   b. suffix, prefix
   c. suffix, root
   d. prefix, root

3. The cardiovascular system distributes blood through the body in
   a. arteries and capillaries.
   b. arteries, capillaries, and veins.
   c. veins and arteries.
   d. veins, glands, and arteries.

4. Blood pressure records two phases. Label the correct phase in this reading: 140/90.
   a. 140 = conductive   90 = inductive
   b. 140 = inductive   90 = conductive
   c. 140 = systole   90 = diastole
   d. 140 = diastole   90 = systole

5. Chemicals that assist in regulating body functions are called
   a. antibodies.
   b. hormones.
   c. proteins.
   d. catalysts.

6. The gland in the endocrine system that regulates body metabolism is the
   a. thyroid gland.
   b. adrenal gland.
   c. pituitary gland.
   d. thymus gland.

7. Insulin and glucagon are produced in the
   a. kidney.
   b. liver.
   c. pancreas.
   d. pituitary gland.

8. The hepatic and cystic ducts carry bile to
   a. the liver.
   b. the esophagus.
   c. the duodenum.
   d. the pharynx.

9. A disease of the gastrointestinal tract is
   a. anorexia.
   b. gastritis.
   c. hepatitis.
   d. all of the above

10. Which gland(s) is(are) part of the integumentary system?
   a. adrenal glands
   b. pituitary gland
   c. thyroid gland
   d. mammary glands

11. The top layer of the skin is referred to as the _____ layer.
   a. epidermis
   b. dermis
   c. cutaneous
   d. subcutaneous

12. The integumentary system
   a. regulates the immune response to bacterial infection.
   b. regulates body temperature and defends against disease.
   c. regulates red blood cell production.
   d. provides structural support for the body.

13. The lymph and blood systems are the center of the _____ system of the body?
   a. reproductive
   b. nervous
   c. cardiovascular
   d. immune

14. The spleen is the largest organ in the lymph and blood systems and is the storage organ for
   a. leukocytes.
   b. hepatocytes.
   c. lymphocytes.
   d. monocytes.

15. Skeletal muscles are attached to the bones by
   a. cartilage.
   b. striated muscles.
   c. tendons.
   d. none of the above.

16. Muscle action that is controlled consciously is called _____ movement.
   a. agonist
   b. antagonist
   c. involuntary
   d. voluntary

REVIEW

17. The basic functional unit of the nervous system is the
    a. brain.
    b. cerebrum.
    c. neuron.
    d. meninges.

18. The nerves that branch out from the spinal cord are collectively called the
    a. peripheral nervous system.
    b. autonomic nervous system.
    c. somatic nervous system.
    d. central nervous system.

19. Body functions such as breathing and digestion are controlled by the
    a. cerebrum.
    b. autonomic nervous system.
    c. somatic nervous system.
    d. spinal cord.

20. The bones in the foot are called _____ bones.
    a. carpal
    b. flexor
    c. axial
    d. appendicular

21. Fetal development in the fallopian tubes is called
    a. endometriosis.
    b. dystocia.
    c. salpingocyesis.
    d. mastitis.

22. The major hormone produced by the male reproductive system is _____.
    a. progesterone
    b. testosterone
    c. estrogen
    d. aldosterone

23. The _____ surrounds the lungs and provides lubrication for respiration.
    a. pulmonary cavity
    b. pleural cavity
    c. diaphragm
    d. alveolar sacs

24. The functional unit of the kidney is the
    a neuron.
    b. alveoli.
    c. nephron.
    d. axon.

5

PRESCRIPTIONS

Learning Objectives

At the completion of study, the student will:

➥ understand the prescription process, including each of the steps involved from the creation of a prescription to patient pick up and counseling.

➥ understand the importance of preventing and identifying medication errors at every step of the prescription filling process.

➥ understand the differences in responsibilities between pharmacy technicians and pharmacists, as well as the legal and safety reasons for never assuming pharmacist-only responsibilities.

➥ understand the importance of protecting patient privacy and treating all patients with respect.

Chapter Outline

PRESCRIPTIONS

A prescription is a written order from a practitioner for the preparation and administration of a medicine or a device.

Medical doctors (MD), doctors of osteopathy (DO), dentists (DDS), and veterinarians (DVM) are the primary practitioners that write prescriptions. Opticians and podiatrists are also allowed to write prescriptions for drugs relative to their field of practice. In most states, nurse practitioners, physicians assistants and/or pharmacists are also allowed to prescribe medications based on predetermined protocols (specific guidelines for practice) and in collaboration with one of the primary practitioners mentioned above.

Prescriptions are subject to many federal and state rules and regulations.

These regulations have been developed to protect the patient and to provide for certain minimum standards of practice. The rules and regulations that govern both community and hospital pharmacy practice are continually evaluated and updated as new technologies, new medications, and new protocols are developed and adopted.

Community pharmacists dispense directly to the patient and the patient is expected to administer the medication according to the pharmacist's directions.

This requires clear communication between the pharmacist and the patient. The pharmacist counsels the patient or the patient's representative when the prescription is purchased. In addition, the patient receives information on the prescription label as well as from an information sheet supplied with the medication.

In institutional settings, nursing staff generally administer medications to patients.

As a result, the rules and regulations that govern prescription dispensing in institutional settings are quite different from those that apply to community practice. Labeling is also different and many medications are packaged in individual doses.

Prescription Products

Prescriptions are usually written for commercially available products that are specified by brand or generic name, strength, and route of administration. The prescription may be filled with that exact product or, if allowed, a product that is determined to be equivalent may be dispensed. Prescriptions sometimes require the pharmaceutical preparation of a medication from raw or individual ingredients (**extemporaneous compounding**).

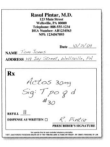

1. A prescription is written by a prescriber.

A physician/practitioner determines that a medication is necessary and communicates the details in the written form known as a prescription.

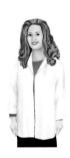

10. Pharmacist provides counseling.

As required by OBRA '90 and other state or provincial statutes, the pharmacist is called to the counter to provide counselling on all new prescriptions and on refilled prescriptions as per protocol.

9. Patient receives the prescription.

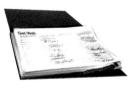

A technician completes his/her final safety and accuracy check by ensuring the correct patient receives the correct drug. The patient or patient's representative signs the insurance log. If the patient has not yet signed the pharmacy's notice of HIPAA compliance, they are given a copy and asked to sign the log. Then the technician rings the sale through the cash register and calls the pharmacist for a consultation, as per protocol.

A B C D *prescription* a written, verbal, or electronic order from a practitioner for the preparation and administration of a drug or device.

extemporaneous compounding the on-demand preparation of a drug product according to a physician's prescription, formula, or recipe.

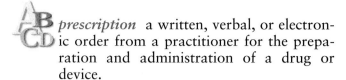

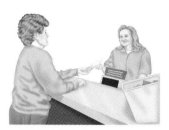

2. The written prescription is presented at the pharmacy.

The patient or a representative presents the written prescription at the pharmacy counter.

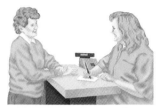

3. Prescription information is checked.

A technician checks the prescription for completeness (e.g., prescriber information, drug name, strength, dosage form, directions) and availability of the drug.

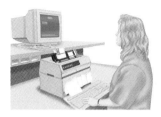

4. Patient and prescription data is entered into system.

A technician collects or confirms the patient's name, address, insurance and allergy information, scans the prescription into the computer system, and keys in the prescription information.

5. Insurance and billing information is processed.

The computer system evaluates the data against stored information and processes any third party billing online. Messaging may be returned regarding drug utilization review (DUR) edits or the insurance claim.

THE PRESCRIPTION PROCESS

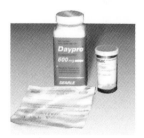

8. The pharmacist checks the prescription.

A pharmacist performs a final check to make sure the prescription is as prescribed and to evaluate any clinical issues.

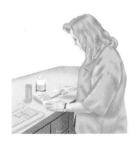

7. Prescription is prepared.

A technician selects the correct product, measures the prescribed amount, places it into a suitable container, and attaches the label. Child-proof containers are required by law unless the patient has on file a request for easy-open caps.

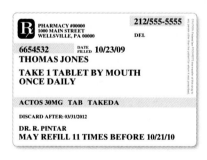

R PHARMACY #00000 1000 MAIN STREET WELLSVILLE, PA 00000	212/555-5555 DEL
6654532 DATE FILLED **10/23/09**	

THOMAS JONES

TAKE 1 TABLET BY MOUTH ONCE DAILY

ACTOS 30MG TAB TAKEDA

DISCARD AFTER: 03/31/2012

DR. R. PINTAR
MAY REFILL 11 TIMES BEFORE 10/21/10

6. Label is generated.

Once the prescription and third-party billing is confirmed, the computer prints the label and receipt. The label includes member copayment or coinsurance information.

PHARMACY ABBREVIATIONS

COMMON ABBREVIATIONS

Abbreviations are regularly used in the pharmacy to communicate essential information such as the dosage form, dosage regimen, and route of administration. To be safe and efficient, technicians must memorize these abbreviations and understand their meaning.

	Abbreviation	Meaning	Abbreviation	Meaning
Route of Administration	a.d.	right ear	top.	topically, locally
	a.s., a.l.	left ear	p.r.	rectally, into the rectum
	a.u.	each ear	p.v.	vaginally, into the vagina
	o.d.	right eye	i.m., IM	intramuscular
	o.s., o.l.	left eye	i.v., IV	intravenous
	o.u.	each eye	i.v.p., IVP	intravenous push
	p.o.	by mouth	IVPB	intravenous piggyback
	S.L.	sublingually, under the tongue	SC, subc, subq	subcutaneously
	per neb	by nebulizer		
Dosage Form	tab.	tablet	syr.	syrup
	cap	capsule	liq.	liquid
	SR, XR, XL	slow/extended release	supp.	suppository
	sol	solution	crm	cream
	susp	suspension	ung., oint	ointment
Timing of Administration	q.d.	every day	prn	as needed
	bid	twice a day	a.c.	before food, before meals
	tid	three times a day	p.c.	after food, after meals
	qid	four times a day	stat.	immediately
	a.m.	morning	q__h	every__ hour(s)
	p.m.	afternoon or evening	qod	every other day
	h.s.	at bedtime		
Measurement	$\dot{\text{i}}$, $\ddot{\text{ii}}$	one, two, etc.	mcg., μg	microgram
	$\overset{..}{\text{ss}}$	one-half	mg.	milligram
	gtt.	drop	g., G., gm.	gram
	ml., mL	milliliter, millilitre	mEq.	milliequivalent
	tsp.	teaspoon (= 5 mL)	a.a. or aa	of each
	tbsp.	tablespoon (= 15 ml)	ad	to, up to
	fl. oz.	fluid ounce (= 30 mL)	aq. ad	add water up to
	l, L	liter/Litre	qs, q.s. ad	add sufficient quantity to make
Other	UTD	as directed	c, w/	with
	NR, ø	no refill	$\bar{\text{s}}$, w/o	without

Note that some prescribers will leave out periods in written abbreviations, and that some may use capital letters, while others may not.

R_x is an abbreviation of the Latin word "recipe," which means "take." Today it is commonly associated with the word "prescription."

LESS COMMON ABBREVIATIONS

Abbreviation	Meaning	Abbreviation	Meaning
aq, aqua	water	per g. button	by/through gastric button
BSA	body surface area	per n.g.t.	by/through naso-gastric tube
c.c.	cubic centimeter (1 cc $\simeq$ 1 ml)	Sig.	write, label
c.c.	with food; with meals	SOB	shortness of breath
D5W	Dextrose 5% in water	troche	lozenge
gr.	grain (1 gr $\simeq$ 65 mg)	tuss.	cough
NS	normal saline		

EXAMPLES

Drug	Rx	Label Directions
Diovan® 80 mg tablets	$\dot{\text{i}}$ po qd	➡ Take one tablet by mouth once daily.
cephalexin 250 mg capsules	$\ddot{\text{ii}}$ stat, $\dot{\text{i}}$ po QID x 10d	➡ Take two capsules by mouth now, then take one capsule four times daily for ten days.
Alphagan-P® 0.1% eye drops	$\dot{\text{i}}$ q 8h ou	➡ Instill one drop into each eye every 8 hours.
Strattera® 25 mg capsules	$\dot{\text{i}}$ q a.m.	➡ Take one capsule by mouth every morning.
Enbrel® 50 mg SC injection	$\dot{\text{i}}$ q week	➡ Inject the contents of one syringe, subcutaneously, once weekly.*

Check with your pharmacist—sometimes "as directed" is added for complex drug products such as injections.

 safety you should know

To help prevent costly and potentially tragic medication errors, technicians must be on alert throughout the prescription filling process to identify any possible prescribing or filling errors. For example, ask yourself, "Does the route of administration make sense for this drug? What about the dosage form and the timing of doses?" Never guess—the patient, the doctor, and your supervising pharmacist are all depending on you to put quality control and safety first. Ask your supervising pharmacist when in doubt.

PRESCRIPTION INFORMATION

The written prescription has stringent requirements designed to inform the pharmacist and protect the patient.

Prescription regulations vary from state to state and province to province, but generally a prescription for a community pharmacy will contain the information illustrated below.

ELEMENTS OF THE PRESCRIPTION

Prescriber information: Name, title, office address, and telephone number

Drug Enforcement Agency (DEA) registration number of prescriber: Required for all controlled substances)

Name and address of patient

Other patient information such as date of birth or weight is optional, but may be important in verifying the correct patient and/or dosing of the medication.

Note: If a compound is prescribed, a list of ingredients and directions for mixing is included.

Refill instructions

DAW/PSC: Dispense As Written/Product Select Code—generic substitution instructions (optional)

National Provider Identifier (NPI): Prescriber's unique national identification number

Date: The date the prescription is written

Inscription: Name (brand or generic), strength of medication and quantity

Signa: This comes from the latin word signa, meaning "to write." It is abbreviated to **Sig** or **S** (or left out entirely) and indicates the directions for use and the administration route (e.g., p.o., p.r., sc).

Signature of prescriber: Required on written prescriptions

Rasul Pintar, M.D.
123 Main Street
Wellsville, PA 00000
Telephone: 888-555-1234
DEA Number: AB1234563
NPI: 1234567893

Date _10/21/09_

NAME _Tom Jones_

ADDRESS _149 Ivy Street, Wellsville, PA_

Rx

Actos 30mg

Sig: T po g d

_#30_

REFILL _II_

DISPENSE AS WRITTEN ☐

R. Pintar

PRESCRIBER'S SIGNATURE

Use separate form for each controlled substance prescription.
THEFT, UNAUTHORIZED POSSESSION AND/OR USE OF THIS FORM INCLUDING ALTERING OR FORGERY. ARE CRIMES PUNISHABLE BY LAW.

Note: Prescriptions may be hand written or electronically produced.

Additional Information

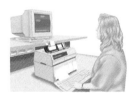

In addition to the above, the information at right must be added to the prescription in the pharmacy. This information is stored in the computer and is printed out with the prescription label. Some data are automatically assigned by the computer (e.g., prescription number), while other information is added by the pharmacist or pharmacy technician as they input the data necessary for the proper filling of the prescription (e.g., the product selected).

➡ Date the product is dispensed.
➡ Identity of the product by manufacturer and NDC (National Drug Code)—DIN (Drug Identification Number) in Canada.
➡ Prescription and/or transaction number.
➡ Insurance information for the patient.
➡ Price charged.
➡ Initials of the technician and pharmacist involved in the filling of the prescription.
➡ Signature of the pharmacist receiving the prescription if it is a verbal order.

Although the prescription shown at left is hand written, many prescribers use computers and hand-held devices to document and produce prescriptions. These prescriptions may be transmitted electronically from the prescriber to the pharmacy.

PRESCRIPTION INFORMATION CHECKLIST

Consider these factors	Take this action

➡ Is the patient's full name clearly written on the prescription? Has a nickname or initial been used?

✔ **Determine the exact name** so that multiple files are not created for one patient.

➡ Is the patient's date of birth, street address, telephone number, insurance information, preference for brand or generic drugs, and allergy information already on file in the pharmacy?

✔ **Always confirm the information on file is current.** Record the patient's date of birth on the prescription to use as a double check when filling the prescription.

➡ Is the medication for an over-the-counter product that the patient can receive without a prescription?

✔ **Check with the pharmacist on all OTC prescriptions.** Only the pharmacist should recommend an OTC medicine or determine which OTC medicine is requested on the prescription.

➡ Is the prescription for a Schedule II drug? **Schedule II drugs** have a high potential for abuse and are subject to special prescription requirements (e.g., tamper-proof prescription blanks and short expiration dates).

✔ **Check with the pharmacist on all Schedule II prescriptions.** Complete Schedule II perpetual inventory log, as appropriate.

➡ When was the prescription written? How many days or weeks has it been since it was written?

✔ **Check with the pharmacist to determine if the prescription can be filled if it is more than a few days old.** Some prescriptions may be valid for months, but others must be verified if they are more than a few days old.

➡ Is the drug available in the pharmacy in the quantity written? Does it require compounding?

✔ **Inform the patient if there may be a delay in filling the prescription.**

➡ Is the prescription suspicious in any way? Is it written on a legitimate prescription blank and all in the same hand writing and with the same ink? Are there any signs of alteration of quantities, strength, or the name of the drug? Is this a possible drug of abuse and if so do the quantities and directions seem appropriate?

✔ **Alert the pharmacist to any potential forgeries.** Let the pharmacist follow through with the patient, the prescriber, and law enforcement, if necessary.

 signa the directions for use to be printed on the prescription label.

Schedule II drugs drugs that have a high potential for abuse or addiction but that also have safe and accepted medical uses; they require special handling.

THE FILL PROCESS

Once prescription information is finalized in the computerized prescription system, a label and receipt are printed out.

At this point, the correct medication must be selected from pharmacy stock and the prescribed amount measured or counted and packaged. If the prescription calls for a compounded product, the technician must follow pharmacy policy in its preparation.

The pharmacy technician completes the fill process by placing the correct amount of medication into an appropriate container and labeling it correctly.

This includes placing the computer-generated label on the container so it sticks firmly, is straight, and is easy to read. It also includes placing the appropriate auxiliary labels on the container. These are the additional warning labels that are placed on filled prescription containers. For more information on auxillary labels, see page 93.

A pharmacist must check the final product and the label.

When finished with preparation, the technician initials the pharmacy copy of the label and organizes the finished product, prescription order, and the stock bottle that the medication was taken from for the pharmacist to check and verify. If the prescription is correctly filled, the pharmacist initials the pharmacy copy of the label information to indicate that the prescription was correctly filled. The prescription may then be released to the patient.

℞ safety you should know: common errors

If a technician is unsure about any aspect of a prescription, he or she must ask the pharmacist for direction. Never dispense guesswork! The careful screening of prescription orders by the technician can prevent medication errors and other errors. Medication errors can be very serious. They include, but are not limited to the dispensing of:

✔ the wrong medication;

✔ the wrong strength, dosage form, or quantity;

✔ the wrong directions;

✔ the medication to the wrong patient;

✔ a medication on a forged or altered prescription.

An awareness that medication errors exist and that they are very serious is the first step in preventing medication errors from happening.

CONSIDERATIONS

The technician should consider these factors when filling prescriptions:

Are the fill instructions clear and reasonable?

Are the directions, quantity, and strength typical for this medication? Check for possible areas of confusion. For example, is the dosing schedule q.i.d. or q.d.? Does the Sig. read: 4 ml or .4 ml?

Are the administration directions clear?

Are the directions clearly translated in an unambiguous fashion in order to avoid any misinterpretation by the patient. For example, does "Take two tablets daily" mean "Take one tablet twice daily" or "Take two tablets once daily"?

Are there look-alike names?

Are there any look-alike drug names that could be confused with the intended medication? For example, did the prescriber write Metadate® 10 mg or Methadone 10 mg, Lamictal® or Lamisil®?

Don't add information!

Never add information based on what you assume the prescriber meant. The prescriber has knowledge of the patient's condition that you don't. Adding directions that you assume to be correct may not be appropriate.

Pay attention to warnings!

When warning screens appear regarding potential insurance claim errors, dosing irregularities, or drug interactions, **call a pharmacist to evaluate each warning.** An ignored warning might result in the patient being over-billed, under-medicated, or hospitalized due to a severe drug-drug interaction. Only a pharmacist may determine which warnings require intervention and which are for informational purposes.

Check against the original!

During the fill process, always refer to the original prescription first and then refer to the label.

A number of drugs have moved from prescription-only to over-the-counter status. Many insurance companies have responded by agreeing to pay for select OTC medications with a valid prescription. Examples of over-the-counter medications that were previously available by prescription only are: Claritin®, OTC Zantac®, Prevacid OTC®, and Zaditor® eye drops.

THE PHARMACY TECHNICIAN'S ROLE

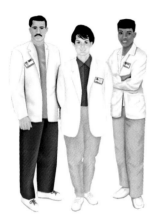

The pharmacy technician's responsibilities include:

✔ assisting the pharmacist in routine, technical aspects of prescription filling;

✔ treating each patient, their personal information, and their medications with respect;

✔ accepting new prescriptions from patients, obtaining all necessary information, and keying it into the computer in an efficient, and accurate manner;

✔ requesting the advice of a pharmacist whenever a warning screen appears while filling a prescription;

✔ faxing or telephoning refill and clarification requests to prescribers;

✔ consulting formularies and responding appropriately to third-party adjudication messaging such as: non-preferred drug, prior authorization or step-edit required;

✔ quickly locating the correct medication for dispensing, calculating quantities, re-packaging medication, and locating the corresponding patient medication guide;

✔ compounding a prescription under supervision;

✔ recording the dispensing of controlled drugs;

✔ checking the work of other technicians, as instructed by a pharmacist;

✔ referring patients to a pharmacist for counseling on the use of prescription and over-the-counter medications, or any other question requiring judgement as per your job description;

✔ ALWAYS ensuring the accuracy and safety of the prescription by incorporating quality control checks into every step in the process.

THE PHARMACIST'S ROLE

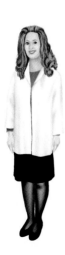

The pharmacist uses his/her expertise to ensure physicians' orders are carried out accurately and safely by checking that:

✔ the correct medication, strength, and dosage form is dispensed to the correct patient;

✔ the directions for the patient are clear, accurate, and unambiguous;

✔ the patient knows how to take the medication and how and when to refill it;

✔ there are no potential problems with drug allergies, drug-drug, or drug-disease interactions;

✔ the patient understands the expected beneficial effects of the medication and any potential side effects the patient should be aware of;

✔ the prescriber has been contacted regarding the prescription if appropriate;

✔ the prescription has been accurately billed to the patient and/or the appropriate third party.

In addition,

✔ only a pharmacist may counsel patients on the use of OTC medications;

✔ only a pharmacist may receive telephone requests for new prescriptions.

LABELS

The prescription label provides information to the patient regarding the dispensed medication and how to take it. Additionally, the label includes information about the pharmacy, the patient, the prescriber, and the prescription or transaction number assigned to the prescription.

As with prescriptions, requirements for prescription labels vary from state to state (and in Canada from province to province). Generally, however, a prescription label contains the information indicated below.

the name, address, and telephone number of the pharmacy

a prescription and/or transaction number

the name of the patient for whom the medication is dispensed

directions for use that are clear, accurate and unambiguous

the name, quantity, strength, manufacturer, and dosage form of the medication dispensed

expiration date of the medication

the name of the prescriber

the date dispensed

the initials of the person who keyed the information into the computer and often the handwritten initials of the pharmacist who checked the prescription

refill information

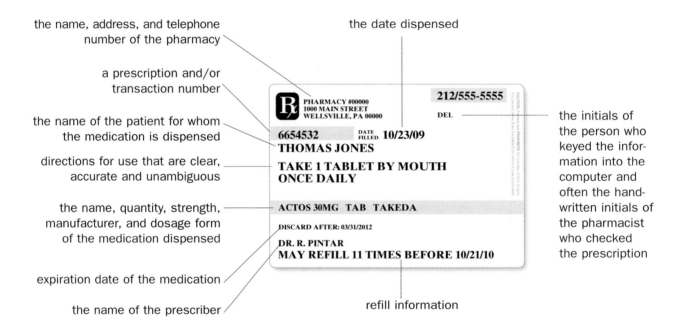

PHARMACY #00000
1000 MAIN STREET
WELLSVILLE, PA 00000

212/555-5555

DEL

6654532   DATE FILLED 10/23/09
THOMAS JONES

TAKE 1 TABLET BY MOUTH
ONCE DAILY

ACTOS 30MG   TAB   TAKEDA

DISCARD AFTER: 03/31/2012

DR. R. PINTAR
MAY REFILL 11 TIMES BEFORE 10/21/10

DIRECTIONS FOR USE

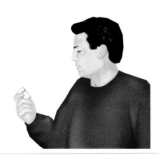

✔ **Directions should start with a verb** (take, instill, inhale, insert, apply) **and completely, clearly, and accurately describe the administration of the medication.**

✔ **Indicate the route of administration.** For example, "take one capsule by mouth," "apply to affected area," "insert rectally," "place one tablet under the tongue," etc.

✔ **Use whole words, not abbreviations.** For example, use "tablets" not "tabs."

✔ **Use familiar words, especially in measurements.** For example, use "two teaspoonfuls" or "10 ml" as most measuring droppers and spoons are calibrated in teaspoons and ml. Double check that the units listed on the label match the units on the measuring spoon or dropper supplied.

OTC drugs drugs that are available for sale without a prescription; however, they may also be ordered on a prescription since some insurance companies cover prescriptions for over-the-counter drugs.

AUXILIARY LABELS

Colored auxiliary labels may be applied to the prescription container to provide additional information to the patient (e.g., Shake Well, Keep Refrigerated, Take With Food or Milk). Many computer-ized prescription systems will automati-cally print out the appropriate labels to use.

Prescriptions for controlled substances from Schedules II, III and IV must carry the following warning:

Caution: Federal law prohibits the transfer of this drug to any person other than the patient for whom it was prescribed.

This warning is pre-printed on many labels.

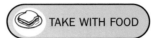
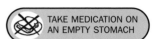
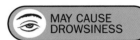
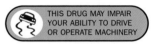
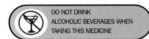
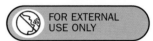
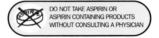
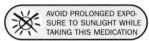

PLACING THE LABEL

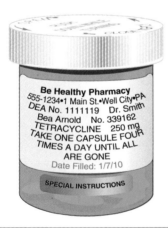

Labeling the container correctly includes:

✔ placing the computer-generated label on the container so it is parallel to the edges of the container, easy to locate, and easy to read;

✔ making sure the label sticks adequately to the container and is without creases. (Some pharmacies place transparent tape over the label to protect the label from spills and prevent acci-dental smudging.);

✔ placing the appropriate auxiliary labels on the container;

✔ placing labels on prescription vials containing eye drops, ear drops and eye ointments;

✔ in some states, placing the label on the actual container rather than the box in which it is packaged.

INSTITUTIONAL LABELS

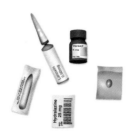

Unit dose packaging is widely used in institutional pharmacy. Al-though rules for institutional pharmacy prescription labels vary by institution, they often contain only the name, strength, manufactur-er, lot number, expiration date, and dosage form of the medication. Since the condition of a patient in an institutional setting may change relatively quickly, patient medication orders are regularly updated. As a result, the nursing staff refer to the most recent physician's instructions in the patient's chart to verify prescribing information.

EXAMPLES

PRESCRIPTION TO LABEL

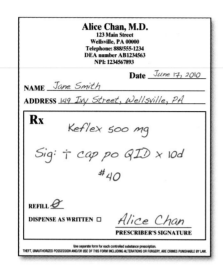

➡ Keflex® is a brand name for Cephalexin.
➡ 500 mg is the strength.
➡ ⅰ cap means "take one capsule."
➡ p.o. means "by mouth."
➡ QID means "four times a day."
➡ x10d means "for ten days."
➡ #40 means a "quantity of 40."
➡ there are no refills; generic substitution may be used.

Therefore, the prescription is for a ten day supply of Cephalexin 500 mg capsules: 40 capsules, one capsule to be taken four times daily for ten days.

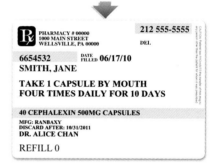

➡ The drug is Neurontin®.
➡ 300 mg is the strength.
➡ ⅰ cap means "take one capsule."
➡ p.o. means "by mouth."
➡ TID means "three times daily"
➡ #90 means a "quantity of 90."
➡ there are 2 refills; dispense as written; generic substitution not allowed.

Therefore, the prescription is for a 30 day supply of Neurontin® 300 mg capsules: 90 capsules, one capsule to be taken three times daily, with two refills.

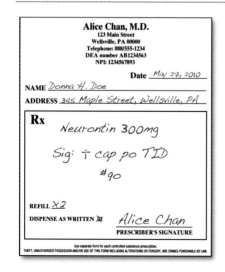

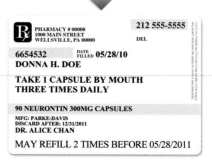

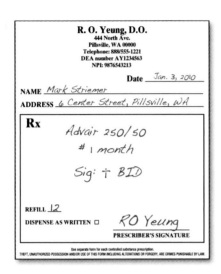

➡ The drug is Advair® Diskus Inhaler.

➡ It is a combination of two drugs and the strength is 250 mcg of one ingredient and 50 mcg of the other.

➡ #1 month means "dispense a one month supply."

➡ Sig means "The directions are..."

➡ ⊤̄ BID means "Inhale the contents of one blister twice daily."

➡ Note: There are 60 "blisters" in the diskus. Each blister is punctured just before use and the contents are inhaled.

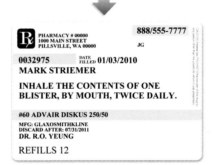

➡ The drug is Nitro-DUR® Transdermal Patches.

➡ The strength is 0.2 mg/h.

➡ The directions are to apply one patch in the morning, and to remove the patch at bedtime.

➡ #30 means a "quantity of 30."

➡ There is one refill.

➡ "As directed" is added to the label to encourage the patient to ask for more information if they are unclear about how to apply the patch.

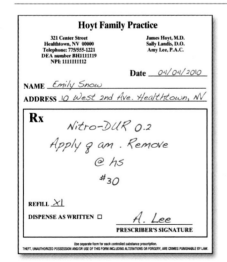

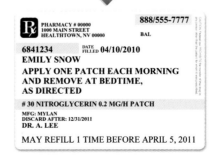

EXAMPLES (cont'd)

MEDICATION ORDERS

There are various formats used for medication orders in institutional settings. Some common aspects of the medication order are:

➡ patient identification information (name, ID#, date of birth)
➡ patient allergy information
➡ patient location (room and bed number)
➡ multiple orders are written on one sheet
➡ date and time of day are indicated, with the most recent entry listed last
➡ orders are often read from the bottom up so as to read the most recent information first
➡ orders may also include requests for lab work, physiotherapy or drug items stocked in the nursing station

These and other aspects of medication orders reflect the special characteristics of the institutional environment.

DOCTOR'S ORDERS

PATIENT IDENTIFICATION
O99999999   675-01
SMITH, JOHN
12/06/1950
DR. P. JOHNSON

DATE	TIME	DOCTOR'S ORDERS 1	DATE/TIME INITIALS	DATE/TIME INITIALS
1/31/10	2200	Admit patient to 6ᵗʰ floor		
		Pneumonia, Dehydration		
		All: PCN- Rash		
		Order CBC, chem-7, blood cultures stat		
		NS @ 125ml/hr IV		
		Dr Johnson x2222		

DATE	TIME	DOCTOR'S ORDERS 2	DATE/TIME INITIALS	DATE/TIME INITIALS
2/01/10	200	Tylenol 650mg po q4-6 hrs PRN for Temp>38°C		
		Verbal Order Dr Johnson/ Jane Doe, RN		

DATE	TIME	DOCTOR'S ORDERS 3	DATE/TIME INITIALS	DATE/TIME INITIALS
2/01/10	600	Start Clarithromycin 500mg po q12°		
		Multivitamin po qd		
		Order CXR for this a.m.		
		Dr Johnson x2222		

LANGRUTH COUNTY HOSPITAL
Medication Administration Record

Room/Bed: 675-01
Patient: SMITH, JOHN
Account #: 099999999
Sex: M
Age: 48Y
Doctor: JOHNSON, P.

From 0730 on 02/01/10 to 0700 on 02/02/10

Diagnosis: PNEUMONIA; DEHYDRATION
Height: 5'11" weight: 75KG

Verified By: Susie Smith, RN

Allergies: PENICILLIN-->RASH

	0730–1530	1600–2300	2330–0700
0.9% SODIUM CHLORIDE 1 LITER BAG DOSE 125 ML/HR IV ORDER #2	800 JD	1600 SS	2400
MULTIVITAMIN TABLET DOSE: 1 TABLET P.O. QD ORDER #4	1000 Gwen® 9AM JD		
CLARITHROMYCIN 500 MG TABLET DOSE: 500MG P.O. Q 12 HRS ORDER #5	1000 JD	2200 SS	
ACETAMINOPHEN 325 MG TABLET DOSE: 650 MG P.O. Q 4-6 H P.R.N. FOR TEMP>38°C ORDER # 17	1200 JD		

Init / Signature	Init / Signature
SS / Susie Smith, RN	____ /
JD / Jane Doe, RN	____ /
____ /	____ /

 There are rules for written information on institutional documents. For example, red ink may be required for some information such as patient allergies.

HIPAA

HIPAA: The Health Insurance Portability and Accountability Act

The Health Insurance Portability and Accountability Act (HIPAA) of 1996 has wide reaching consequences for health care professionals. HIPAA is a large statute that primarily concerns the continuation of health insurance coverage for workers who leave their jobs. However, there are a number of regulations that all health care providers ("covered entities"), including pharmacies, must follow.

HIPAA requires the use of a National Provider Identifier (NPI) for all health care providers. The NPI is a ten-digit number, with a check digit in the last position to help detect keying errors. Each provider may receive only one unique NPI, which is expected to stay with that provider for life. HIPAA mandates that all covered entities, such as health plans, physicians and pharmacies, must use their NPI for all standard transactions covered by HIPAA.

Rules also have been established to regulate how and when pharmacies and other covered entities may use and disclose a patient's protected health information. Other rules require administrative, physical and technical safeguards to prevent illicit access to patient information while it is stored or transmitted electronically. Examples of PHI are name and address, date of birth, social security number, payment history, account number, name and address of health care provider and/or health plan, and medical/prescription drug histories.

Under HIPAA, pharmacies and other covered entities are required to provide a written notice of their privacy practices to their patients. This notice must describe the pharmacy's privacy procedures and patients' privacy rights, and must describe how the pharmacy intends to use and disclose patients' PHI. Each pharmacy must make a good faith effort to have every patient sign an "acknowledgement" that the patient has received its notice of privacy practices. This acknowledgement may be signed when the patient picks up his or her medication. The acknowledgement must be maintained separately from the consultation log that all patients sign when picking up their medication. Acknowledgement signatures must remain on file for six years from the last date of service to the patient.

HIPAA also states that a pharmacy may disclose PHI, without patient approval, to business associates that perform services on behalf of the patient. Examples of such business associates would be physicians' offices and pharmacy benefits management (prescription insurance) companies. However, these disclosures must follow the "minimum necessary" requirement which means that covered entities may use, disclose and request only the minimum necessary amount of PHI to other covered entities.

All personnel who have access to PHI must be formally trained regarding HIPAA. This includes pharmacists, pharmacy technicians, pharmacy clerks, and any other employee who may come into contact with PHI. Even the computer specialists who come to the pharmacy to service computers must be HIPAA trained and HIPAA compliant.

Health Insurance Portability and Accountability Act (HIPAA) a federal act that, among other things, protects the privacy of individuals and the sharing of protected health information.

REVIEW

KEY CONCEPTS

PRESCRIPTIONS

✔ A prescription is a written or verbal order from a practitioner for the preparation and administration of a medicine or a device.

✔ Medical doctors (MD), doctors of osteopathy (DO), dentists (DDS), and veterinarians (DVM) are the primary practitioners who write prescriptions. Podiatrists and optometrists are also allowed to write prescriptions. All practitioners must write within the scope of their practice.

✔ In many states, nurse practitioners, physicians assistants and/or pharmacists are also allowed limited rights to prescribe medications.

✔ In community pharmacies, pharmacy technicians generally receive the prescription, collect patient data (correct spelling of name, address, allergy and insurance information, etc.) and enter them into a computerized prescription system.

PRESCRIPTION INFORMATION

✔ The pharmacist should be consulted on all OTC and Schedule II prescriptions.

✔ The prescription is entered into the computer and drug-drug, drug-disease, and drug-allergy information is automatically checked by the pharmacy software. If third party billing is involved, this is done online simultaneously.

THE FILL PROCESS

✔ Once the prescription and third-party billing is confirmed by the online computer system, the label and receipt are printed and the prescription is prepared.

✔ Since the patient is expected to self-administer the medication, the label's directions for use must be clear, unambiguous and concise.

✔ Pharmacists must provide counseling to patients on all new prescriptions and on any refilled prescriptions where clarification is required. A patient may refuse counseling.

✔ In institutional settings, nursing staff generally administer medications to patients.

✔ Technicians must request the advice of the pharmacist whenever judgment is required.

LABELS

✔ Many computerized prescription systems will automatically indicate which auxiliary labels to use with each drug.

HIPAA

✔ The Health Insurance Portability and Accountability Act (HIPAA) contains regulations related to privacy and protected health information (PHI).

✔ Examples of PHI are name and address, date of birth, social security number, payment history, account number, name and address of health care provider and/or health plan, and medical or prescription history.

✔ Under HIPAA, pharmacies and other covered entities are required to provide a written notice of their privacy practices to their patients.

✔ A pharmacy may disclose PHI to business associates that perform services on behalf of the patient.

✔ All personnel who have access to PHI must be formally trained regarding HIPAA.

SELF TEST

MATCH THE TERMS: I *the answer key begins on page 511*

1. DAW ____

2. DEA number ____

3. extemporaneous compounding ____

4. HIPAA ____

5. National Provider Identifier (NPI) ____

6. OTC drugs ____

7. prescription ____

8. Schedule II drugs ____

9. signa, sig ____

a. a written, verbal, or electronic order from a practitioner for the preparation and administration of a medicine or a device.

b. medications that do not require a prescription but may be filled with a prescription.

c. unique national identification number required for all health care providers.

d. required on all controlled drug prescriptions; identifies the prescriber.

e. the directions for use on a prescription that should be printed on the label.

f. a federal act that, among other things, protects the privacy of individuals and the sharing of protected health information.

g. mechanism by which a prescriber may indicate that the brand product, and not the equivalent generic, must be dispensed.

h. drugs that have been shown to be subject to abuse and require special handling.

i. the on-demand preparation of a drug product according to a physician's prescription, formula, or recipe.

MATCH THE TERMS: II *the answer key begins on page 511*

1. subcutaneously ____

2. drop ____

3. twice a day ____

4. right ear ____

5. four times a day ____

6. as needed ____

7. each eye ____

a. prn

b. gtt

c. pc

d. bid

e. hs

f. SL

g. qd

8. under the tongue ____

9. at bedtime ____

10. microgram ____

11. vaginally ____

12. every day ____

13. every 12 hours ____

14. after food, after meals ____

h. sc

i. qid

j. q 12h

k. ad

l. mcg, μg

m. pv

n. ou

REVIEW

CHOOSE THE BEST ANSWER

the answer key begins on page 511

1. _____ are allowed to write some prescriptions in some states, as determined by protocols and collaboration with a primary prescriber.
   a. Medical doctors
   b. Doctors of osteopathy
   c. Pharmacists, nurse practitioners, and/or physician assistants
   d. Doctors of veterinary medicine

2. Counseling, as required by OBRA '90, is provided by
   a. physicians.
   b. pharmacy technicians.
   c. pharmacists.
   d. nurses.

3. Child-proof containers are
   a. not required for liquid dosage.
   b. required by law on all prescriptions with no exceptions.
   c. not required for patients aged 65 and over.
   d. none of the above.

4. When the directions for a prescription are unclear, the pharmacy technician should
   a. fax the doctor for clarification.
   b. ask the pharmacist.
   c. ask the patient.
   d. do their best to fill the prescription without assistance.

5. The directions on a medication are: $\dot{\text{i}}$ gtt ou hs. This medication is
   a. an eye drop.
   b. dosed twice a day.
   c. taken in the morning.
   d. used by injection.

6. For the prescription: Glucophage XR® 500 mg, $\overline{\text{ii}}$ BID x 90 days, how many tablets are dispensed?
   a. 90
   b. 180
   c. 360
   d. not enough information is given to fill the prescription.

7. If a prescription is written for Zoloft® 100 mg D.A.W., this means that
   a. the insurance may require the patient to receive the generic.
   b. the patient may switch to generic for refills.
   c. the patient may choose the generic.
   d. the brand name must be dispensed.

8. The unique identifying number of a drug is the
   a. DEA.
   b. PHI.
   c. DAW.
   d. NDC.

9. For the prescription: Clarithromycin 500 mg #20 $\dot{\text{i}}$ b.i.d., what is the Sig?
   a. $\dot{\text{i}}$ b.i.d
   b. 500
   c. Clarithromycin 500 mg
   d. #20

10. A medication error may involve
   a. the wrong dosage form.
   b. the wrong directions.
   c. the wrong patient.
   d. all of the above.

11. The two drug names Accupril® 40 mg and Accutane® 40 mg exemplify
    a. Signa.
    b. extemporaneous compounding.
    c. look-alike names.
    d. OTC medications.

12. Which of the following may be performed only by a pharmacist?
    a. accepting a return call from a prescriber's office approving refills
    b. accepting a return call from a prescriber's office clarifying a prescription
    c. calling a prescriber's office on behalf of a patient to request refills
    d. calling an insurance company to verify a patient's eligibility

13. All of the following duties may be performed by a pharmacy technician except
    a. requesting PHI from a patient such as date of birth, address, allergy and insurance information.
    b. selecting an OTC product for a patient.
    c. inputting and updating patient information in the computer.
    d. placing the medication in a vial and attaching the prescription label to it.

14. Directions for use should start with a/an
    a. adjective.
    b. verb.
    c. noun.
    d. adverb.

Questions 15–17 are based on this information from a prescription:

Amoxil®   250 mg/5ml
Sig: ī tsp tid x10d
M: qs

15. The medication should be taken
    a. twice daily.
    b. every 10 hours.
    c. three times daily.
    d. none of the above.

16. The amount of medication to be dispensed is:
    a. 100 ml.
    b. 150 ml.
    c. 250 ml.
    d. the amount of medication is not indicated.

17. The following auxiliary label should be placed near the medication label:
    a. shake well and refrigerate
    b. may cause drowsiness
    c. do not take with milk or other dairy products
    d. discard unused portion after 5 days

18. For the prescription "methotrexate 2.5 mg tab v̈i po q week # 24", the day's supply is
    a. 28 days.
    b. 34 days.
    c. 42 days.
    d. 90 days.

REVIEW

19. For the prescription

    prednisone 5 mg tab

    Sig: 5 bid x 2 days, 4 bid x 2 days, 3 bid x 2 days, 2 bid x 2 days, 1 bid x 2 days, then stop

    M: qs

    the number of tablets to dispense is
    a. 15.
    b. 30.
    c. 45.
    d. 60.

20. For the prescription "ProAir HFA® # 1, Sig: $\overline{ii}$ puff q 6h prn" there are 200 doses in one inhaler. The day's supply would be
    a. 15.
    b. 25.
    c. 30.
    d. 50.

21. The directions on a prescription read "1 tbsp QID, ac and hs." The quantity to be dispensed for a 30 day supply is
    a. 600 ml.
    b. 1000 ml.
    c. 1800 ml.
    d. 2000 ml.

22. Medication orders in institutional settings may
    a. be administered by nursing staff.
    b. contain only one request per sheet.
    c. not be used in place of label directions for dosing information.
    d. all of the above

23. All of the following are examples of PHI except the
    a. patient's insurance identification number.
    b. patient's address.
    c. pharmacy address.
    d. patient's date of birth.

24. All of the following pharmacy personnel must be formally trained regarding HIPAA except
    a. the pharmacist.
    b. the pharmacy technician.
    c. custodial personnel.
    d. none of the above

6

CALCULATIONS

LEARNING OBJECTIVES

At the completion of study, the student will:

→ define numerator, denominator, and fractions.

→ perform mathematical operations to solve problems with fractions.

→ perform mathematical operations to solve problems with decimals and percents.

→ describe measurement systems used in pharmacy.

→ perform mathematical operations to solve problems that involve different units of measurement.

→ use ratio and proportion to solve problems in pharmacy.

→ use the alligation method to solve problems in pharmacy that involve two different strengths of the same ingredient.

→ describe how powder volume is used to solve problems with powders for constitution.

→ describe considerations for children's doses of medications.

→ perform basic calculations associated with the business aspect of pharmacy.

NUMBERS

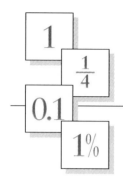

The amount of a drug in its manufactured or prescribed form is always stated numerically—that is, with numbers.

Knowing how to work with numbers is essential to the proper handling of drugs and preparation of prescriptions. This involves understanding the different number forms, measurement units, and mathematical operations that are regularly used. In pharmacy we use two different number systems: Arabic (such as 1, 1/2, 0.5, or 50%) and Roman (such as I, V, X, L, C, D, or M). Most of the time we use Arabic numerals, although Roman numerals are often used to indicate quantities in prescription order writing.

ROMAN NUMERALS

Roman numerals are letters that represent numbers. They were originally developed and used by the Roman Empire. They can be capital or lower case letters, and are:

ss = $\frac{1}{2}$	L or l = 50
I or i = 1	C or c = 100
V or v = 5	D or d = 500
X or x = 10	M or m = 1000

When grouped together, these few letters can express a large range of numbers, using a simple **positional notation**. That means the position of the letters has a mathematical importance, as determined by these rules:

When the second of two letters has a value equal to or smaller than that of the first, their values are to be added.

EXAMPLE:

xxx = 30	or	10 plus 10 plus 10
dc = 600	or	500 plus 100
lxvi = 66	or	50 plus 10 plus 5 plus 1

When the second of two letters has a value greater than that of the first, the smaller is to be subtracted from the larger.

EXAMPLE:

ix = 9	or	1 subtracted from 10
xxxix = 39	or	30 plus (1 subtracted from 10)
xc = 90	or	10 subtracted from 100

Note: The answers for all the exercises in this chapter can be found in the answer key beginning on page 511.

—I V X L C D M—

PRACTICE PROBLEMS—ROMAN NUMERALS

Write the following in Roman numerals:

1. 18 _____
2. 64 _____
3. 72 _____
4. 126 _____
5. 100 _____
6. 7 _____
7. 28 _____

Write the following in Arabic numbers:

8. xxxiii _____
9. CX _____
10. mc _____
11. iss _____
12. XIX _____
13. xxiv _____

Interpret the quantity in each of these phrases taken from prescriptions:

14. Caps. no. xiv. _____
15. Gtts. ix. _____
16. Tabs. no. XLVIII. _____
17. Tabs. no. xxi

positional notation a system used in Roman Numerals whereby the the position of the numeral signifies its mathematical value.

FRACTIONS

$$\frac{1}{4}$$

FRACTIONS

Fractions are commonly used in the Arabic system. A fraction is a numerical representation (as 3/4, 5/8, 3.234) indicating there is part of a whole. A fraction also represents the division of two numbers.

Numerators and Denominators

In a fraction, the **denominator** (number below the bar) tells us how many parts the whole is divided into, and the **numerator** (number above the bar) tells us how many of those parts exist.

In a fraction, the numerator can be zero, but the denominator cannot be zero. Division by zero is undefined, therefore no denominator can be zero.

One way to think of a fraction is as division that hasn't been completed.

Fractions can be used to indicate equal parts of a whole unit.

EXAMPLE

We can read $\frac{2}{5}$ as two-fifths, two over five or two divided by five.

Every fraction can be converted to a decimal by dividing. Using a calculator to divide 2 by 5:

$$\frac{2}{5} \quad = \quad 0.4$$

Here are some other fractions and their decimal equivalents. Remember, you can find the decimal equivalent of any fraction by dividing.

$$\frac{1}{8} \quad = \quad 0.125$$

$$\frac{1}{2} \quad = \quad 0.5$$

$$\frac{3}{4} \quad = \quad 0.75$$

denominator the bottom or right number in a fraction.

numerator the top or left number in a fraction.

Reciprocals

Reciprocals are two different fractions that equal 1 when multiplied together. Every fraction has a reciprocal (except those fractions with zero in the numerator). The easiest way to find the reciprocal of a fraction is to switch the numerator and denominator, or just turn the fraction over.

To find the reciprocal of a whole number, just put 1 over the whole number.

EXAMPLE:

The reciprocal of 2 is $\frac{1}{2}$

EXAMPLE:

The reciprocal of 3 is $\frac{1}{3}$

EXAMPLE:

The reciprocal of 4 is $\frac{1}{4}$

EXAMPLE:

The reciprocal of 2/3 is $\frac{3}{2}$

PRACTICE PROBLEMS—NUMERATORS, DENOMINATORS, AND RECIPROCALS

Use a calculator to convert the following fractions to decimals:

1. $\frac{1}{3}$ = _____

2. $\frac{1}{2}$ = _____

3. $\frac{1}{4}$ = _____

4. $\frac{3}{10}$ = _____

5. $\frac{1}{10}$ = _____

Determine the reciprocal of the following fractions:

6. $\frac{1}{5}$ is _____

7. $\frac{2}{3}$ is _____

8. $\frac{2}{5}$ is _____

9. $\frac{2}{9}$ is _____

10. $\frac{1}{15}$ is _____

FRACTIONS (cont'd)

$$\frac{1}{4}$$

ADDING AND SUBTRACTING FRACTIONS

In order to add or subtract fractions the fractions must have the same denominator or common denominators. Addition and subtraction of like fractions is easy. To add or subtract like fractions just add or subtract the numerators and write the sum or difference over the common denominator.

To add or subtract fractions with different denominators, you must first find equivalent fractions with common denominators: First find the smallest multiple for the denominator of both numbers. Then rewrite the fractions as equivalent fractions with the smallest multiple of both numbers as the denominator. (The smallest multiple of both numbers is called the **least common denominator**.)

EXAMPLE: $\frac{1}{3} + \frac{3}{5}$

The smallest multiple for the denominator of both numbers is 15.

$$\frac{1}{3} = \frac{1 \times 5}{3 \times 5} = \frac{5}{15}$$

$$\frac{3}{5} = \frac{3 \times 3}{5 \times 3} = \frac{9}{15}$$

The problem can now be rewritten:

$$\frac{5}{15} + \frac{9}{15}$$

Since the denominators are equal, we only have to add the numerators to get the answer:

$$\frac{5 + 9}{15} = \frac{14}{15}$$

PRACTICE PROBLEMS—ADDING AND SUBTRACTING FRACTIONS

Add or subtract the following fractions.

1. $\frac{1}{4} + \frac{1}{4} =$ _____

2. $\frac{3}{8} + \frac{5}{8} =$ _____

3. $\frac{2}{5} - \frac{1}{5} =$ _____

4. $\frac{7}{8} - \frac{3}{8} =$ _____

5. $\frac{2}{5} + \frac{3}{5} =$ _____

6. $\frac{1}{8} + \frac{3}{8} =$ _____

7. $\frac{1}{4} + \frac{1}{5} =$ _____

8. $\frac{4}{15} + \frac{1}{5} =$ _____

9. $\frac{1}{4} + \frac{3}{16} =$ _____

10. $\frac{5}{8} - \frac{1}{4} =$ _____

least common denominator smallest possible denominator for an equivalent fraction so that two fractions can be added or subtracted and have the same denominator.

 Multiplying fractions is frequently stated by using the word "of." If you must determine 1/2 of 10, you would multiply 1/2 X 10. 1/2 X 10 = 5.

MULTIPLYING AND DIVIDING FRACTIONS

To multiply fractions, first multiply the numerators of the fractions to get the new numerator. Then multiply the denominators of the fractions to get the new denominator.

EXAMPLE: $\frac{2}{3}$ of 24

Multiply $\frac{2}{3}$ X $\frac{24}{1}$

= $\frac{48}{3}$

$\frac{48}{3}$ can be reduced to 16.

To divide a number by a fraction multiply the number by the reciprocal of the fraction.

EXAMPLE: 24 DIVIDED BY $\frac{1}{3}$

Find the reciprocal of the fraction:

The reciprocal of $\frac{1}{3}$ is 3.

Multiply the number by the reciprocal of the fraction:

24 X 3 = 72

EXAMPLE: Divide $\frac{1}{3}$ by 8.

First, find the reciprocal of the fraction:

The reciprocal of 8 is $\frac{1}{8}$.

Second, multiply the number by the reciprocal of the fraction:

$\frac{1}{3}$ X $\frac{1}{8}$ = $\frac{1}{24}$

PRACTICE PROBLEMS—MULTIPLYING AND DIVIDING FRACTIONS

Multiply the following fractions:

1. $\frac{1}{4}$ of $\frac{1}{4}$ = _____

2. $\frac{1}{3}$ of $\frac{3}{8}$ = _____

3. $\frac{2}{3}$ of $\frac{1}{3}$ = _____

4. $\frac{3}{8}$ of $\frac{5}{8}$ = _____

Divide the following fractions:

5. $\frac{1}{3}$ divided by $\frac{1}{2}$ = _____

6. $\frac{1}{4}$ divided by $\frac{3}{4}$ = _____

7. $\frac{2}{5}$ divided by $\frac{1}{5}$ = _____

8. $\frac{3}{8}$ divided by $\frac{3}{8}$ = _____

DECIMAL NUMBERS

ADDING AND SUBTRACTING DECIMALS

To add decimal numbers, first put the numbers in a vertical column, aligning the decimal points Then add each column of digits, starting on the right and working left. If the sum of a column is more than ten, "carry" digits to the next column on the left. Place the decimal point in the answer directly below the decimal points in the terms.

EXAMPLE: Add 324.5678 to 1.2345

Step 1:

$$324.5678$$
$$\underline{1.2345}$$
$$3 \text{ (carry the 1)}$$

Step 2:

$$324.5678$$
$$\underline{1.2345}$$
$$23 \text{ (carry the 1)}$$

Step 3:

$$324.5678$$
$$\underline{1.2345}$$
$$023 \text{ (carry the 1)}$$

Step 4:

$$324.5678$$
$$\underline{1.2345}$$
$$.8023$$

Step 5:

$$324.5678$$
$$\underline{1.2345}$$
$$5.8023$$

Step 6:

$$324.5678$$
$$\underline{1.2345}$$
$$25.8023$$

Step 7:

$$324.5678$$
$$\underline{1.2345}$$
$$325.8023$$

PRACTICE PROBLEMS—ADDING DECIMALS

Add the following decimal fractions:

1. 0.6 + 0.4 + 0.3   = _____

2. 4 + 3.1 + 0.3   = _____

3. 0.39 + 3.92 + 0.03   = _____

4. 3.365 + 15.432 + 5.001   = _____

5. 37.02 + 25 + 6.4 + 3.89 = _____

6. 4.0086 + 0.034 + 0.6 + 0.05 = _____

7. 43.766 + 9.33 + 17 + 206 = _____

8. 354.2312
    +5.1092

9. 224.0021
    +6.4444

10. 5223.2312
    +65.3217

When adding and subtracting decimals it is very important to line up the terms so that all the decimal points are in a vertical line.

To subtract decimal numbers, first put the numbers in a vertical column, aligning the decimal points. Then subtract each column, starting on the right and working left. If the digit being subtracted in a column is larger than the digit above it, "borrow" a digit from the next column to the left. Place the decimal point in the answer directly below the decimal points in the terms.

EXAMPLE: Subtract 1.203 from 32.255

Step 1:

```
  32.255
   1.203
       2
```

Step 2:

```
  32.255
   1.203
      52
```

Step 3:

```
  32.255
   1.203
    .052
```

Step 4:

```
  32.255
   1.203
   1.052
```

Step 5:

```
  32.255
   1.203
  31.052
```

PRACTICE PROBLEMS—SUBTRACTING DECIMALS

Subtract the following decimal fractions:

1. 3.2 - 3.36   =   _____

2. 14.33 - 5.7   =   _____

3. 25.5 - 11.21   =   _____

4. 1.0026 - 0.03   =   _____

5. 75.013 - 3.048   =   _____

6. 30.313 - 15.721   =   _____

7.   254.2311
          -3.1082

8.   24.0032
         -3.3333

9.   523.2309
         -63.3467

10.   372.21
          -3.89

DECIMAL NUMBERS
(cont'd)

MULTIPLYING DECIMALS

To multiply decimal numbers, first multiply the numbers just as if they were whole numbers. Then line up the numbers on the right (do not align the decimal points). Next, starting on the right, multiply each digit in the top number by each digit in the bottom number. Then add the products.

Finally, place the decimal point in the answer by starting at the right and moving the point the number of places equal to the sum of the decimal places in both numbers that were multiplied together.

EXAMPLE: Multiply 47.2 by 5.5

```
      47.2    (has 1 decimal place)
   x   5.5    (has 1 decimal place)
      2360
      2360
    259.60    (has 2 decimal places)
```

EXAMPLE: Find the product (9.683)(6.1)

```
     9.683    (has 3 decimal places)
   x   6.1    (has 1 decimal place)
     9683
    58098
    59.0663   (has 3 + 1 = 4 decimal places)
```

PRACTICE PROBLEMS—MULTIPLYING DECIMALS

Multiply the following decimals:

1. $(0.5)(0.7)$ = _____

2. $(0.4)(0.8)$ = _____

3. $(0.3)(0.3)$ = _____

4. $(0.5)(0.3)$ = _____

5. $6(3.7)$ = _____

6. $5.3(0.03)$ = _____

7. $7.2(0.02)$ = _____

8. $0.22(0.12)$ = _____

9.
```
     25.24
   x 23.02
```

10.
```
   123.444
   x    3.1
```

SIGNIFICANT FIGURES

SIGNIFICANT FIGURES

In pharmacy, we usually use a calculator to perform our calculations. Calculators are useful because they help us to avoid mathematical errors. We use decimal fractions when we use calculators.

In pharmacy, we also often perform calculations using measured amounts (for example, we may need to measure 80 mL of water to prepare an oral suspension). The actual value that we can use in our calculations that contain measured amounts depends on the sensitivity of the measuring device. When we multiply and divide decimal fractions using calculators, we must be careful to *include only the significant figures in our calculations* and answers. That is to say, we must be careful to keep in mind the sensitivity of the measuring device that is used when we perform the calculations.

A significant figure (or significant digit) is one that is actually measured using the measuring device. For instance, in the example above to measure 80 mL of water, if the sensitivity of the graduate used to measure the water measures to the nearest mL, the measurement should be expressed as 80 mL and not 80.0 mL. Numbers that are not measured (for example 30 capsules) are not affected by the sensitivity of a measuring device, and therefore are not subject to the rules of significant figures. When a calculation (addition, subtraction, multiplication, etc.) involves several measurements, and each measurement has a different number of significant digits, the final answer should have the same number of significant figures as the measured term that has the least number of significant figures. Also, if a calculation contains both numbers that are measured and numbers that are not measured, only the numbers that are measured should be considered when determining the number of significant figures for the answer.

There are four rules for assigning significant figures:

1. Digits other than zero are always significant.

2. Final zeros after a decimal point are always significant.

3. Zeros between two other significant digits are always significant.

4. Zeros used only to space the decimal are never significant.

EXAMPLE

1.40 gm of hydrocortisone powder are needed to compound a prescription. How many significant figures are in this measured amount?

Since final zeros after a decimal point are always significant, the number of significant figures is 3.

MEASUREMENT

There are different systems of measurement used in pharmacy: metric, English, apothecary, and Avoirdupois.

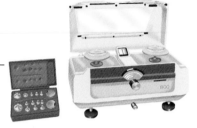

The metric system is the primary system used. Within these systems there are different measurements for weight, volume, and length, as well as for liquids and solids. There are also different measurement systems for temperature. It is necessary to know how to perform **conversions**—i.e., how to convert one type of measurement to another so that both amounts are equal.

METRIC SYSTEM

The major system of weights and measures used in medicine is the metric system. It was developed in France in the late 18th century and is based on a decimal system. That is, *different measurement units are related by measures of ten*. Technicians need to know metric measures for both liquids and solids.

Liquids

Liquids (including lotions) are measured by volume. The most widely used metric volume measurements are liters or milliliters.

Unit	Symbol	Liquid Conversions		
liter	L	1 L	= 10 dl	= 1000 ml
deciliter	dl	1 dl	= 0.1 L	= 100 ml
milliliter	ml	1 ml	= 0.001 L	= 0.01 dl

Note: deciliters are rarely used in pharmacy, but are included here for reference and to illustrate the decimal relationship of these measures.

Solids

Solids (pills, granules, ointments, etc.) are measured by weight.

Unit	Symbol	Solid Conversions		
kilogram	kg	1 kg	= 1,000 g	
gram	g	1 g	= 0.001 kg	= 1000 mg
milligram	mg	1 mg	= 0.001 g	= 1000 mcg
microgram	mcg or μg	1 mcg	= 0.001 mg	= 0.000001 g

 Milliliters are sometimes referred to as cubic centimeters (cc). They are not precisely the same but are quite close and are sometimes used interchangeably. Milliliter is the preferred usage for pharmacy.

To convert milligrams to grams, move the decimal 3 places to the left (1 mg = 0.001 g).

AVOIRDUPOIS SYSTEM

The Avoirdupois system is the system of weight (ounces and pounds) that we commonly use. However, one Avoirdupois unit used in pharmacy is rarely used elsewhere. It is the grain.

Unit	Symbol	Conversions		
pound	lb	1 lb	=	16 oz
ounce	oz	1 oz	=	437.5 gr
grain	gr	1 gr	=	64.8 mg

THE GRAIN

The grain is the same weight in several different measurement systems: Apothecary, Avoirdupois, and Troy. It is said to have been established as a unit of weight in 1266 by King Henry III of England when he required the English penny to weigh the equivalent of 32 dried grains of wheat. On the metric scale, one grain equals 64.8 milligrams. However, this is often rounded to 65 milligrams.

APOTHECARY SYSTEM

The Apothecary system is sometimes used in prescriptions, primarily with liquids. It includes the fluid ounce, pint, quart, and gallon. Although there are Apothecary weight units, they are generally not used, with the exception of the grain. The fluid ounce is a volume measure and is different than the weight ounce. It is always indicated by "fl oz."

Unit	Symbol	Conversions		
gallon	gal	1 gal	=	4 qt
quart	qt	1 qt	=	2 pt
pint	pt	1 pt	=	16 fl oz
ounce	fl oz	1 fl oz	=	8 fl dr
fluid dram	fl dr	1 fl dr	=	60 min
minim	min or M_x			

Note: drams and minims are rarely used in pharmacy today, but are included here for reference.

 conversions changing one unit of measure into another so that both amounts remain equal.

MEASUREMENT (cont'd)

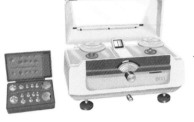

HOUSEHOLD UNITS

The teaspoon and tablespoon are common household measurement units that are regularly used in liquid prescriptions. Note that home teaspoons and tablespoons are not accurate for use in measuring medications.

Unit	Symbol	Conversions
teaspoon	tsp	1 tsp = 5 ml
tablespoon	tbsp	1 tbsp = 3 tsp = 15 ml
cup	cup	1 cup = 8 fl oz

TEMPERATURE

The Centigrade scale, which is also called Celsius, is used to measure temperature. The relationship of Centigrade (C) to Fahrenheit (F) is:

F temperature = ($1\frac{4}{5}$ times number of degrees C) + 32

EXAMPLE $\qquad$ 212°F = 100°C

$\qquad\qquad$ *because* $\qquad$ a) $1\frac{4}{5}$ x 100 = 180

$\qquad\qquad\quad$ *and* $\qquad$ b) 180 + 32 = 212

C temperature = $\frac{5}{9}$ x (number of degrees F - 32)

EXAMPLE $\qquad$ 100°C = 212°F

$\qquad\qquad$ *because* $\frac{5}{9}$ x (212 - 32) = $\frac{5}{9}$ x 180 = 100

Note that the temperature of water freezing is 0°C and 32°F.

Some people find the following formula easier to remember and use:

9C = 5F - 160

CONVERSIONS

Following are some commonly used unit conversions. See page 149 for additional conversions.

1 L	=	33.8 fl oz	1 oz	=	28.35 g
1 pt	=	473.167 ml	1 g	=	15.43 gr
1 fl oz	=	29.57 ml	1 gr	=	64.8 mg
1 kg	=	2.2 lb	1 tsp	=	5 ml
1 lb	=	453.59 g	1 tbsp	=	15 ml

PRACTICE PROBLEMS—METRICS

Provide the abbreviation for these:

1. microgram _____
2. liter _____
3. milliliter _____
4. gram _____
5. milligram _____
6. kilogram _____

Convert these units to equivalents:

7. 1 kg = _____ g
8. 1 mg = _____ mcg
9. 2 gr = _____ mg
10. 1 L = _____ ml
11. 1 ml = _____ L
12. 1 mg = _____ g

PRACTICE PROBLEMS—CONVERSIONS

Convert these numbers using the conversions provided on the preceding pages as well as your knowledge of decimals:

1. 7 mg = _____ mcg
2. 3.2 g = _____ mg
3. 1 gr = _____ g
4. 2 tbsp = _____ ml
5. 0.3 L = _____ ml
6. 7 kg = _____ g
7. 1 oz = _____ gr
8. 0.5 kg = _____ lb
9. 10 ml = _____ tsp
10. 15 ml = _____ tbsp
11. 0°C = _____ °F
12. 250 ml = _____ L

Interpreting Common Pharmacy Sigs for Pharmacy Calculations

Sig	Meaning	Interpret As
i tab q.d.	Take one tablet every day	1 tablet / dose X 1 dose / day = 1 tablet / day
i tab b.i.d.	Take one tablet twice a day	1 tablet / dose X 2 doses / day = 2 tablets / day
i tab t.i.d.	Take one tablet three times a day	1 tablet / dose X 3 doses / day = 3 tablets / day
i tab q.i.d.	Take one tablet four times a day	1 tablet / dose X 4 doses / day = 4 tablets / day
i tab q.o.d.	Take one tablet every other day	1 tablet/dose X 1/2 dose/day = 1/2 tablet/ day
ss tab q.d.	Take one-half tablet every day	1/2 tablet / dose X 1 dose / day = 1/2 tablet / day
i tab a.m.	Take one tablet in the morning	1 tablet / dose X 1 dose / day = 1 tablet / day
i tab h.s.	Take one tablet at bedtime	1 tablet / dose X 1 dose / day = 1 tablet / day
i tab a.c.	Take one tablet before meals	1 tablet / dose X 3 doses / day = 3 tablets / day
i tab p.c.	Take one tablet after meals	1 tablet / dose X 3 doses / day = 3 tablets / day
i tsp q.d.	Take one teaspoonful every day	5 ml / dose X 1 dose / day = 5 ml / day

EQUATIONS & VARIABLES

EQUATIONS AND VARIABLES

In the calculations of Pharmacy related problems there is often an unknown value that needs to be determined. To solve the unknown value involves setting up a mathematical statement between the known amounts and the unknown. This statement is called an equation. The unknown fact in an equation is called a **variable.** The variable is often indicated by the letter x.

> **An equation is a mathematical statement in which two terms are equal.**

Equations use the equal sign (=) to indicate equivalence. The following are equations:

$$1 = \tfrac{1}{2} + \tfrac{1}{2}$$
$$1 = \tfrac{1}{2} \times 2$$

EXAMPLE

You have a prescription for 120 ml of Theophylline liquid and want to know how many fluid ounces is equal to 120 ml. In this case, the number of ounces is the variable x that you want to determine. Since there are 29.57 ml in each fluid ounce, one way to state this problem mathematically is the following equation:

x fl oz = (total prescribed ml) ÷ (ml/fl oz conversion rate)

or

$$x \text{ fl oz} = \frac{\text{total prescribed ml}}{\text{ml/fl oz conversion rate}}$$

$$x \text{ fl oz} = \frac{120 \text{ ml}}{29.57 \text{ ml}}$$

x fl oz = 4 (approximately)

variable an unknown value in a mathematical equation.

EXAMPLE—FILLING A CAPSULE PRESCRIPTION

You have a prescription for amoxicillin 250 mg, one capsule orally, three times a day for seven days. You want to know how many capsules will be needed to fill this prescription. In this case capsules needed is the unknown fact or variable that you are trying to solve for.

x (capsules needed) = (capsules per dose) x (doses per day) x (days)

x = (1 capsule per dose) x (3 doses per day) x (7 days)

x = 21

You need 21 capsules of amoxicillin 250 mg to fill the prescription.

EXAMPLE—INTRAVENOUS SOLUTION

You are preparing an intravenous solution (IV) that requires the addition of potassium chloride (KCl). You have a vial of KCl containing a concentration of 20 mEq per 10 ml. How many ml of this solution should you add to the IV if the IV should have a total of 50 mEq of KCl in it? This is made easier by first solving for the number of KCl per ml:

20 mEq divided by 10 ml = 2 mEq per ml

x (mL of KCl solution) = mEq KCl needed ÷ mEq KCl per mL

x = (50 mEq) ÷ (2 mEq/mL)

x = 25 mL

You need to add 25 ml of KCl solution to the IV.

RATIO & PROPORTION

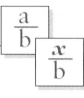

RATIO AND PROPORTION

Understanding ratios and proportions is important for pharmacy technicians. If you understand ratios and proportions, you will be able to perform most of the calculations necessary for your job.

Ratio

A ratio states **a relationship between two quantities**. The ratio of **a** to **b** can be stated as:

$$\frac{a}{b}$$

Proportion

Two equal ratios form a proportion: $\frac{a}{b} = \frac{c}{d}$

EXAMPLE

An example of this is the equation: $\frac{1}{2} = \frac{2}{4}$

$\frac{1}{2}$ and $\frac{2}{4}$ are equivalent ratios. 1 has the same relationship to 2 as 2 has to 4. Therefore, the equation is a proportion.

EXAMPLE

If one person has a bottle containing 5 tablets and another has 3 bottles each containing 5 tablets, one may have more tablets than the other but they both have the same proportion of tablets to bottles.

$$\frac{5 \text{ tablets}}{1 \text{ bottle}} = \frac{15 \text{ tablets}}{3 \text{ bottles}}$$

Each person has fives times as many tablets as bottles. The ratios are equivalent.

EXAMPLE

A solution of 5 g of a substance in 100 ml of water is equivalent to 50 g of the same substance in 1000 ml of water.

$$\frac{5 \text{ g}}{100 \text{ ml}} = \frac{50 \text{ g}}{1000 \text{ ml}}$$

Both numerators can be divided into their denominators twenty times. Therefore, the ratios are equivalent.

Solving Ratio and Proportion Problems

In a proportion equation, all four terms are related to each other and the relationship of each term to the others can be stated in different ways:

➤ $\dfrac{a}{b} = \dfrac{c}{d}$ *can be stated as* $\dfrac{b}{a} = \dfrac{d}{c}$

You can also state the equation for any one term by multiplying both sides of the equation by one of the other terms. For example:

➤ $b \times \dfrac{a}{b} = b \times \dfrac{c}{d}$ ➤ $\cancel{b} \times \dfrac{a}{\cancel{b}} = b \times \dfrac{c}{d}$

➥ *cancel out equal values*

➤ $a = \dfrac{bc}{d}$

These are also true: $b = \dfrac{ad}{c}$ $c = \dfrac{ad}{b}$ $d = \dfrac{bc}{a}$

Therefore, if three of the four terms in a proportion problem are known, an unknown fourth term *(x)* can also be calculated.

EXAMPLE

When you know the values of three of the four terms in a proportion equation, the unknown term is indicated by *x*, and the proportion equation can be written as:

$\dfrac{x}{b} = \dfrac{c}{d}$ ➡ *ratio you want = ratio you have*

Multiplying both sides of the equation by the value of **b** will then establish the relationship of the known terms to *x*.

$b \text{ times } \left(\dfrac{x}{b}\right) = b \text{ times } \left(\dfrac{c}{d}\right)$

⬇

$\cancel{b} \text{ times } \dfrac{x}{\cancel{b}} = b \text{ times } \dfrac{c}{d}$ ➤ $x = \dfrac{bc}{d}$

➥ *cancel out equal values*

You can then solve for the value of *x* by simple multiplication and division of the known values of b, c, and d.

x = (b times c) divided by d

RATIO & PROPORTION
(cont'd)

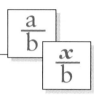

In one bottle there are 30 capsules. If every bottle contains the same number of capsules, how many capsules are in six bottles?

Steps

1. **Define the variable and the correct ratios.**

   a. define the unknown variable ➡ x (total capsules)

   b. establish the known ratio ➡ 30 capsules/1 bottle

   c. establish the unknown ratio ➡ x capsules/6 bottles

2. **Set up the proportion equation $\left(\frac{x}{b} = \frac{c}{d}\right)$.**

$$\frac{x \text{ capsules}}{6 \text{ bottles}} = \frac{30 \text{ capsules}}{1 \text{ bottle}}$$

   Note that the units must be the same in both the numerator and denominator:

   numerator: capsules
   denominator: bottles

3. **Establish the x equation.**

$$6 \text{ bottles times } \frac{x \text{ capsules}}{6 \text{ bottles}} = 6 \text{ bottles times } \frac{30 \text{ capsules}}{1 \text{ bottle}}$$

$$6 \text{ bottles times } \frac{x \text{ capsules}}{6 \text{ bottles}} = 6 \text{ bottles times } \frac{30 \text{ capsules}}{1 \text{ bottle}}$$

   ➡ *cancel out equal values and units*

$$x \text{ capsules} = 6 \text{ times } 30 \text{ capsules}$$

4. **Solve for x.**

$$x \text{ capsules} = 180 \text{ capsules}$$

5. **Express solution in correct units.**

   There are **180 capsules** in the six bottles.

> CONDITIONS FOR USING RATIO AND PROPORTION
>
> 1. Three of the four values must be known.
>
> 2. Numerators must have the same units.
>
> 3. Denominators must have the same units.

EXAMPLE—A PRESCRIPTION FOR TABLETS

You receive a prescription for KTabs® one tablet BID x 30 days. How many tablets are needed to fill this prescription correctly?

Steps

1. **Define the variable and correct ratios.**

   a. define the unknown variable ➡ x = total tablets needed

   b. establish the known ratio ➡ 2 tablets / 1 day

   c. establish the unknown ratio ➡ x tablets / 30 days

2. **Set-up the proportion equation.**

$$\frac{x \text{ tablets}}{30 \text{ days}} = \frac{2 \text{ tablets}}{1 \text{ day}}$$

3. **Establish the x equation.**

$$x \text{ tablets} = 30 \text{ days times} \frac{2 \text{ tablets}}{1 \text{ day}}$$

4. **Solve for x.**

$$x \text{ tablets} = 30 \; \cancel{\text{days}} \text{ times} \frac{2 \text{ tablets}}{1 \; \cancel{\text{day}}} = 60 \text{ tablets}$$

$$x \text{ tablets} = 60 \text{ tablets}$$

5. **Express solution in correct units.**

   60 tablets of KTabs® are needed to fill the prescription.

RATIO & PROPORTION (cont'd)

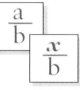

EXAMPLE—A LIQUID PRESCRIPTION

You receive a prescription for Amoxicillin 75 mg four times a day for ten days. You have available Amoxicillin 250 mg/5 ml 150 ml.

A. What is the correct individual dose?

   1. Define the variable and correct ratios.

   a. define the unknown variable ➡ x = ml per dose
   b. establish the known ratio   ➡ 5 ml / 250 mg
   c. establish the unknown ratio ➡ x ml / 75 mg

   2. Set-up the proportion equation.

   x ml / 75 mg = 5 ml / 250 mg

   3. Establish the x equation.

   $$x \text{ ml} = 75 \text{ mg times } \frac{5 \text{ ml}}{250 \text{ mg}}$$

   4. Solve.

   $$x \text{ ml} = 75 \text{ mg times } \frac{5 \text{ ml}}{250 \text{ mg}} = \frac{375 \text{ ml}}{250} = 1.5 \text{ ml}$$

   5. Express solution in correct units.

   The dose is 1.5 ml of amoxicillin.

B. How many mls of amoxicillin do you need to last for ten days? A simple equation can determine this. Note that it is often useful to state the equation first in words, and then restate it in numbers. Using words to describe mathematical operations helps you to visualize and better understand the mathematics involved.

   Word Equation:
   amount needed = dose amount x doses day x number of days

   amoxicillin needed = 1.5 ml times 4 times 10 = 60 ml

C. Double check your answer.

   $$1.5 \text{ ml of } \frac{250 \text{ mg}}{5 \text{ ml}} = 75 \text{ mg}$$

EXAMPLE—A MIXTURE DOSE

If an antidiarrheal mixture contains 3 ml of Paregoric in each 30 ml of mixture, how many ml of Paregoric would be contained in a teaspoonful dose of mixture?

conversion: 1 tsp = 5 ml

1. Define the variable and correct ratios.

 a. define the unknown variable ➡ x ml of Paregoric

 b. establish the known ratio ➡ 3 ml / 30 ml (mix)

 c. establish the unknown ratio ➡ x ml /5 ml (mix)

2. Set-up the proportion equation.

 x ml Paregoric / 5 ml mix = 3 ml Paregoric/ 30 ml mix

3. Establish the x equation.

$$x \text{ ml} = 5 \text{ ml mix times } \frac{3 \text{ ml Paregoric}}{30 \text{ ml mix}}$$

4. Solve.

$$x \text{ ml Paregoric} = 5 \text{ ml mix times } \frac{3 \text{ ml Paregoric}}{30 \text{ ml mix}} =$$

$$\frac{15 \text{ ml Paregoric}}{30 \text{ ml mix}} = 0.5 \text{ ml Paregoric}$$

5. Express solution in correct units.

There are 0.5 ml of paregoric in a teaspoon.

USING CALCULATORS

Though most of these examples can be solved without the use of a calculator, the use of calculators is essential in the correct computation of many dosage calculations. Their answers are precise and provided in decimals. Since it is relatively easy to make entry mistakes on a calculator, always recheck answers. Also, use judgment. If an answer doesn't appear to make sense, check it.

RATIO & PROPORTION
(cont'd)

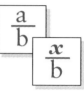

EXAMPLE—IV FLOW RATE

In the pharmacy setting, you may be asked to provide information on **flow rate** or **rate of administration** for an IV solution. Flow rates are calculated using ratio and proportion equations. They are generally done in ml/hour, but for pumps used to dispense IV fluids to the patient, the calculation may need to be done in ml/min.

For example, if you have an order for KCl 10 mEq and K Acetate 15 mEq in D5W 1000 ml to run at 80 ml/hour, you would determine the administration rate in ml/minute as follows:

1. **Define the variable and correct ratios.**

   a. define the unknown variable ➡ x = ml

   b. establish the known ratio ➡ 80 ml / 60 min

   c. establish the unknown ratio ➡ x ml / 1 min

2. **Set-up the proportion equation.**

   x ml / 1 min = 80 ml / 60 min

3. **Establish the x equation.**

   x ml = 1 min times $\dfrac{80\ ml}{60\ min}$

4. **Factor and solve.**

   x ml = 1 ~~min~~ times $\dfrac{80\ ml}{60\ \text{~~min~~}}$ = 1.33 ml

   ➡ *80 divided by 60 = 1.33*

5. **Express solution in correct units.**

   The flow rate would be 1.33 ml/minute.

Note: IV Flow Rate calculations may involve *drops per ml* or *drops per minute* or involve calculating the amount of time before an IV bag will empty and require replacement. Using simple ratio and proportion equations will solve these problems.

 flow rate the rate (in ml/hour or ml/minute) at which a solution is administered to a patient; also known as *rate of administration*.

STEPS FOR SOLVING PROPORTION PROBLEMS

1. Define the variable and correct ratios.
2. Set-up the proportion equation
3. Establish the x equation
4. Solve for x.
5. Express solution in correct units.

PRACTICE PROBLEMS—RATIO AND PROPORTION

Use the space below the problem (and the rules you've learned from the preceding pages) to work out the answer.

1. A prescription calls for 100 mg of a drug that you have in a 250 mg/5 ml concentration. How many ml of the liquid do you need?

2. A prescription calls for 400 mg of a drug that you have in a 50 mg/ml concentration. How many ml of the liquid do you need?

3. A prescription calls for 10 mg of a drug that you have in a 2 mg/15 ml concentration. How many ml of the liquid do you need?

4. KCl 10 mEq and K Acetate 15 mEq in D5W 1000 ml is ordered to be administered over 8 hours. What would the rate be in ml/min?

5. A prescription calls for 0.24 mg of a drug that you have in a 50 mcg/ml concentration. How many ml of the liquid do you need?

PERCENTS & SOLUTIONS

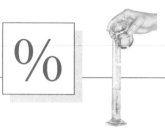

PERCENTS & SOLUTIONS

Percents are used to indicate the amount or **concentration** of something in a solution. Concentrations are indicated in terms of weight to volume or volume to volume.

Weight to Volume: grams per 100 milliliters   ➡   g/100mL

Volume to Volume: milliliters per 100 milliliters ➡   mL/100mL

EXAMPLE—IV SOLUTION

If there is 50% dextrose in a 1000 ml IV bag, how many grams of dextrose are there in the bag? You can solve this by developing a proportion equation. Since 50% dextrose means there are 50 grams of dextrose in 100 ml, the equation would be:

x g divided by 1000 ml   =   50 g divided by 100 ml

The x equation:

$$x \text{ g } = \text{ 1000 } \cancel{ml} \text{ times } \frac{50 \text{ g}}{100 \ \cancel{ml}} = 10 \text{ times } 50 \text{ g} = \mathbf{500 \text{ g}}$$

➡ *1000 divided by 100 = 10*

Answer: There are 500 grams of dextrose in the bag.

Another way to solve this is to **convert the percent to a decimal.** In a 50% solution, there are .5 g per ml:

50 g/100 ml = 0.5 g/ml

You can then multiply 0.5 g by the total number of milliliters.

x = 0.5 g times 1000 = 500 g

Now how many ml will give you a 10 g of Dextrose?

The proportion equation:

x ml/10 g = 100 ml /50 g

The x equation:

$$x \text{ ml } = \text{ 10 } \cancel{g} \text{ times } \frac{100 \text{ ml}}{50 \ \cancel{g}} = \frac{1000 \text{ ml}}{50} = \mathbf{20 \text{ ml}}$$

Answer: 20 ml of 50% solution contain 10 g of dextrose.

concentration the strength of a solution as measured by the weight-to-volume or volume-to-volume of the substance being measured.

PRACTICE PROBLEMS—PERCENTS

Convert the following fractions to percents:

1. 60/100 = _____ %
2. 80/100 = _____ %
3. 12/100 = _____ %

Convert the following percents to decimals:

4. 50% = _____
5. 12.5% = _____
6. 99% = _____

You have a 70% dextrose solution. How many grams in:

7. 50 ml of solution

8. 75 ml of solution

9. 20 ml of solution

You have a 50% dextrose solution, how many ml will give you:

10. 25 g of dextrose

11. 35 g

12. 10 g

13. You have a liquid that contains 12 mg /10 ml. What percent is this liquid?
(Hint: To solve, you will need to convert mg to g per 100 ml using decimals.)

PERCENTS & SOLUTIONS
(cont'd)

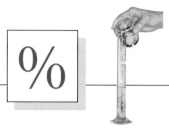

A PERCENT SOLUTION FORMULA

It is possible to set up a proportion equation specifically to convert concentrations for preparation of special intravenous solutions known as hyperalimentation or **total parenteral solutions (TPNs)**.

$$\frac{x \text{ volume needed}}{\text{want \%}} = \frac{\text{volume prescribed}}{\text{have \%}}$$

EXAMPLE—A DILUTION

The physician wants a 35% solution of dextrose 1000 ml. You have a 50% solution of dextrose 1000 ml. How will you make up what the physician wants?

The terms for the formula are:

volume needed	➡ **x** ml
want %	➡ 35% dextrose
volume prescribed	➡ 1000 ml
have %	➡ 50% dextrose

The formula is:

x ml / 35% = 1000 ml / 50%

The **x** equation is:

$$x \text{ ml} = 35\% \text{ times } \frac{1000 \text{ ml}}{50\%} = 35 \text{ times } 20 \text{ ml} = \textbf{700 ml}$$

➥ *1000 divided by 50 = 20*

700 ml of dextrose 1000 ml will give you the 350 g of dextrose you will need in your solution. However, you will still need to add sterile water qs ad until you have a total solution of 1000 ml as ordered by the physician. (**qs ad** means quantity needed to make total volume).

Total Volume	1000 ml
Dextrose 50% Solution	-700 ml
Sterile Water (qs ad)	300 ml

Answer: You need to add 300 ml of sterile water to 700 ml of 50% dextrose to create 1000 ml of 35% dextrose.

total parenteral nutrition administration of all nutrients intravenously; also known as hyperalimentation.

qs ad the quantity needed to make a prescribed amount.

In order to calculate mEq for an electrolyte, the atomic weight and valence of the electrolyte must first be known. The weight is then divided by the valence.

MILLIEQUIVALENTS: mEq

Electrolyte solutions are often used in hospitals. Electrolytes are substances which conduct an electrical current and are found in the body's blood, tissue fluids, and cells. Salts are electrolytes and saline solutions are commonly used electrolyte solutions.

COMMON ELECTROLYTES:

NaCl	Sodium Chloride
MgSO4	Magnesium Sulfate
KCl	Potassium Chloride
K Acetate	Potassium Acetate
Ca Gluconate	Calcium Gluconate
Na Acetate	Sodium Acetate

The concentration of electrolytes is expressed as milliequivalents (mEq) per milliliter or milliequivalents per liter.

A **milliequivalent** is a specific unit of measurement that cannot be converted into the metric system. A 0.9% solution of one electrolyte will have a different mEq value than a 0.9% solution of another because mEq values are different for different electrolytes. Milliequivalents are based on each electrolyte's atomic weight and electron properties known as **valence**.

EXAMPLE

A solution calls for 5 mEq of sodium that you have in a 1.04 mEq / ml solution of NaCl. How many ml of it do you need?

x ml / 5 mEq = 1 ml/1.04 mEq

x ml = 5 ~~mEq~~ times $\dfrac{1 \text{ ml}}{1.04 \text{ ~~mEq~~}} = \dfrac{5 \text{ ml}}{1.04} = 4.8$ ml

Answer: 4.8 ml of the solution is needed.

COMMON SALINE SOLUTIONS:

0.9% NaCl	Normal Saline
0.45% NaCl	1/2 Normal Saline
0.2% NaCl	1/4 Normal Saline
3% NaCl	Hypertonic Saline

 milliequivalent (mEq) the unit of measure for electrolytes in a solution.

valence the number of positive or negative charges on an ion.

PERCENTS & SOLUTIONS (cont'd)

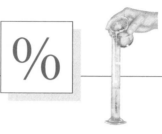

EXAMPLE—TOTAL PARENTERAL NUTRITION

A TPN order calls for the amounts on the left (including additives) to be made from the items on the right. The total volume is to be 1000 ml. How much of each ingredient do you need to prepare this TPN?

TPN Order	On Hand
Aminosyn 4.25%	Aminosyn 8.5% 1000 ml
Dextrose 25%	Dextrose 70% 1000 ml

Additives:

KCl	20 mEq	KCl 2mEq / ml 10 ml
MVI	10 ml	MVI 10 ml
NaCl	24 mEq	NaCl 4.4mEq / ml 20 ml

Aminosyn

Using Percent Solutions Formula:

x ml / 4.25% = 1000 ml / 8.5%

$$x \text{ ml} = 4.25\% \text{ times } \frac{1000 \text{ ml}}{8.5\%} = 1000 \text{ ml times } 0.5$$

➥ *4.25 divided by 8.5 = 0.5*

x ml = 500 ml

500 ml of aminosyn 8.5% is needed.

Dextrose

Using Percent Solutions Formula:

x ml / 25% = 1000 ml / 70%

$$x \text{ ml} = 25\% \text{ times } \frac{1000 \text{ ml}}{70\%} = \frac{25000 \text{ ml}}{70}$$

x ml = 357.14 ml dextrose ➡ 357 ml

357 ml of dextrose 70% is needed.

 safety you should know

Generally, amounts less than 0.5 are rounded down and amounts greater than 0.5 are rounded up. However, some drugs may be rounded and others may not. You will need to know when you must be precise and when you may round for each drug.

132

KCl

Use a proportion equation:

x ml / 20mEq = 1 ml / 2 mEq

x ml = 20 ~~mEq~~ times $\dfrac{1\ ml}{2\ mEq}$ = 10 ml KCl

10 ml KCl are needed.

MVI

Add the 10 ml MVI on hand.

NaCl

Use a proportion equation:

x ml / 24 mEq = 1 ml / 4.4 mEq

x ml = 24 ~~mEq~~ times $\dfrac{1\ ml}{4.4\ mEq}$ = 5.45 ml

5.45 ml of NaCl is needed.

Sterile Water

Add as needed (qs ad) for a volume of 1000 ml.

Word Equation:
water needed = 1000 ml minus (other ingredients)

Other ingredients:

Aminosyn	500 ml
Dextrose	357 ml
KCl	10 ml
MVI	10 ml
NaCl	5.45 ml
total	882.45 ml

water needed = 1000 minus 882.45 = 117.55

117.55 ml sterile water is needed to fill the TPN order.

PERCENTS & SOLUTIONS
(cont'd)

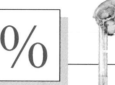

%

PERCENT SOLUTION FORMULA

$$\frac{x \text{ volume needed}}{\text{want \%}} = \frac{\text{volume prescribed}}{\text{have \%}}$$

PRACTICE PROBLEMS—TPN SOLUTIONS

A TPN order calls for the amounts on the left (including additives) to be made from the items on the right. The total volume is to be 250 ml. How much of each ingredient do you need to prepare this TPN?

TPN Order	What you have
Aminosyn 2.5%	Aminosyn 8.5% 500 ml
Dextrose 7.5%	Dextrose 50% 1000 ml

Additives:

KCl 4 mEq	KCl 2 mEq/ml 10 ml
Ca Gluconate 2 mEq	Ca Gluconate 4.4 mEq/ml 25 ml
Ped MVI 5 ml	Ped MVI 10 ml

Use the space to work out the answers.

1. **Aminosyn 8.5%**   Answer: _____ ml

2. **Dextrose 50%**   Answer:_____ ml

3. KCl 2 mEq/ml   Answer: _____ ml

4. Ca Gluconate 4.4 mEq/ml   Answer: _____ ml

5. Pediatric MVI 10 ml   Answer: _____ ml

6. Sterile Water (qs ad)   Answer: _____ ml

ALLIGATION

ALLIGATION

Alligation is a way to solve problems associated with mixing preparations of two different strengths of the same ingredient to obtain a strength in between the starting preparation. The problems could also be solved using algebra, but using the alligation method is often easier.

To use the alligation method set up a grid with three rows and three columns. Place the strength of the lower strength component in the upper left corner, place the strength of the higher strength component in the lower left corner, and place the desired strength of the product in the middle.

Strength of lower strength component (L)		
	Desired strength of product (P)	
Strength of higher strength component (H)		

Then subtract the lower value from the higher value on each diagonal to find the amounts needed of the lower strength (L) and higher strength (H) components:

Strength of lower strength component (L)		$H - P =$ Relative amount of L needed to prepare P
	Desired strength of product (P)	
Strength of higher strength component (H)		$P - L =$ Relative amount of H needed to prepare P

EXAMPLE

What are the relative amounts of 70% alcohol and 40% alcohol needed to prepare 60% alcohol? (In this example, since the value of P is higher than that of L, you will be subtracting L from P rather than P from L.)

Strength of lower strength component (L): 40		70 - 60 (H - P) = 10 parts needed of L
	Desired strength of product (P): 60	
Strength of higher strength component (H): 70		60 - 40 (P - L) = 20 parts needed of H

In the above example, the proportion of each component in the final product is found by first adding the part values in the right-hand column (10 + 20) to get the total part value of the product (30) and then dividing each part value by the total part value. Thus the amount of 70% alcohol will be 20/30 of the product and the amount of 40% alcohol will 10/30.

In practice, it is necessary to know how to convert relative amounts to real values that can be measured. This requires using addition, subtraction, multiplication, division, and fractions.

EXAMPLE

Using the alligation above, how many mL of 70% alcohol should be mixed with how many mL of 40% alcohol to prepare 300 mL of 60% alcohol?

To solve for the volume of H

300 mL P x 20 mL H / 30 mL P = 200 mL H

To solve for the volume of L:

300 mL P x 10 mL L / 30 mL P = 100 mL L

So, when 200 mL of 70% alcohol are mixed with 100 mL of 40% alcohol, the resulting solution is 300 mL of 60% alcohol.

ALLIGATION (cont'd)

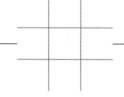

EXAMPLE

How many grams of 1% hydrocortisone cream and 5% hydrocortisone cream to prepare 30 grams of 2.5% hydrocortisone cream?

1 (L)		5 - 2.5 (H - P) = 2.5 parts of L
	2.5 (P)	
5 (H)		2.5 - 1 (P - L) = 1.5 parts of H

To solve for total parts of P:

   2.5 (L) + 1.5 (H) = 4 total parts of P

To solve for grams of 5% hydrocortisone cream:

   30 g P x 1.5 g H / 4 g P = 11.25 g H

To solve for grams of 1% hydrocortisone cream:

   30 g P x 2.5 g L / 4 g P = 18.75 g L

So, when 11.25 g of 5% hydrocortisone cream are mixed with 18.75 g of 1% hydrocortisone cream, the resulting product is 30 g of 2.5% hydrocortisone cream.

EXAMPLE

How many grams of 20% zinc oxide ointment and petrolatum should be mixed to prepare to prepare 60 grams of 3% zinc oxide ointment? (Hint: petrolatum has 0% zinc oxide.)

```
0 (L)                          20 - 3
                               (H - P)
                               = 17 parts
                                 of L

              3 (P)

20 (H)                         3 - 0
                               (P - L)
                               = 3 parts of
                                 H
```

To solve for total parts P:

17 + 3 = 20 total parts P

To solve for grams of 20% zinc oxide ointment:

60 g P x 3 g H / 20 g P = 9 g H

To solve for grams of petroleum:

60 g P x 17 g L / 20 g P = 51 g L

So, when 9 g of 20% zinc oxide ointment are mixed with 51 g of petrolatum, the resulting product is 60 g of 3% zinc oxide ointment.

POWDER VOLUME

POWDER VOLUME

Some medications that are dispensed in liquid dosage form are manufactured and provided to the pharmacy as powders. The powders are then constituted or mixed with a specific volume of liquid to produce a desired strength of the liquid dosage form.

There may be a need to perform two different types of calculations with powders for constitution:

1. Determining the strength or concentration of a product when different volumes of diluent are added.
2. Determining how to change the concentration or strength of the constituted dosage form by varying the amount of diluent.

For either type of calculation, it is necessary to make an assumption that when the powder is constituted or mixed, the volume occupied by the powder portion of the final product is a constant. The portion of the volume of the final mixed product that is attributed to the powder is called the *powder volume*.

For calculations with powders for constitution, the following relationship exists:

The final volume of the constituted product (FV)
=
The volume of the diluent (D) + the powder volume (PV)

Or

FV = D + PV

Additionally, it is important to keep in mind the total amount of drug in the manufacturer's bottle remains constant no matter how much diluent is added. For example, if a manufacturer packages 7500 mg of a drug in a bottle for constitution, the amount of drug in the bottle will always be 7500 mg (unless some medication is removed from the bottle).

EXAMPLE

The directions for mixing a liquid antibiotic state when 80 mL of water are added to the contents of the bottle, the resulting volume is 150 mL. Determine the powder volume.

$$FV = D + PV$$
$$150 \text{ mL} = 80 \text{ mL} + PV$$
$$PV = 150 \text{ mL} - 80 \text{ mL} = 70 \text{ mL}$$

EXAMPLE

The directions for mixing a 250 mg / 5 mL liquid antibiotic state when 80 mL of water are added to the contents of the bottle, the resulting volume is 150 mL. Determine the concentration of drug in mg / 5 mL if only 40 mL of water were added.

In order to solve this problem, you need to first determine the total mg of drug in the bottle and then determine the volume of the new product (NP) when only 40 mL of water was added.

First, determine the total mg of drug in the bottle (recall, this amount is a constant):

250 mg drug /5 mL FV x 150 mL FV = 7500 mg drug

Next, determine the powder volume for the drug in the bottle:

FV = D + PV

150 mL = 80 mL + PV

PV = 150 mL – 80 mL

PV = 70 mL

Now that we know the value for PV, we can determine the volume of the new product (NP):

(NP) = D + PV

NP = 40 mL + 70 mL

NP = 110 mL

So the new concentration is:

Total mg drug in bottle / Volume of the new product (NP)

7500 mg / 110 mL = 6.82 mg / mL = 341 mg / 5 mL

CHILDREN'S DOSES

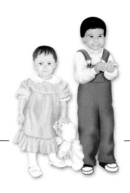

CALCULATION OF CHILDREN'S DOSES

The average doses in the U.S.P. (United States Pharmacopoeia) and other drug reference sources are for adults. Doses for drugs that can be taken by a child are often provided by the manufacturer. When children's doses are not provided, the adult dose needs to be lowered. One formula for this is:

CLARK'S RULE

$$\frac{\text{weight of child}}{\text{150 lb}} \text{ x adult dose = dose for child}$$

150 lbs is considered an average weight for an adult. This is not a very precise way to calculate pediatric doses as there are many factors besides weight which may need to be taken into account: height, age, condition, etc. Another approach is based upon multiplying the adult dose by a ratio of the child's size to that of an average adult:

BODY SURFACE AREA FORMULA

$$\frac{\text{child bsa times adult dose}}{\text{average adult bsa}} = \text{child's dose}$$

The **body surface area** of a person is based on their height and weight. It is always given in square meters (m^2). 1.73 m^2 is commonly used as an average bsa for adults. A chart called a **nomogram** has been traditionally used to manually calculate bsa. Body surface area nomograms contain three columns of numbers: height, body surface, and weight. The bsa is identified by the intersection of a line drawn between the weight and height columns with the bsa column, which is in the middle. Now, bsa formulas are generally solved by computer. (There are a number that can be found on the Internet, for example.) For a comparison to the average bsa for adults (1.73 m^2), a bsa for a nine year old child that was 44" tall and weighing 50 lbs would be about .92 m^2.

Because of the many variables, however, conversion formulas for pediatric doses are not always appropriate and can lead to incorrect doses with some medications. *Although doses are generally given by the physician, pharmacy should always check children's doses to make sure they are appropriate by using a suitable drug information resource.* Children's doses are stated by kg of body weight (dose/kg). Since 1 kg = 2.2 lb, you can solve for the prescribed dose by using a proportion equation if you know the child's body weight. See the example at right.

body surface area a measure used for dosage that is calculated from the height and weight of a person and measured in square meters.

nomogram a chart showing relationships between measurements.

EXAMPLE—INFANT DOSE

An antibiotic IV is prescribed for an infant. The dose is to be 15mg/kg twice a day. The baby weighs 18 lbs. How much drug is to be given for one dose? First you need to calculate the infant's weight in kilograms.

$$x \text{ kg} / 18 \text{ lb} = 1 \text{ kg} / 2.2 \text{ lb}$$

$$x \text{ kg} = 18 \text{ lb} \text{ times } \frac{1 \text{ kg}}{2.2 \text{ lb}} = \frac{18 \text{ kg}}{2.2} = 8.18 \text{ kg}$$

You can also easily solve this with a calculator:

- ➡ enter   18
- ➡ press   divide (/) key
- ➡ enter   2.2
- ➡ press   equal (=) key
- ➡ answer   8.18

You can solve the next part of this problem with a proportion equation or you can set up a simple word equation.

one dose = (amount of drug) times (number of kg of infant weight)

$$\text{one dose} = \frac{15 \text{ mg}}{\text{kg}} \text{ times } 8.18 \text{ kg}$$

With a calculator:

- ➡ enter   15
- ➡ press   multiplication (*) key
- ➡ enter   8.18
- ➡ press   equal (=) key
- ➡ answer   122.7 mg

CALCULATIONS FOR BUSINESS

$

USUAL AND CUSTOMARY PRICE

The usual and customary price (U&C) is the lowest price charged if a patient pays cash, on that day, for that drug. Usual and customary prices are usually determined at the corporate level, although pharmacy prices are sometimes determined when the prescription is filled using a formula. Pharmacy computers are usually programmed to automatically calculate the usual and customary price when a prescription is filled.

EXAMPLE

If prescription prices are determined using the following formula:

average wholesale price (AWP) + professional fee = selling price of prescription

and the professional fee is determined using the following chart:

AWP	Professional Fee
less than $20.00	$4.00
$20.01–$50.00	$5.00
$50.01 and higher	$6.00

and the AWP for 30 capsules of amoxicillin 250 mg is $3.50, what will be the retail price of the prescription?

Since the AWP for the prescription is less than $20.00, the professional fee is $4.00. Using the formula

AWP + professional fee = selling price of prescription,

$$\$3.50 + \$4.00 = \$7.50$$

Some pharmacies sell certain medications at a price lower than the acquisition cost. Therefore, the usual and customary price may be less than the average wholesale price (AWP) or less than the acquisition cost. Many third party plans reimburse the pharmacies based on the lowest amount: AWP, acquisition cost, or U&C, since the third parties do not want to pay more for a prescription than a patient would pay by cash.

PRACTICE PROBLEMS—USUAL AND CUSTOMARY

Calculate the retail price of the following prescriptions using the formula AWP + professional fee = retail price of prescription if the professional fee is determined using the chart in the example above:

1. Verapamil SR Tabs #30 AWP/100 $135.85   retail price _____

2. Glyburide 5 mg Tabs #30 AWP/1000 $480.15   retail price _____

3. Dexamethasone 4 mg Tabs #12 AWP/100 $62.50   retail price _____

4. Danazol 200 mg Caps #100 AWP/100 $322.38   retail price _____

5. Doxepin 150 mg Caps #30 AWP/100 $73.50   retail price _____

usual and customary price (U&C) the price charged for a prescription if there are no discounts or third parties paying for the prescription.

DISCOUNTS

Pharmacies sometimes give a 5 or 10% discount on the price of prescriptions to certain patients such as senior citizens that do not participate in third party programs. State pharmacy regulations or third party contractual agreements may prohibit discounting prescriptions that are covered by third party programs. Sometimes the discount is restricted to prescriptions purchased on certain days of the week.

EXAMPLE

A senior citizen is paying for a prescription for amoxicillin 250 mg #30. The usual and customary price is $8.49; however this patient qualifies for a 10% discount. How much will the patient pay?

$$\$8.49 - 10\%(\$8.49) = \$8.49 - (0.1)(\$8.49) = \$8.49 - \$0.85$$
$$= \$7.64$$

PRACTICE PROBLEMS—DISCOUNTS

Calculate how much the patient will pay for the following prescriptions if the patient qualifies for a 5% discount

1. Retail prescription price is $8.99   patient price after 5% discount _____

2. Retail prescription price is $18.41   patient price after 5% discount _____

3. Retail prescription price is $39.20   patient price after 5% discount _____

4. Retail prescription price is $99.90   patient price after 5% discount _____

5. Retail prescription price is $128.52   patient price after 5% discount _____

Calculate how much the patient will pay for the following prescriptions if the patient qualifies for a 10% discount

6. Retail prescription price is $8.99   patient price after 10% discount _____

7 .Retail prescription price is $18.49   patient price after 10% discount _____

8. Retail prescription price is $39.30   patient price after 10% discount _____

9. Retail prescription price is $9.90   patient price after 10% discount _____

10. Retail prescription price is $180.55   patient price after 10% discount _____

CALCULATIONS FOR BUSINESS (cont'd)

$

GROSS PROFIT AND NET PROFIT

Gross Profit

The gross profit is the difference between the selling price and the acquisition cost. For cash prescriptions, the selling price is the usual and customary price for prescriptions paid by cash customers. To calculate gross profit, there is no consideration for any of the expenses associated with filling the prescription.

Gross profit = Selling price - acquisition cost

The gross profit can be expressed as a percent.

EXAMPLE

A prescription for amoxicillin 250 mg #30 has a usual and customary price of $8.49. The acquisition cost of amoxicillin 250 mg #30 is $2.02. What is the gross profit?

Gross profit = Selling price - Acquisition cost

Gross profit = $8.49 - $2.02 = $6.47

Net Profit

The net profit is the difference between the selling price of the prescription and the sum of all the costs associated with filling the prescription. All the costs associated with filling the prescription include the cost of the medication, the cost of the container, the cost of the label, the cost of the bag, the cost of the labor to dispense the prescription, a portion of the rent, etc. For practical purposes, all the other costs can be grouped together and considered as a dispensing fee. Since the costs associated with operation of a pharmacy vary, the dispensing fee can vary.

Net profit = Selling price - Acquisition cost - Dispensing fee

or

Net profit = Gross profit - Dispensing fee

Net profit can also be expressed as a percent.

EXAMPLE

A prescription for amoxicillin 250 mg #30 has a usual and customary price of $8.49. The acquisition cost of amoxicillin 250 mg #30 is $2.02. What is the net profit if the dispensing fee/professional fee is $5.50?

Net profit = Selling price - Acquisition cost - Dispensing fee

Net profit = $8.49 - $2.02 - $5.50 = $0.97

PRACTICE PROBLEMS—GROSS PROFIT AND NET PROFIT

Use this table to determine the dispensing/professional fee

AWP	Professional Fee
less than $20.00	$4.00
$20.01–$50.00	$5.00
$50.01 and higher	$6.00

and then calculate the gross profit and the net profit for the following prescriptions.

1. **Zocor® 5 mg, 60 tablets**
   acquisition cost = $85.47   AWP = $106.84   selling price = $109.93
   Gross profit = _____   Net profit = _____

2. **Prilosec® 20 mg, 30 cap.**
   acquisition cost = $99.20   AWP = $108.90   selling price = $116.38
   Gross profit = _____   Net profit = _____

3. **Norvasc® 5 mg, 90 tablets**
   acquisition cost = $97.92   AWP = $125.66   selling price = $117.82
   Gross profit = _____   Net profit = _____

4. **Procardia® XL 30 mg, 100 tab.**
   acquisition cost = $105.05   AWP = $131.31   selling price = $134.36
   Gross profit = _____   Net profit = _____

5. **Vasotec® 10 mg, 100 tab.**
   acquisition cost = $85.56   AWP = $102.94   selling price = $109.19
   Gross profit = _____   Net profit = _____

6. **Relafen® 500 mg, 100 tab.**
   acquisition cost = $88.88   AWP = $111.10   selling price = $120.27
   Gross profit = _____   Net profit = _____

7. **Zoloft® 50 mg, 100 tab.**
   acquisition cost = $172.44   AWP = $215.55   selling price = $226.50
   Gross profit = _____   Net profit = _____

8. **Fosamax® 10 mg, 30 tablets**
   acquisition cost = $50.91   AWP = $51.88   selling price = $57.62
   Gross profit = _____   Net profit = _____

9. **Cardizem CD® 240 mg, 90 tablets**
   acquisition cost = $154.10   AWP = $165.42   selling price = $179.69
   Gross profit = _____   Net profit = _____

10. **Ticlid® 250 mg, 60 tablets**
   acquisition cost = $99.44   AWP = $108.90   selling price = $122.07
   Gross profit = _____   Net profit = _____

REVIEW

ROMAN NUMERALS

When the second of two letters has a value equal to or larger than that of the first, their values are to be subtracted.

When the second of two letters has a value equal to or smaller than that of the first, their values are to be added.

CONDITIONS FOR USING RATIO AND PROPORTION

1. Three of the four values must be known.

2. Numerators must have the same units.

3. Denominators must have the same units.

STEPS FOR SOLVING PROPORTION PROBLEMS

1. Define the variable and correct ratios.

2. Set-up the proportion equation

3. Establish the x equation

4. Solve for x.

5. Express solution in correct units.

PERCENT SOLUTION FORMULA

$$\frac{x \text{ volume needed}}{\text{want \%}} = \frac{\text{volume prescribed}}{\text{have \%}}$$

CONVERSIONS

Liquid Metric

1 L	=	10 dl	=	1000 ml
1 dl	=	0.1 L	=	100 ml
1 ml	=	0.001 L	=	0.01 dl

Solid Metric

1 kg	=	1,000 g		
1 g	=	0.001 kg	=	1,000 mg
1 mg	=	0.001 g	=	1,000 mcg
1 mcg	=	0.001 mg		

Avoirdupois

1 lb	=	16 oz
1 oz	=	437.5 gr
1 gr	=	64.8 mg (0.0648 g)

Apothecary

1 gal	=	4 qt
1 qt	=	2 pt
1 pt	=	16 fl oz
1 fl oz	=	8 fl dr
1 fl dr	=	60 m

Household

1 tsp	=	5 ml		
1 tbsp	=	3 tsp	=	15 ml
1 cup	=	8 fl oz		

Temperature

$$9C = 5F - 160$$

Conversions Between Systems

1 L	=	33.8 fl oz	1 lb	=	453.59 g
1 pt	=	473.167 ml	1 oz	=	28.35 g
1 fl oz	=	29.57 ml	1 g	=	15.43 gr
1 kg	=	2.2 lb	1 gr	=	64.8 mg

REVIEW

SELF TEST

MATCH THE TERMS   *the answer key begins on page 511*

1. body surface area ____

2. concentration ____

3. conversions ____

4. denominator ____

5. flow rate ____

6. least common denominator ____

7. milliequivalent (mEq) ____

8. nomogram ____

9. numerator ____

10. positional notation ____

11. qs ad ____

12. total parenteral nutrition ____

13. usual and customary (U&C) ____

14. valence ____

15. variable ____

a. a system used in Roman Numerals whereby the position of a numeral signifies its value.

b. the bottom (or right) number in a fraction; it indicates how many parts the whole is divided into.

c. the top (or left) number in a fraction; it indicates how many parts of the whole exist.

d. the change from one unit of measure to another so that both amounts are equal.

e. an unknown value in a mathematical equation.

f. the rate (in ml/hour or ml/minute) at which a solution is administered to a patient; also known as rate of administration.

g. the strength of a solution as measured by the weight-to-volume or volume-to-volume of the substance being measured.

h. administration of all nutrients intravenously; also known as hyperalimentation.

i. adding a sufficient quantity to make the prescribed amount.

j. the unit of measure for electrolytes in a solution.

k. the number of positive or negative charges on an ion.

l. a measure used for dosage that is calculated from the height and weight of a person and measured in square meters.

m. a chart showing relationships between measurements.

n. the price charged for a prescription if there are no discounts or third parties paying for the prescription.

o. smallest possible denominator for an equivalent fraction so that two fractions can be added or subtracted and have the same denominator.

CHOOSE THE CORRECT ANSWER   *the answer key begins on page 511*

1. A solution of Halperidol (Haldol®) contains 2 mg/ml of active ingredient. How many grams would be in 473 ml of this solution?
   a. 9.46 grams
   b. 0.946 grams
   c. 0.0946 grams
   d. 0.00946 grams

2. The physician orders Ferrous Sulfate 500 mg po qd x 30 days. You have on the shelf Ferrous Sulfate 220 mg/5 ml 473 ml. How many ml is required for one dose?
   a. 5.4 ml
   b. 8.4 ml
   c. 11.4 ml
   d. 13.4 ml

3. Using the information from the previous problem, approximately how many ml are required to completely fill this prescription?
   a. 162 ml
   b. 252 ml
   c. 342 ml
   d. 402 ml

4. The infusion rate of an IV is over twelve hours. The total volume is 1000 ml. What would the infusion rate be in ml per minute?
   a. 83.3 ml / minute
   b. 8.3 ml / minute
   c. 16.7 ml / minute
   d. 1.4 ml / minute

5. You have a 70% solution of Dextrose 1000 ml. How many kg of Dextrose is in 400 ml of this solution?
   a. 280 kg
   b. 28 kg
   c. 2.8 kg
   d. 0.28 kg

6. You receive an order for Vancomycin (Vancocin®) 10 mg/kg 500 ml to be infused over 90 minutes. The patient is five foot eleven inches tall and weighs 165 lb. What dose is needed for this patient?
   a. 750 mg
   b. 500 mg
   c. 250 mg
   d. 125 mg

7. The doctor orders 1/2 gr Codeine. How many milligrams is this equivalent to?
   a. 15 mg
   b. 30 mg
   c. 60 mg
   d. 90 mg

8. You receive a prescription for Metronidazole (Flagyl®) 250 mg/5 ml po qid 240 ml. You find that you will have to compound this using 500 mg tablets. How many tablets will be needed to fill this order completely?
   a. 22 tablets
   b. 24 tablets
   c. 42 tablets
   d. 48 tablets

9. You are asked by the Pharmacist to add 45 mEq of Ca Gluconate in an IV bag of D5%W 1000 ml. You have a concentrated vial of Ca Gluconate 4.4 mEq/ml 50 ml. How many ml of this concentrated vial needs to be added to the IV bag?
   a. 1.2 ml
   b. 10.2 ml
   c. 0.12 ml
   d. 2.4 ml

10. A patient is taking 2 teaspoonfuls of sucralfate suspension four times a day. How much suspension will the patient use in 72 hours?
    a. 3 oz
    b. 100 ml
    c. 4 oz
    d. 150 ml

11. What volume of solution that is 25 mg/ml should be measured to deliver a dose of 20 mg?
    a. 1.25 ml
    b. 0.8 ml
    c. 0.20 ml
    d. 0.25 ml

12. Phos-Flur® Rinse contains sodium fluoride 0.044% (w/v). How many mg of sodium fluoride are in a 10 ml dose?
    a. 0.044 mg
    b. 0.44 mg
    c. 4.4 mg
    d. 44 mg

REVIEW

13. If 0.44 mg of sodium fluoride is equal to 0.2 mg of fluoride, how many mg of fluoride are in 2.2 mg of sodium fluoride?

   a. 1 mg
   b. 2 mg
   c. 5 mg
   d. 20 mg

14. How much hydrocortisone powder is needed to compound 60 g of hydrocortisone cream 1%?

   a. 0.6 mg
   b. 600 mg
   c. 0.06 g
   d. 6 mg

15. You have an ampule of digoxin injection that contains 500 mcg in 2 ml. What volume is needed to deliver a dose of 0.125 mg?

   a. 0.124 ml
   b. 0.25 ml
   c. 0.5 ml
   d. .75 m

16. An IV contains 5 mg of drug per ml and the patient needs to receive 50 mg per hour. What is the infusion rate in ml/hr?

   a. 5 ml/hr
   b. 10 ml/hr
   c. 16.7 ml/hr
   d. 0.167 ml/hr

17. The doctor changes a prescription for 150 ml of amoxicillin 250 mg/5 ml to 250 mg chewable tablets. How many chewable tablets should be dispensed?

   a. 15 tablets
   b. 30 tablets
   c. 45 tablets
   d. 60 tablets

18. A child's dose for cefadroxil is 30 mg/kg body weight once a day for 14 days. What is the smallest bottle that will provide enough medication to last 14 days if the child weighs 44 pounds?

   a. 50 ml bottle of 125 mg/5 ml
   b. 50 ml bottle of 250 mg/5 ml
   c. 75 ml bottle of 500 mg/5 ml
   d. 100 ml bottle of 500 mg/5 ml

19. You have diluted 40 ml of a 50% dextrose solution with water so the volume of the resulting solution is 100 ml. What is the concentration of dextrose in the resulting solution?

   a. 12%
   b. 20%
   c. 24%
   d. 40%

20. What is the cost for 30 tablets of a drug if the cost for 100 tablets is $75.00?

   a. $19.65
   b. $21.83
   c. $22.50
   d. $24.23

21. The retail price for a prescription is $37.50. What amount should be charged if the patient is to receive a 10% discount?

   a. $34.50
   b. $34.00
   c. $33.75
   d. $31.95

22. If the dose of a drug is 500 mg and the drug is available as 400 mg/5 ml, how many teaspoonfuls are needed for the required dose?

   a. 1.25 teaspoonfuls
   b. 2.5 teaspoonfuls
   c. 4 teaspoonfuls
   d. 5 teaspoonfuls

23. How many tablets should be dispensed if a prescription is written as follows:
Tabs iss b.i.d. for 10 days
   a. 10 tablets
   b. 15 tablets
   c. 30 tablets
   d. 45 tablets

24. How many ounces of medication are needed to last 8 days if the dose of medication is one and one-half teaspoonfuls four times a day?
   a. 4 oz
   b. 6 oz
   c. 8 oz
   d. 12 oz

25. How many 4 oz bottles can be filled from a gallon of Coke™ Syrup?
   a. 32 bottles
   b. 48 bottles
   c. 64 bottles
   d. 72 bottles

26. If the temperature in the refrigerator is 45° Fahrenheit, to the nearest whole degree, what is the temperature in degrees Centigrade?
   a. 5° Centigrade
   b. 6° Centigrade
   c. 7° Centigrade
   d. 10° Centigrade

27. The mixing instructions for a liquid antibiotic call for 45 mL of water for constitution to make a 150 mL suspension. The final concentration of the suspension is 250 mg/5 mL. What is the powder volume?
   a. 45 mL
   b. 90 mL
   c. 105 mL
   d. 205 mL

28. How many mL of 70% alcohol should be mixed with 20 mL of 20% alcohol to prepare 50% alcohol?
   a. 20 mL
   b. 30 mL
   c. 40 mL
   d. 50 mL

29. How many grams of 1% hydrocortisone cream should be mixed with 30 g of 2.5% hydrocortisone cream to make 2% hydrocortisone cream?
   a. 10 g
   b. 15 g
   c. 20 g
   d. 30 g

CONVERT THE FOLLOWING:

the answer key begins on page 511

1. 5 g   = _____ mg

2. 10 kg   = _____ g

3. 300 ml   = _____ L

4. 600 mg   = _____ g

5. 120 mcg = _____ mg

6. 102 kg   = _____ lb

7. 2.2 kg   = _____ g

8. 473ml   = _____ L

9. 145 lb   = _____ kg

10. 0.01 kg = ——— mg

REVIEW

SOLVE THE FOLLOWING PROBLEMS IN THE SPACE PROVIDED.   *the answer key begins on page 511*

1. Oral Polio Virus Vaccine (Poliovax®) should be stored in a temperature not to exceed 46 degrees Fahrenheit. What is this temperature in Centigrade?

2. A prescription reads for Erythromycin 100 mg every six hours for ten days. You have on hand Erythromycin 250 mg/5 ml. How much Erythromycin is needed for one dose?

3. You have an IV that needs $MgSO_4$ (Magnesium Sulfate) 10 mEq. You have on hand a bottle of $MgSO_4$ 4 mEq/ml. How much $MgSO_4$ do you need to inject into this IV bag?

4. You have an order for 20% Dextrose 500 ml. You have a 1000 ml bag of Dextrose 70%. How much of the Dextrose 70% do you need to use to make Dextrose 20% 500 ml? How much sterile water do you need?

ROUTES & FORMULATIONS

ROUTES & FORMULATIONS

The way in which the body absorbs and distributes drugs varies with the route of administration and the dosage form used. Drugs are contained in dosing units called formulations or dosage forms. There are many dosage forms and many different routes to administer them.

Routes of administration are classified as enteral or parenteral.

Enteral refers to anything involving the alimentary tract, i.e., from the mouth to the rectum. This tract is involved with digesting foods, absorbing nutrients, and eliminating unabsorbed wastes. There are four enteral routes of administration: oral, sublingual, buccal, and rectal.

Any route other than oral, sublingual, buccal, or rectal is considered a parenteral administration route.

The term parenteral means next to, or beside the enteral. It refers to any sites of administration that are outside of or beside the alimentary tract.

For each route of administration, there are various formulations used to deliver the drug via that route.

Different dosage forms affect onset times, duration of action, or concentrations of a drug in the body. Some drugs are formulated in more than one dosage form, each of which produces different characteristics. A consideration for selecting a particular route of administration or dosage form is the type of effect desired. A **local effect** occurs when the drug activity is at the site of administration (e.g., eyes, ears, nose, skin). A **systemic effect** occurs when the drug is introduced into the circulatory system from the route of administration and carried by the blood to the site of activity.

local effect when drug activity is at the site of administration.

systemic effect when a drug is introduced into the venous (circulatory) system and carried to the site of activity.

DOSAGE FORMS

Enteral Route	Dosage Form
Oral	Tablets
	Capsules
	Bulk powders
	Solutions
	Suspensions
	Elixirs
	Syrups
	Emulsions
Buccal	Tablets
	Solutions
Sublingual	Tablets
	Lozenges
Rectal	Solutions
	Ointments
	Suppositories

Parenteral Route	Dosage Form
Intraocular	Solutions
	Suspensions
	Ointments
	Inserts
Intranasal	Solutions
	Suspensions
	Ointments
	Gels
Inhalation	Solutions
	Aerosols
	Powders
Intravenous **Intramuscular** **Intradermal**	Solutions
	Suspensions
	Colloids
	Emulsions
Dermal	Solutions
	Tinctures
	Collodions
	Liniments
	Suspensions
	Ointments
	Creams
	Gels

ROUTES OF ADMINISTRATION

Enteral Routes are in red. Parenteral routes are in blue.
The term is followed by the organ(s) of absorption.

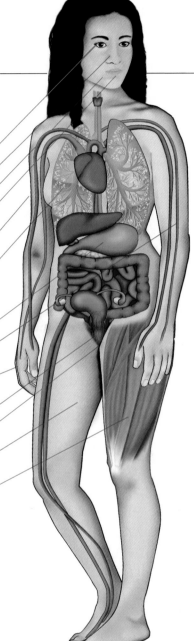

Intraocular	Eye
Intranasal	Nose
Buccal	Inside the cheek
Sublingual	Under the tongue
Dermal	Through or on the skin*
Inhalation	Lungs
Oral	Stomach and intestine
Intravenous	Venous circulatory system
Intradermal	Dermal layer of the skin*
Vaginal	Vagina
Rectal	Rectum
Subcutaneous	Subcutaneous layer of the skin*
	Muscle*
Intramuscular	

this route has various administration sites

Parenteral Route	Dosage Form
Dermal (cont'd)	Lotions
	Pastes
	Plasters
	Powders
	Aerosols
	Transdermal patches
Subcutaneous	Solutions
	Suspensions
	Emulsions
	Implants
Vaginal	Solutions
	Ointments
	Creams

Parenteral Route	Dosage Form
Vaginal (cont'd)	Aerosol foams
	Powders
	Suppositories
	Tablets
	IUDs

ORAL FORMULATIONS

Oral administration is the most frequently used route of administration.

Oral dosage forms are easy to carry, use, and administer. The term used to specify oral administration is peroral or PO (per os). This indicates that the dosage form is to be swallowed and that absorption will occur primarily from the stomach and the intestine.

When formulations are orally administered, they enter the stomach, which is very acidic.

The stomach has a **pH** around 1–2. Certain drugs cannot be taken orally because they are degraded (chemically changed to a less effective form) or destroyed by stomach acid and intestinal enzymes. Additionally, the absorption of many drugs is affected by the presence of food in the stomach.

Drugs administered in liquid dosage forms generally reach the circulatory system faster than drugs formulated in solid dosage forms.

This is because the processes of **disintegration** and **dissolution** are not required. Oral liquids include solutions, suspensions, gels, and emulsions. Solid oral dosage forms include tablets, capsules, and bulk powders.

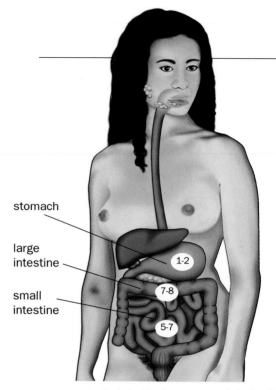

gastrointestinal organs and their pH

Gastrointestinal Action

The disintegration and dissolution of tablets, capsules, and powders generally begins in the stomach, but will continue to occur when the stomach content empties into the intestine. Enteric coated tablets are used when the drug can be degraded by the stomach acid. The enteric coating will not let the tablet disintegrate until it reaches the higher pHs of the intestine.

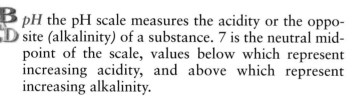

pH the pH scale measures the acidity or the opposite (alkalinity) of a substance. 7 is the neutral midpoint of the scale, values below which represent increasing acidity, and above which represent increasing alkalinity.

Most oral dosage forms are intended for systemic effect, but not all. For example, antacids have a local effect confined to the gastrointestinal tract.

Inactive Ingredients

Oral formulations contain various ingredients beside the active drug. These include binders, lubricants, fillers, diluents, and disintegrants. They are added to help manufacture the formulation and to help the dosage form disintegrate and dissolve when administered. A sample breakdown of ingredients is illustrated at right. (Note, however, that the breakdown for each formulation is different.)

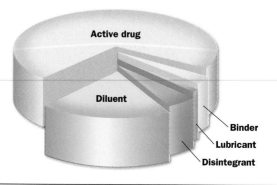

disintegration the breaking apart of a tablet into smaller pieces.

dissolution when the smaller pieces of a disintegrated tablet dissolve in solution.

SOLID FORMULATIONS

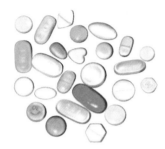

Tablets are hard formulations in which the drug and other ingredients are machine compressed under high pressure into a shape. Tablets vary in size, weight, hardness, thickness, and disintegration and dissolution characteristics, depending upon their intended use. Most tablets are manufactured for oral use, and many are coated on the formulation to give an identifying color or logo. Sugar-coated tablets are coated with a sweet glaze. Film-coated tablets are coated with a non-sweet coating. Multiple compressed tablets contain one drug in an inner layer and another drug (or the same drug) compressed at a lower pressure around it as an outer layer. A multiple compressed tablet can also have the two layers adjacent to each other. Repeat action tablets initially release one dose of the drug and then release a second dose sometime later. Other popular tablets are chewable and effervescent.

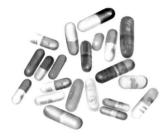

Capsules contain the drug and the other ingredients packaged in a gelatin shell. There are several capsule sizes. The capsule size used in any formulation is based on the amount of material to be placed inside the capsule. The gelatin shell dissolves in the stomach and releases the contents of the capsule. The freed contents must still undergo disintegration and dissolution before the drug is absorbed into the circulatory system. There are some capsule formulations that contain liquid instead of powders inside the gelatin shell; these are called "soft" or "soft-gel" capsules. The active drug is already dissolved in the liquid.

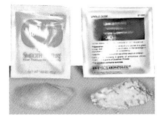

Bulk powders (e.g., Goody's BC powders) contain the active drug in a small powder paper or foil envelope. The patient empties the envelope into a glass of water or juice and drinks the contents. Most of the drug and ingredients dissolve in the water before the patient takes it.

MODIFIED RELEASE FORMULATIONS

Several oral formulations release the drug so that a longer duration of action is achieved compared to a conventional tablet, capsule, or powder. These are called modified release drug products. The primary goal of these products is to reduce the number of doses a patient needs to take during a day (i.e., reduce the frequency of dosing). Some modified release products also control the blood concentrations of the drug better than conventional dosage forms.

Through the years, many terms have been used to identify these kinds of products. Some of these include sustained release (SR), sustained action (SA), extended release (ER or XR), prolonged action (PA), controlled release or continuous release (CR), time release (TR), and long acting (LA).

ORAL FORMULATIONS (cont'd)

LIQUID FORMULATIONS

Solutions

A solution is a clear liquid (not necessarily colorless) made up of one or more ingredients dissolved in a solvent. A solvent is a liquid that can dissolve another substance to form a solution. Aqueous solutions are the most common of the oral solutions. Aqueous means that water was used as the solvent. Although water is the most common solvent for oral solutions, alcohol, glycerin, propylene glycol (or combinations of these) can be used.

Syrups are concentrated or nearly saturated solutions of sucrose (i.e., sugar) in water. They are more viscous (thicker) than water, and contain less than 10% alcohol. Syrups containing flavoring agents are known as flavoring syrups (e.g., Wild Cherry Syrup), and medicinal syrups are those which contain drugs (e.g., Guaifenesin Syrup).

Nonaqueous solutions are those solutions which predominately contain solvents other than water, either alone or in addition to water. Only a few nonaqueous solvents such as glycerin, alcohol, and propylene glycol can be used in oral solutions.

Elixirs are clear, sweetened, hydroalcoholic liquids intended for oral use. They can contain either alcohol soluble or water soluble drugs. Elixirs are usually less sweet and less viscous than syrups, and are generally less effective in masking taste. Their alcohol content ranges from 5–40% (10–80 proof), though a few commercial elixirs contain no alcohol.

Spirits or **essences** are alcoholic or hydroalcoholic solutions of volatile substances (usually volatile oils) with alcohol contents ranging from 62–85% (124–170 proof). They are most frequently used as flavoring agents (e.g., Peppermint Spirit) but some spirits are used for their medicinal effect.

Tinctures are alcoholic or hydroalcoholic solutions of nonvolatile substances. Tinctures of potent drugs have 10 grams of the drug in each 100 ml of tincture; they are called 10% tinctures. Tincture of nonpotent tinctures generally have 20 grams of the drug per 100 ml of tincture.

Suspensions

Suspensions are formulations in which the drug does not completely dissolve in the solvent. The drug particles are suspended in the formulation. Since they are intended for oral administration, suspensions are sweetened and flavored.

The primary concern in formulating suspensions is that they tend to settle over time leading to a lack of dose uniformity. A well-formulated suspension will remain suspended or settle very slowly, and can be easily redispersed with shaking.

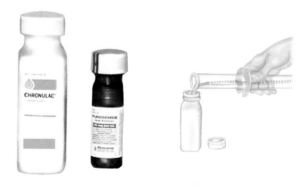

Some commercial suspensions are packaged as lyophilized powder. Water is added to the container, and the suspension is made. This process is called reconstitution.

Advantages of Solutions	Disadvantages of Solutions
➥ Completely homogenous doses	➥ Drugs and chemicals are less stable in solution than in dry dosage forms
➥ Immediately available for absorption	➥ Some drugs are not soluble in solvents that are acceptable for therapeutic use
➥ For patients who cannot swallow tablets or capsules	➥ May require special additives or techniques to mask objectionable taste
➥ Doses can be easily adjusted	➥ More difficult to handle, transport, and store because of bulk and weight
	➥ Solutions in bulk containers require dosage measurement devices

Emulsions

It is well known that "oil and water don't mix." Yet, some formulations contain both aqueous and oleaginous (oil based) components. These two non-mixable components can be formulated into a homogenous mixture when an emulsifying agent (emulsifier) is used. Emulsifiers enable one of the components to be dispensed in the other in the form of tiny droplets or globules. If the oleaginous component is present as droplets, the emulsion is called an oil-in-water (o/w) emulsion. If the aqueous component is present as droplets, the emulsion is called a water-in-oil (w/o) emulsion.

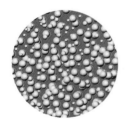

droplets in an emulsion

Emulsions are used in many routes of administration. Oral administration can be used, but patients generally object to the oily feel of emulsions in the mouth. But sometimes emulsions are the formulation of choice to mask the taste of a very bitter drug or when the oral solubility or bioavailability of a drug is to be dramatically increased. More typically, emulsions are used for topical administration as creams, lotions, or ointment bases.

Emulsions used for oral administration are physically unstable and tend to separate into two distinct phases over time. Creaming occurs when dispersed droplets merge and rise to the top or fall to the bottom of the emulsion. A creamed emulsion can be easily redispersed by shaking. Coalescence (breaking or cracking) is the irreversible separation of the dispersed phase.

Gels

Gels are made using substances called gelling agents that increase the viscosity (or thickness) of the medium in which they are placed. The gelling agents form an interlacing three-dimensional network of particles that restricts the movement of the solvent.

There are many gelling agents. Some of the common ones are acacia, alginic acid, Carbopols® (now known as carbomers), gelatin, methylcellulose, tragacanth, and xanthan gum. Though each gelling agent has some unique properties, there are some generalizations that can be made.

➡ Most gelling agents require 12–24 hours to reach maximum viscosity and clarity.

➡ Gelling agents are used in concentrations of 0.5% up to 10% depending on the agent.

➡ It is easier to add the active drug before the gel is formed if the drug doesn't interfere with the gel formation.

➡ Only Carbopol® 934P, methylcellulose, hydroxypropylmethylcellulose, and sodium caboxymethylcellulose are recommended for oral administration.

 emulsions mixture of two liquids that do not mix with each other in which one liquid is dispersed through the other by using a stabilizer called an emulsifier.

Advantages of Suspensions

➡ Can orally administer drugs that are insoluble in acceptable solvents

➡ Can be taken or administered to patients who cannot swallow tablets or capsules

➡ Masks objectionable taste of some drugs

➡ Drugs are chemically more stable than in solution

Disadvantages of Suspensions

➡ Tend to settle over time leading to a lack of dose uniformity

➡ Unpleasant oral texture

SUBLINGUAL & BUCCAL

The mouth is the route of administration for certain drugs when a rapid action is desired.

Formulations used in the mouth are generally fast dissolving uncoated tablets which contain highly **water soluble** drugs. These tablets are placed under the tongue (**sublingual** administration). When the drug is released from the tablet, it is quickly absorbed into the circulatory system since the membranes lining the mouth are very thin and there is a rich blood supply to the mouth.

Nitroglycerin is the best known example of a sublingual tablet formulation.

Nitroglycerin is sublingually administered since it is degraded in the stomach and intestine. Nitroglycerin is also available in a translingual aerosol that permits a patient to spray droplets of nitroglycerin under the tongue. There are also some steroid sex hormones that are sublingually administered.

Sublingual administration has certain limitations.

For instance, the bitter taste of most drugs makes holding a tablet in the mouth for almost any period time unpleasant, so lozenges, which are generally formulated with sweetening agents, are sometimes used instead of tablets for sublingual administration. For various reasons (including the condition of the mouth, the patient, etc.), other routes of administration are considered more convenient for many drugs that would otherwise be candidates for sublingual administration.

The *buccal* cavity is also in the mouth and refers to the insides of the cheek.

Buccal tablets and lozenges are placed in the pouch between the cheeks and the teeth to dissolve. Like the sublingual administration route, the buccal cavity allows for rapid absorption of drugs and bypasses first-pass metabolism in the liver.

Using Sublingual Tablets

Sublingual tablets are highly water soluble, so patients should first take a sip of water to wet their mouth if it is dry.

The tablet is then placed far under the tongue and the mouth is closed and must remain closed until the tablet dissolves and is absorbed. No food or beverages should be placed in the mouth until the drug is fully absorbed.

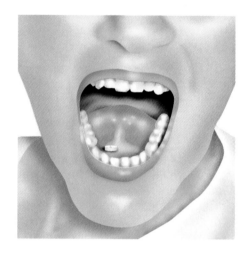

 Like many medical terms, *sub, trans, and lingua* are Latin words. They mean under, across or over, and tongue respectively.

water soluble the property of a substance being able to dissolve in water.

sublingual under the tongue.

buccal pouch between the teeth and cheek in the mouth.

RECTAL

Drugs are administered via the rectum either for a local effect or to avoid degradation after oral administration.

Local effects may include the soothing of inflamed **hemorrhoidal** tissues or promoting laxation. Rectal administration for systemic activity is preferred when the drug is degraded by stomach acid or intestinal enzymes, or if oral administration is unavailable (if the patient is vomiting, unconscious, or incapable of swallowing oral formulations). Rectal administration is used to achieve a variety of systemic effects including asthma control, antinausea, motion sickness, and anti-infective therapy.

The most common rectal administration dosage forms are suppositories, solutions, and ointments.

Suppositories are semisolid dosage forms that dissolve or melt when inserted into the rectum. Suppositories are manufactured in a variety of shapes and are used in other routes of administration such as vaginal or urethral. Most rectal solutions are used as enemas or cleansing solutions. Rectal ointments are intended to be spread around the anal opening and are most often used to treat inflamed hemorrhoidal tissues.

Rectal dosage forms have certain significant disadvantages.

They are not preferred by most patients. They are inconvenient. Moreover, rectal absorption of most drugs is frequently erratic and unpredictable.

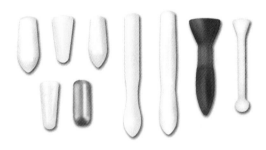

various suppository sizes and shapes

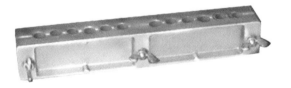

aluminum mold for making suppositories

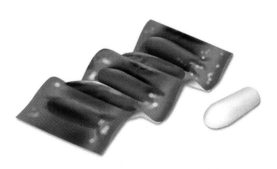

suppository in plastic mold

Enemas

Enemas create an urge to defecate due to the placement of fluid into the rectum. A cleansing enema uses water or a cleansing solution. A retention enema uses an oil that is held in the rectum to soften the stool. Frequent use of enemas is discouraged as it can have significant adverse effects.

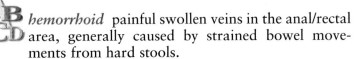

hemorrhoid painful swollen veins in the anal/rectal area, generally caused by strained bowel movements from hard stools.

PARENTERAL ROUTES

Parenteral routes of administration are used for a variety of reasons.

If an orally administered drug is poorly absorbed, or is degraded by stomach acid or intestinal enzymes, then a parenteral route may be indicated. Some parenteral routes are also preferred when a rapid drug response is desired, as in an emergency situation. Parenteral routes of administration are also useful when a patient is uncooperative, unconscious, or otherwise unable to take a drug by an enteral route.

There are disadvantages to giving formulations by parenteral routes.

One is cost. Many parenterals are more expensive than enteral route formulations. Another is that many parenterals require skilled personnel to administer them. A third disadvantage is that once a parenteral drug is administered, it is most difficult to remove the dose if there is an adverse or toxic reaction. Finally, some types of parenteral administration have risks associated with invading the body with a needle (e.g., infection, thrombus, etc.).

Several parenteral routes require a needle and some type of propelling device (syringe, pump) to administer a drug.

Some of these routes of administration are the intravenous, intramuscular, intradermal, and subcutaneous routes. These injectable routes have several characteristics in common. The formulations that can be used are limited to solutions, suspensions, and emulsions. Any other dosage formulation cannot pass through a syringe. These formulations must be **sterile** (bacteria-free) since they are placed in direct contact with the internal body fluids or tissues where infection can easily occur. The pH of the formulation must also be carefully maintained. This is commonly done by adding ingredients to the formulation to create a **buffer system**. A fourth characteristic is that limited volumes of formulation can be injected. Too much volume can cause pain and increased cell death (**necrosis**).

PARENTERAL ROUTES OF ADMINISTRATION

Injection Independent

ophthalmic
intranasal
inhalation
dermal
vaginal
otic

Injection Dependent

intravenous
intramuscular
intradermal
subcutaneous
epidural
intrathecal

Route of Administration	Needle Gauge	Needle Length
Intravenous (IV)	16–20	1–1.5″
Intramuscular (IM)	19–22	1–1.5″
Subcutaneous (SC)	24–27	3/8–1″
Intradermal (ID)	25–26	3/8″

syringe needle recommendations for injection dependent routes of administration

sterile a sterile condition is one which is free of *all* microorganisms, both harmful and harmless.

buffer system ingredients in a formulation designed to control the pH.

necrosis increase in cell death.

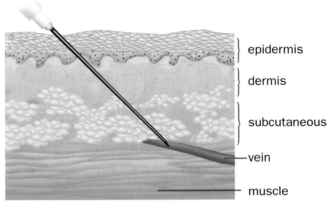

epidermis

dermis

subcutaneous

vein

muscle

Intravenous

Intravenous injections are administered directly into veins. They may be large volume, slow infusions with aqueous solutions such as D5W (dextrose 5% in water) or NS (0.9% sodium chloride in water), or small volume single injections (e.g., furosemide, metoprolol, or morphine). Fat emulsions, blood transfusions, and patient-controlled analgesia (PCA) solutions are also administered by IV administration.

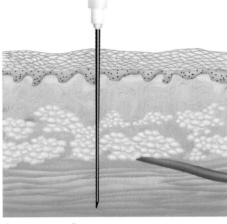

Intramuscular

Intramuscular injections are administered into muscle tissue and generally result in a slower onset but longer duration of action compared to IV administration. Drugs that can be given by IM administration include haloperidol, prochlorperazine, iron dextran, olanzapine, ziprasidone, and metoclopramide.

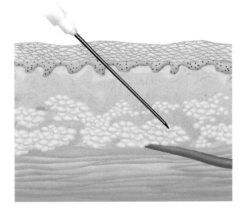

Subcutaneous

Subcutaneous injections are administered into the subcutaneous tissue of the skin. Subcutaneous administration generally provides slower absorption compared to IM administration, but faster absorption compared to oral administration. It is also the preferred route of administration for implants. Common drugs given by SC administration include the insulins, heparin, enoxaparin, and several vaccines.

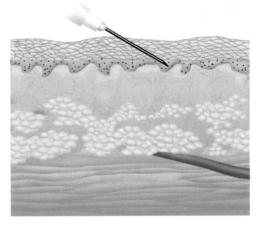

Intradermal

Intradermal injections are administered into the top layer of the skin at a slight angle using short needles. Most of the drugs administered by this route are for diagnostic determinations, desensitization, or immunization.

INTRAVENOUS FORMULATIONS

Intravenous dosage forms are administered directly into a vein and therefore the circulating blood.

It takes about 20 seconds for intravenously administered drugs to circulate throughout the body. Solutions are the most common intravenously administered formulations. Most solutions are **aqueous**, but they may also have glycols, alcohols, or other nonaqueous solvents in them.

Injectable suspensions are difficult to formulate because they must possess suitable syringeability and injectability.

Syringeability refers to the ease with which the suspension can be drawn from a container into a syringe. **Injectability** refers to the properties of the suspension while being injected, such as flow evenness, freedom from clogging, etc.

Emulsions are formulations that contain both aqueous and nonaqueous (oil) components.

Fat emulsions in total parenteral nutrition (TPN) solutions are used to provide triglycerides, fatty acids, and calories for patients who cannot absorb them from the gastrointestinal tract.

Dry powder formulations are manufactured for intravenous use, but they must be reconstituted with a suitable diluent to make a liquid formulation.

Many drugs that are not stable in liquid form can be lyophilized (freeze-dried) into a powder. The powder is reconstituted just prior to use with a solvent called a **diluent**. The most common diluents are Sterile Water for Injection and Bacteriostatic Water for Injection. A drug product's package insert will indicate the appropriate diluent to use.

COMPLICATIONS

There are a number of complications that can occur from intravenous administration such as thrombus formation, phlebitis, air emboli, and particulate material.

➡ Thrombus (blood clot) formation can result from many factors: extremes in solution pH, particulate material, irritant properties of the drug, needle or catheter trauma, and selection of too small a vein for the volume of solution injected.

➡ Phlebitis, or inflammation of the vein, can be caused by the same factors that cause thrombosis.

➡ Air emboli occur when air is introduced into the vein. The human body is generally not harmed by very small amounts of air injected into the venous system, but *excess air injected into the veins can be fatal,* so it is necessary to remove all air bubbles from formulation and administration sets before use.

➡ Particulate material can include small pieces of glass that chip from the product's vial or rubber pieces that comes from the closure on the vials. Although great care is taken to eliminate the presence of particulate material, a final filter in the administration line just before entering the venous system is an important precaution.

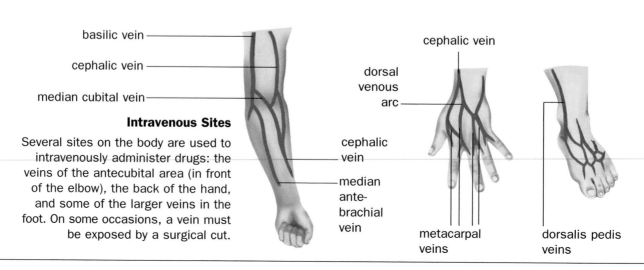

basilic vein

cephalic vein

median cubital vein

Intravenous Sites

Several sites on the body are used to intravenously administer drugs: the veins of the antecubital area (in front of the elbow), the back of the hand, and some of the larger veins in the foot. On some occasions, a vein must be exposed by a surgical cut.

cephalic vein

median antebrachial vein

cephalic vein

dorsal venous arc

metacarpal veins

dorsalis pedis veins

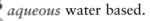 *aqueous* water based.

syringeability the ease with which a suspension can be drawn from a container into a syringe.

diluent a solvent that dissolves a freeze-dried powder or dilutes a solution.

injectability the ease of flow when a suspension is injected into a patient.

DEVICES

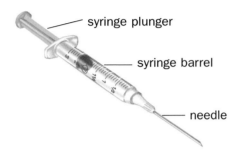

syringe plunger

syringe barrel

needle

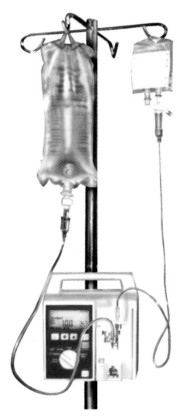

a solution bag and a minibag connected to an infusion pump

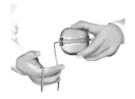

an elastomeric pump

Syringes

Simple syringe and needle setups can be used to inject formulations over a short period of time (generally up to 2 minutes). There are a variety of syringe sizes and needle sizes; syringe size is selected based on the volume of the formulation to inject. The needle size is generally based on the route of administration being used (IV, IM, SC, ID). Some products come from the manufacturer with syringes and needles already assembled and prefilled.

Infusion

Infusion is the gradual intravenous injection of a volume of fluid into a patient. The infusion solution is generally a large volume (500 ml to 1,000 ml) of electrolyte solution such as D5W (dextrose 5% in water) or 1/2NS (one-half normal saline, 0.45% sodium chloride in water). It is infused at a rate of 2 ml to 3 ml per minute.

The solution bag has two ports: an administration set port and a medication port. The administration set provides the connection between the solution bag and the needle in the patient. The administration set may also be connected to an infusion pump to control the flow rate. A simple syringe and needle may be used to inject a drug through the medication port into the solution bag. Sometimes a second small bag containing the drug (called a minibag) can be piggybacked onto the administration set or through an infusion pump.

Infusion Pumps

Administration devices that are dependent upon gravity flow have been shown to have a variable delivery rate. To ensure a constant delivery rate, controlled rate infusion pumps are used. Beginning in the late 1980s, patients were allowed to operate these pumps for occasional self administration of analgesics. The term patient controlled analgesia (PCA) was coined to describe this practice.

Elastomeric Pumps

Elastomeric pumps are useful for intermittent or very slow, continuous infusions. They are balloon-like reservoirs filled with medication that is forced out of the reservoir through a flow restrictor.

INTRAMUSCULAR

Drugs are often given by the intramuscular route to patients unable to take them by oral administration.

This route is also used for drugs that are poorly absorbed from the gastrointestinal tract. It is generally considered less hazardous and easier to use than the intravenous route. However, patients generally experience more pain from intramuscular administration than intravenous administration.

Intramuscular (IM) injections are made into the muscle fibers that are under the subcutaneous layer of the skin.

Needles used for the injections are generally 1 inch to 1.5 inches long, and are generally 19 to 22 gauge in size. The principal sites of injection are the gluteal maximus (buttocks), deltoid (upper arm), and vastus lateralis (thigh) muscles. When giving intramuscular injections into the gluteus maximus, one must be aware of the thickness of gluteal fat, particularly in female patients, and an appropriate size needle must be used. Otherwise, the injection will not reach the muscle.

The site of injection should be as far as possible from major nerves and blood vessels to avoid nerve damage and accidental intravenous administration.

Injuries that can occur following intramuscular injection are abscesses, cysts, embolism, hematoma, skin sloughing, and scar formation. To avoid injury when a series of injections are given, the injection site is changed or rotated. Generally only limited volumes can be given by intramuscular injection: 2 ml in the deltoid and thigh muscles, and up to 5 ml in the gluteus maximus.

Intramuscular injections usually result in lower but longer lasting blood concentrations than with intravenous administration.

Part of the reason is that intramuscular injections have an absorption step which delays the time to peak concentration. Also, when a formulation is injected, a **depot** forms inside the muscle tissue where the drug is injected. Absorption from this depot is dependent on many factors such as muscle exercise, particle size of the drug, and the salt form of the drug used in the formulation.

FORMULATIONS

Drugs for intramuscular injection are formulated as:

➡ solutions;
➡ suspensions;
➡ **colloids** in aqueous and oleaginous (oil-based) solvents;
➡ oil-in-water emulsions;
➡ water-in-oil emulsions.

Colloids and suspensions both contain insoluble particles in solution, but the particles in colloids are about 100 times smaller than those in suspensions.

Emulsions are mixtures of two liquids, one aqueous and the other oleaginous, which are not miscible in each other. One liquid is dispersed through the other by using a stabilizing agent called an emulsifier.

Different salt forms of the drug may also be used to take advantage of a slower dissolution rate or a lower solubility.

So, particle size, the type of emulsion, and the salt form of the drug can all be varied to achieve the desired absorption rate. In general, aqueous solutions have a faster absorption rate than oleaginous solutions. Both have a faster absorption rate than colloids or suspensions.

 depot the area in the muscle where the formulation is injected during an intramuscular injection.

colloids particles up to a hundred times smaller than those in suspensions that are, however, likewise suspended in a solution.

INJECTION SITES

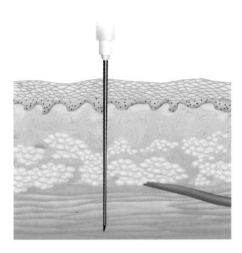

When administering intramuscular injections, it is necessary to adjust the needle size for any layers of body fat (especially in the gluteal area) and to use a size of needle that will penetrate to the muscle.

Z-Tract Injection

This is a technique used for medications that stain the skin (e.g., iron dextran injection) or irritate tissues (e.g., diazepam). The skin is pulled to one side prior to injection. Then the needle is inserted and the injection is performed. Once the needle is removed, the skin is released so that the injection points in the skin and muscle are no longer aligned. This keeps the drug from entering the subcutaneous tissue and staining or irritating the skin. A Z-track injection is generally 2 to 3 inches deep.

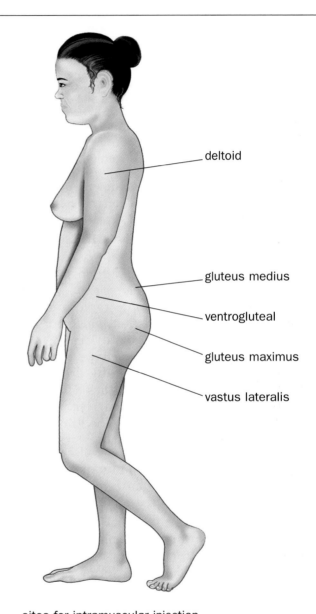

deltoid

gluteus medius

ventrogluteal

gluteus maximus

vastus lateralis

sites for intramuscular injection

 Intramuscular injections are generally more painful than intravenous injections.

SUBCUTANEOUS

The subcutaneous (SC, SQ) route is a versatile route of administration that can be used for both short term and very long term therapies. The injection of a drug or the implantation of a device beneath the surface of the skin is made in the loose tissues of the upper arm, the front of the thigh, and the lower portion of the abdomen. The upper back also can be used as a site of subcutaneous administration. The site of injection is usually rotated when injections are given frequently. The maximum amount of medication that can be subcutaneously injected is about 2 ml. Needles are generally 3/8 to 1 inch in length and 24 to 27 gauge.

Absorption of drugs from the subcutaneous tissue is influenced by the same factors that determine the rate of absorption from intramuscular sites.

However, there are fewer blood vessels in the subcutaneous tissue than in muscle, and absorption may be slower than with intramuscular administration. On the other hand, absorption after subcutaneous administration is generally more rapid and predictable than with oral administration. There are several additional ways to change the absorption rate. Using heat or massaging the site have been found to increase absorption rates of many drugs. Also, there are various co-administered drugs which have been shown to increase absorption rate. By contrast, epinephrine decreases regional blood flow, which in turn decreases the absorption rate.

Many different solution and suspension formulations are given subcutaneously, but insulin is the most common drug routinely administered by this route.

Insulin comes in many different formulations each having a characteristic rate of absorption. The rate is controlled by the same factors used for intramuscular formulations: slowly soluble salt forms, suspensions versus solutions, differences in particle size, **viscosity** (thickness) of the media, etc. Other drugs commonly administered by subcutaneous injection include heparin and enoxaparin.

In spite of the advantages of this route of administration, there are some precautions to observe.

Drugs which are irritating or in very viscous (thick) suspensions may produce serious adverse effects (including abscesses and necrosis) and be painful to the patient.

INJECTION SITES

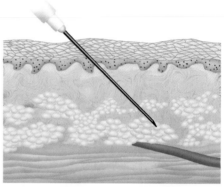

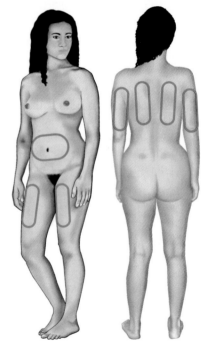

Subcutaneous injection sites are:
➤ lower abdomen;
➤ front of thigh;
➤ upper back;
➤ back of upper arm.

 viscosity the thickness of a liquid. A measure of a liquid's resistance to flow.

Intradermal injections involve small volumes that are injected into the top layer of skin.

They are used for diagnostic reasons, desensitization, or immunization. Their effects are generally local rather than systemic.

An intradermal injection forms a *wheal*, or raised blister-like area, from which the drug will slowly be absorbed into the dermis.

The dermis is the layer of the skin just beneath the epidermis. It contains more blood vessels than the epidermis but fewer than most other injection sites. As a result, absorption is gradual.

The usual site for intradermal injections is the anterior surface of the forearm.

Needles are generally 3/8 inches long and 25 to 26 gauge. The needle is inserted horizontally into the skin with the bevel facing up. The injection is made when the bevel just disappears into the skin. For this route of administration, 0.1 ml of solution is the maximum volume that can be administered.

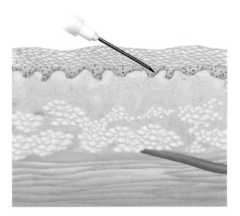

IMPLANTS

One of the most popular ways to achieve very long term drug release is to place the drug in a delivery system or device that is implanted into the body tissue. The subcutaneous tissue is the ideal tissue for implantation of such devices. Implantation generally requires a surgical procedure or a specialized injection syringe. The fact that the device will be in constant contact with the subcutaneous tissue requires that the implant materials be **biocompatible** (i.e., not irritating) and won't promote infection or sterile abscess. An advantage of the subcutaneous tissue for the site of implantation is that the device can be easily removed if necessary.

There are many devices that are used in subcutaneous implantation. Viadur™ Duros® implants are made of titanium alloy and are capable of delivering a drug for up to 1 year. Supprelin LA® implants last one year and are used to treat prostrate cancer. Implanon® releases a drug for three years and is used to prevent pregnancy. Other devices include degradable microspheres, vapor pressure devices for morphine delivery, osmotic pressure devices for insulin delivery, and magnetically activated pellets.

Sometimes ports and pumps are placed in subcutaneous tissue and an attached delivery catheter is placed in a vein, cavity, artery, or CNS system. This allows for the injection of chemotherapy agents, or antibiotics.

ABCD *biocompatibility* not irritating; does not promote infection or abscess.

wheal a raised blister-like area on the skin caused by an intradermal injection.

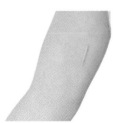

a subcutaneous implant

OPHTHALMIC FORMULATIONS

Drugs are administered to the eye for local treatment of various eye conditions and for anesthesia.

Formulations that are used include aqueous solutions, aqueous suspensions, ointments, and implants. *Every ophthalmic product must be manufactured to be sterile in its final container.* Also, because of the sensitivity of the eye, various elements of the formulation, including pH and viscosity, must be carefully controlled.

A major problem of ophthalmic administration is the immediate loss of a dose by natural spillage from the eye.

The normal volume of tears in the eye is estimated to be 7 microliters, and if blinking occurs, the eye can hold up to 10 microliters without spillage. The normal commercial eyedropper dispenses 50 microliters of solution. As a result, *about 80% of a dose will be lost from the eye by overflow.* The ideal volume of drug solution to administer would be 5 to 10 microliters. However, microliter dosing eye droppers are not generally available to patients.

Other problems include lacrimal (tear) drainage and very rapid absorption by the eyelid lining.

Tears that wash the eyeball flow from the **lacrimal gland** across the eye and drain into the **lacrimal canalicula** (tear ducts). In man, the rate of tear production is approximately 2 microliters per minute, and so the entire tear volume in the eye turns over every 2 to 3 minutes. This rapid washing and turnover accounts for loss of an ophthalmic dose in a relatively short period of time. It can also cause systemic absorption because the drug drains into the lacrimal sac and is then emptied into the gastrointestinal tract where it can be absorbed into the blood. A similar and frequently occurring problem is caused by absorption of the drug through the **conjunctiva** (eyelid lining). The drug is then rapidly carried away from the eye by the circulatory system.

 Ophthalmic administration is used to deliver a drug on the eye, into the eye, or onto the conjunctiva. Drug penetration into the eye (**transcorneal transport**) is not considered an effective process because only one-tenth of a dose penetrates into the eye.

OPHTHALMIC ADMINISTRATION

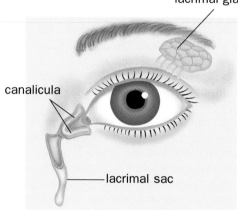

anatomy of the eye

How to Use Ophthalmic Drops

1. Wash your hands thoroughly with soap and warm water.

2. If the product container is transparent, check the solution before using it. If it is discolored or has changed in any way (e.g., particles in the solution, color change), don't use it.

3. If the product container has a depressible rubber bulb, draw up a small amount of medication into the eye dropper by first squeezing, then relieving, pressure on the bulb.

4. Tilt your head back with your chin up, and look toward the ceiling.

5. With both eyes open, gently draw down the lower lid of the affected eye with your index finger.

6. In the "gutter" formed, place one drop of the solution. Hold the drop per or administration tip as close as possible to the lid without actually touching your eye. Do not allow the dropper or administration tip to touch any surface.

7. If possible, hold your eyelid open, and don't blink for 30 seconds.

8. Press your finger against the inner corner of your eye for one minute. This will keep the medication in your eye.

9. Cap the bottle tightly.

℞ Ophthalmic ointment tubes are typically small, holding approximately 3.5 g of ointment and fitted with narrow gauge tips which permit the extrusion of a narrow ribbon of ointment.

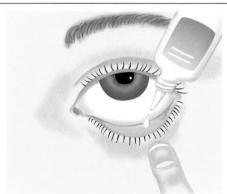
using an eye dropper

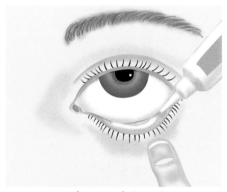
using an ointment

Tips for Using Ophthalmic Drops

➡ Keep in mind that this is a sterile solution. Contamination of the dropper or eye solution can lead to a serious eye infection.
➡ If irritation persists or increases, discontinue use immediately.
➡ Avoid eye make-up while using eye solutions.
➡ Use a mirror when applying the drops, or have someone help instill the eye drops.

Most ophthalmic solutions and suspensions are dispensed in eye dropper bottles.

Because of the unique characteristics of this route, patients must be shown how to properly instill the drops in their eyes, and every effort should be made to emphasize the need for instilling only one drop, not two or three.

To maintain longer contact between the drug and the surrounding tissue, suspensions and ointments have been developed.

Ophthalmic suspensions are aqueous based, with the drug's particle size kept to a minimum to prevent irritation of the eye. Ointments tend to keep the drug in contact with the eye longer than suspensions. Most ophthalmic ointment bases are a mixture of mineral oil and white petrolatum and have a melting point close to body temperature. But ointments tend to blur patient vision as they remain viscous and are not removed easily by the tear fluid. Therefore, ointments are generally used at night as additional therapy to eye drops used during the day.

Contact lenses and soluble inserts can be used to deliver ophthalmic dosages.

Hydrogel contact lenses are placed in a solution containing a drug such as an antibiotic, and the lenses absorb some of the drug. The lenses are then placed in the eye and the drug will be released from the lenses over a period of time. Soluble ophthalmic drug inserts are dried solutions that have been fashioned into a film or rod. These solid inserts are placed between the eyeball and the lower eyelid, and as they absorb tears, they slowly erode away. Lacrisert® is a soluble insert used in the treatment of moderate to severe dry eye syndrome.

 ophthalmic related to the eye.
lacrimal gland the gland that produces tears for the eye.
lacrimal canalicula the tear ducts.
conjunctiva the eyelid lining.
transcorneal transport drug transfer into the eye.

INTRANASAL FORMULATIONS

The adult *nasal cavity* has a capacity of about 20 ml, a very large surface area for absorption, and a very rich blood supply.

The most common drugs used for intranasal administration are used for their decongestant activity on the **nasal mucosa**, the cellular lining of the nose. Other drugs that are typically used are antihistamines and corticosteroids.

The intranasal absorption of some drugs produces blood concentrations similar to when the drug is intravenously administered.

Because of this, intranasal administration is being investigated as a possible route of administration for insulin in the treatment of diabetes mellitus and for glucagon in the treatment of hypoglycemia. Intranasal administration also serves as a possible alternate route for drugs that are seriously degraded or poorly absorbed after oral administration.

Intranasal formulations include solutions, suspensions, ointments, and gels.

Generally solutions or suspensions are administered by drops or as a fine mist from a nasal spray or aerosol container. Nasal sprays are preferred to drops because drops are more likely to drain into the back of the mouth and throat and be swallowed. Plastic squeeze bottles were commonly used to administer nasal mists but have been largely replaced by glass containers with a metered dose inhaler (MDI) actuator.

If the drug is sufficiently volatile, it can be administered in a nasal inhaler.

The **nasal inhaler** is a cylindrical tube with a cap that contains fibrous material impregnated with a volatile drug. The cap is removed and the inhaler tip is placed just inside the nostril. As the patient inhales, air is pulled through the tube and the vaporized drug is pulled into the nasal cavity.

---

nasal mucosa the cellular lining of the nose.

nasal inhaler a device which contains a drug that is vaporized by inhalation.

nasal cavity the cavity behind the nose and above the roof of the mouth that filters air and moves mucous and inhaled contaminants outward and away from the lungs.

DEVICES

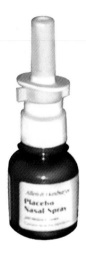

nasal spray with MDI actuator

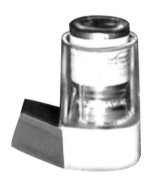

nasal aerosol

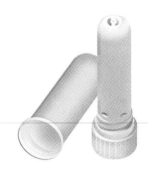

nasal inhaler

USING A NASAL SPRAY

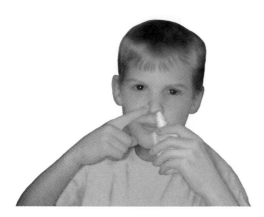

using a nasal spray

How to Use Intranasal Sprays

1. Blow your nose gently to clear the nostrils.

2. Wash your hands with soap and warm water.

3. Hold your head upright.

4. Close one nostril with one finger.

5. With the mouth closed, insert the tip of the spray into the open nostril. Breathe in through the nostril while quickly and firmly squeezing the spray container or activating the MDI actuator.

6. Hold your breath for a few seconds, and then breathe out through your mouth.

7. Repeat this procedure for the other nostril only if directed to do so.

8. Rinse the spray or MDI tip with hot water, and replace the cap tightly on the container.

9. Wash your hands.

There are three ways a dosage can be lost following nasal administration.

The nasal lining contains enzymes which can metabolize and degrade some drugs. In addition, normal mucous flow, which protects the lungs by moving mucus and inhaled contaminants away from the lungs and out of the nostril, will carry the drug with it as well. Finally, nasal administration often causes amounts of the drug to be swallowed. In some cases, enough drug will be swallowed to be equal to an oral dose. This may lead to a systemic effect from the drug even though it is intranasally administered.

Intranasal dosage forms should not be used for prolonged periods.

This may lead to chronic swelling (edema) of the nasal mucosa which aggravates the symptoms the dosage forms were intended to relieve. As a result, intranasal administration should be for short periods of time (no longer than 3 to 5 days). Patients should be advised not to exceed the recommended dosage and frequency of use.

Ways Intranasal Dosage Is Lost

✔ enzymes in the mucosa metabolize certain drugs;

✔ normal mucous flow removes drug;

✔ amounts of the drug are swallowed.

℞ **safety you should know**
Because it can lead to irritation and swelling, intranasal administration is generally kept to limited volumes for short periods of time.

INHALATION FORMULATIONS

Inhalation dosage forms are intended to deliver drugs to the pulmonary system (lungs).

The lungs have a large surface area for absorption and a rich blood supply. This route avoids the problems of degradation and poor absorption found with oral administration. However, there is enough inconsistency in the absorption of drugs from the lungs that this route is not considered an alternative to intravenous administration.

Gaseous or volatile anesthetics are the most important drugs administered via this route.

Other drugs administered affect lung function, act as bronchodilators, or treat allergic symptoms. Examples of drugs administered by this route are adrenocorticoid steroids (beclomethasone), bronchodilators (isoproterenol, metaproterenol, albuterol), and antiallergics (cromolyn sodium).

Most inhalation dosage forms are MDI aerosols that depend on the power of compressed or liquefied gas to expel the drug from a container.

Aerosols are easy to use, and have no danger of contamination. However, they are not very effective in delivering a drug to the respiratory tract. This is not due to poor aerosol design, but to the physical barriers of the airway and lungs that any inhalation dosage form must overcome to be effective.

Particle size is the critical factor with these dosage forms.

Large particles (about 20 microns) hit in the back of the mouth and throat and are eventually swallowed rather than inhaled. Particles from 1 to 10 microns reach the bronchioles. Smaller particles (0.6 micron) penetrate to the **alveolar sacs** of the lungs where absorption is rapid, but retention is limited since a large fraction of the dose is exhaled. The particles that reach the alveolar sacs and remain there are responsible for providing systemic effects. Breathing patterns and the depth of breathing also play important roles in the delivery of drugs into the lung by inhalation aerosols.

ABSORPTION

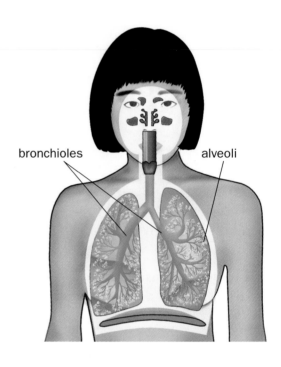

bronchioles   alveoli

For an inhalation dosage to reach the alveoli of the lungs, it has to pass through a series of twists, turns, and increasingly smaller passageways. When the drug reaches the alveoli, it will be absorbed directly into the circulatory system. Because of the difficult route from the mouth to the alveoli, varying amounts of inhaled drug are lost along the way.

ABCD *alveolar sacs (alveoli)* the small sacs of specialized tissue that transfer oxygen out of inspired air into the blood and carbon dioxide out of the blood and into the air for exhalation.

inspiration breathing in.

DEVICES

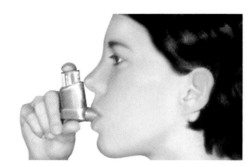

using an MDI aerosol

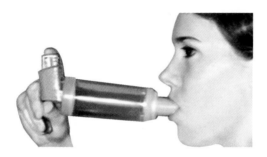

using an MDI aerosol with spacer

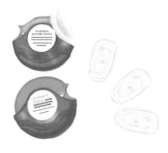

Diskus®

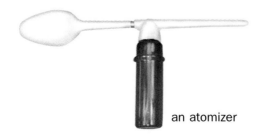

an atomizer

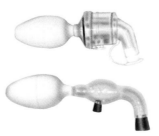

nebulizers

Metered Dose Inhaler (MDI) Aerosols

MDI aerosols used to administer drugs by inhalation have special metering valves that deliver a fixed dose when the aerosol is actuated. The amount of drug released with each actuation is regulated by a valve that has a fixed capacity or fixed dimensions.

Adapters and Spacers

Coordination is required on the part of the patient between breathing in (**inspiration**) and actuation of the aerosol. Extender devices or spacers have been developed to assist patients who cannot coordinate these two processes. The spacer goes between the aerosol's mouthpiece and the patient's mouth. The spacer allows the patient to separate actuation of the aerosol from inhalation by 3 to 5 seconds.

Dry Powder Inhalers

Some drugs are administered in powder form using a special inhalation device. The device automatically releases the drug when the user inhales. The powdered drug is supplied in hard gelatin capsules, cartridges, or disks (e.g., Diskus®) and is loaded into the inhalation device.

Atomizers and Nebulizers

Atomizers are devices which break a liquid up into a spray. One type of atomizer uses a squeeze bulb to blow air across a liquid solution causing the liquid to vaporize. As the liquid vaporizes, the air stream created by the bulb also carries the spray out of the device and into the mouth. A nebulizer contains an atomizing unit inside a chamber. When the rubber bulb is squeezed, the drug solution is drawn up the dip tube and aerosolized by the passing air stream.

DERMAL FORMULATIONS

The skin is the largest and heaviest organ in the body and accounts for about 17% of a person's weight.

It forms a barrier that protects the underlying organ systems from trauma, temperature, humidity, harmful penetrations, moisture, radiation, and micro-organisms. Dosage forms that are applied to the skin are called dermal dosage formulations.

Most dermal dosage forms are used for local effects on or within the skin.

Dermal formulations are used as protectants, lubricants, emollients, or drying agents, or as a delivery vehicle for a drug. Examples of treatments using dermal formulations include minor skin infections, itching, burns, diaper rash, insect stings and bites, athlete's foot, corns, calluses, warts, dandruff, acne, psoriasis, and eczema. Some dermal formulations promote **percutaneous absorption** (i.e., absorption through the skin).

Dermal administration has a number of advantages.

It provides an ease of administration not found in other routes, and usage by patients is generally good. It can also provide continuous drug delivery. In addition, dermal formulations can be easily removed if necessary. The major disadvantage of this route of administration is that the amount of drug that can be absorbed will be limited to about 2 mg/hour. This is often a significant limitation if the route is being considered for systemic therapy.

Basic rules of percutaneous absorption:

➡ More drug is absorbed when the formulation is applied to a larger surface area.

➡ Formulations or dressings that increase the hydration of the skin generally improve absorption.

➡ The greater the amount of rubbing in (inunction) of the formulation, the greater the absorption.

➡ The longer the formulation remains in contact with the skin, the greater will be the absorption.

---

percutaneous absorption the absorption of drugs through the skin, often for a systemic effect.

stratum corneum the outermost cell layer of the epidermis.

hydrates absorbs water.

THE SKIN

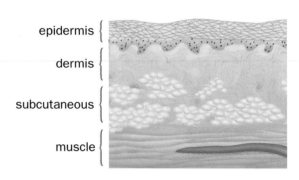

epidermis
dermis
subcutaneous
muscle

The skin is composed of three layers of tissue:

➡ epidermis;
➡ dermis;
➡ subcutaneous tissue.

The skin is generally 3–5 millimeters thick, though it is thicker in the palms and soles of the feet and thinner in the eyelids and genitals. Within the skin are several other structures: hair follicles, sebaceous glands, sweat glands, and nails.

The outer layer of epidermis is called the **stratum corneum**. In normal skin, this layer is continually replaced by new cells from underneath. The turnover time from cell development to shedding of the dead cells (sloughing) is about 21 days.

The stratum corneum is the primary barrier to drug penetration. It is about 10 micrometers thick, but can swell to approximately three times that by absorbing as much as five times its weight in water. When the stratum corneum absorbs water (**hydrates**), it becomes easier for drugs to penetrate. For that reason, certain dressings are designed to hydrate the skin. Also, some skin conditions such as eczema and psoriasis cause the stratum corneum to hydrate and increase the absorption of some drugs.

FORMULATIONS

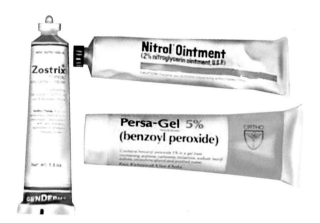

Solutions, Tinctures, Collodions, and Liniments

Dermal solutions and tinctures are generally used as anti-infective agents. Both are generally dispensed in small volumes, and should be packaged in containers that are convenient to use. Dropper bottles (glass bottles with an applicator tip) are most often used. Examples of solutions and tinctures are Coal Tar Solution, Hydrogen Peroxide, Povidone Iodine Tincture, and Compound Benzoin Tincture.

Collodions are liquid preparations of pyroxylin dissolved in a solvent mixture of alcohol and ether. Pyroxylin looks like raw cotton and is slowly but completely soluble in the solvent mixture. When applied to the skin, the solvent rapidly evaporates, leaving a protective film on the skin that contains a thin layer of the drug. Liniments are alcoholic or oleaginous solutions generally applied by rubbing.

Ointments, Creams, Gels, and Lotions

Ointments, creams, gels, and lotions are the most popular dermal formulations. Physically, they appear to be very similar in consistency and texture, but there are differences. Ointments have drugs that have been incorporated into a base. There are several different types of bases ranging from petrolatum to polyethylene glycols. Creams are semisolid emulsions, and are less viscous and softer in texture than ointments. Creams have an added feature in that they "vanish" or disappear with rubbing. Gels are dispersions of solid drugs in a jelly-like vehicle. Lotions are suspensions of solid drugs in an aqueous vehicle.

Pastes, Plasters, and Powders

Pastes are generally used for their protective action and for their ability to absorb secretions from skin lesions. Pastes contain more solid material than ointments, and are stiffer and less penetrating. Plasters are solid or semisolid adhesive masses that are spread on a suitable backing material. They provide prolonged contact at the site of application. Some of the common backing materials used are paper, cotton, felt, linen, muslin, silk, and moleskin. The backing is cut into different shapes appropriate to cover the affected area. Medicinal powders are a mixture of drug and an inert (inactive) base such as talcum or corn starch. Powders have different dusting and covering capability.

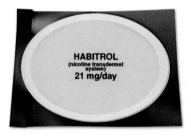

Transdermal Patches, Tapes, and Gauzes

Transdermal systems (patches, tapes, and gauzes) *deliver drugs through the skin for a systemic effect.* The systems can be divided into two kinds: those that control the rate of drug delivery to the skin, and those that allow the skin to control the rate of drug absorption. The first type is for potent drugs that must have their absorption rate controlled by a device. The second type is for less potent drugs. The largest problems with transdermal patches are skin sensitivity experienced by some patients, and technical difficulties associated with the adhesiveness of the systems to different skin types and under various conditions.

Aerosols

Dermal aerosols are generally used to apply anesthetic and antibiotic dosages for local effect.

VAGINAL FORMULATIONS

Vaginal administration has many of the same characteristics found with other parenteral routes of administration.

It avoids the degradation that occurs with oral administration; doses can be retrieved if necessary; and it has the potential of providing long term drug absorption. However, vaginal administration leads to variable absorption since the vagina is a physiologically and anatomically dynamic organ with pH and absorption characteristics changing over relatively short periods of time. Another disadvantage of this route is that administration of a formulation during menstruation could predispose the patient to Toxic Shock Syndrome. There is also a tendency of some dosage forms to be expelled after insertion into the vagina.

Formulations for this route of administration are solutions, powders for solutions, ointments, creams, aerosol foams, suppositories, tablets, and IUDs.

Powders are used to prepare solutions for vaginal douches utilized to cleanse the vagina. The powder is supplied either as bulk or unit dose packages and is dissolved in a prescribed amount of water prior to use. Most douche powders are used for their hygienic effects, but a few contain antibiotics.

 intrauterine device (IUD) an intrauterine contraceptive device that is placed in the uterus for a prolonged period of time.

contraceptive device or formulation designed to prevent pregnancy.

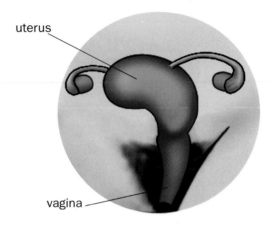

The Vagina

The vagina is a cylinder-like organ that leads from the cervix and uterus to an external opening. It is used for intercourse, releasing menstrual fluids, and is the lower portion of the birth canal.

Toxic Shock Syndrome (TSS)

Toxic Shock Syndrome is a rare and potentially fatal disease that results from a severe bacterial infection of the blood. In women, it can be caused when bacteria natural to the vagina move into the bloodstream. Though primarily associated with the use of superabsorbency tampons, it has also been associated with various vaginal dosage forms. TSS symptoms include a high fever, nausea, skin rash, faintness, and muscle ache. It is treated with antibiotics and other medicines.

FORMULATIONS

Tablets (Inserts)

Vaginal tablets, also called inserts, have the same activity and are inserted in the same manner as vaginal suppositories. Patients should be instructed to dip the tablet into water before insertion. Also, because tablets are generally used at bedtime and can be messy if the formulation is an oleaginous base, it should be recommended to patients that they wear a sanitary napkin to protect nightwear and bed linens. These same instructions should be given to patients receiving vaginal suppositories.

Ointments, Creams, and Aerosol Foams

Vaginal ointments, creams, and aerosol foams typically contain antibiotics, estrogenic hormonal substances, or contraceptive agents.

Creams and foams are placed in a special applicator tube, and the tube is then inserted high in the vaginal tract. The applicator plunger is depressed to deposit the formulation.

Suppositories

Vaginal suppositories are used as **contraceptives**, feminine hygiene antiseptics, bacterial antibiotics, or to restore the vaginal mucosa. They are inserted high in the vaginal tract with the aid of a special applicator. The suppositories are usually globe, egg, or cone-shaped and weigh about five grams.

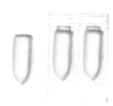

Suppositories are made from a variety of bases. Glycerinated gelatin (70% glycerin, 20% gelatin, 10% water) suppositories are translucent, resilient, and have a soft, rubbery texture. They are the preferred base for vaginal suppositories because they slowly dissolve over about 30 minutes into the vaginal mucous secretions giving a prolonged local effect of the drug. These suppositories require refrigeration.

Polyethylene glycol suppositories also dissolve in vaginal mucous secretions, but do so faster than glycerinated gelatin suppositories. These suppositories can be formulated so that refrigeration is not required.

Intrauterine Devices (IUDs)

Vaginal administration gives the opportunity for long term administration. This potential has been explored in the area of contraception protection using intrauterine devices (IUDs).

Precursors to present day IUDs were first mentioned in scientific literature in the early 1900's. Many of the early prototypes were made of stainless steel and produced high rates of infection and high failure rates. The first plastic T-shaped IUDs were available in the 1970s. These devices had a lower rate of vaginal expulsion due to their similarity to the uterine shape. They also had higher surface areas of copper and were effective at a rate of greater than 99%. ParaGard® is an IUD that has been shown to be effective for up to 12 years.

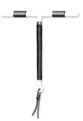

Another category of IUDs are based on the release of the hormone progesterone. Progestasert® was the first hormonal uterine device. It was developed in 1976 and manufactured until 2001. It released an average of 60 micrograms of progesterone per day and had a failure rate of 2% per year.

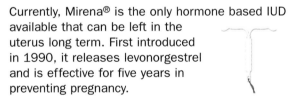

Currently, Mirena® is the only hormone based IUD available that can be left in the uterus long term. First introduced in 1990, it releases levonorgestrel and is effective for five years in preventing pregnancy.

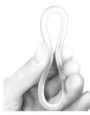

The vaginal ring is also a hormone based IUD, but is used in one month cycles. The ring is inserted in the vagina for 3 weeks, removed for 7 days, and then reinserted. NuvaRing® is an example of such a device.

REVIEW

KEY CONCEPTS

ROUTES AND FORMULATIONS

✔ The way in which the body absorbs and distributes drugs varies with the route of administration and the dosage form used.

✔ Enteral refers to anything involving the alimentary tract from the mouth to the rectum. There are four enteral routes: oral, sublingual, buccal, and rectal.

✔ Parenteral refers to anything next to or beside the enteral route. Some parenteral routes use formulations that are injected. Other parenteral formulations do not require injection.

✔ A local effect occurs when the drug activity is at the site of administration (e.g., eyes, ears, nose, skin).

✔ A systemic effect occurs when the drug is introduced into the circulatory system and carried to the site of activity.

ENTERAL ROUTES AND FORMULATIONS

✔ Oral administration means the dosage form is to be swallowed.

✔ Drugs administered in liquid dosage forms generally reach the circulatory system faster than drugs formulated in solid dosage forms.

✔ The primary goal of modified release dosage forms is to reduce the number of doses a patient must take per day.

✔ The mouth has two enteral routes of administration: sublingual (under the tongue) and buccal (in the cheek pouch).

✔ Rectal administration is used for both systemic and local effects. Suppositories, ointments, and solutions are common dosage forms.

PARENTERAL ROUTES AND FORMULATIONS

✔ Some parenteral routes requiring injection for administration are intravenous, intramuscular, intradermal, and subcutaneous. Intravenous solutions must be sterile (bacteria-free), have an appropriate pH, and be free of particulate material.

✔ Intramuscular injections generally result in lower but longer lasting blood concentrations than with intravenous administration.

✔ The subcutaneous (SC, SQ) route can be used for both short term and very long term therapies. Insulin is the most important drug routinely administered by this route.

✔ Intradermal administration is used for diagnostics, desensitization, and immunization.

✔ Ophthalmic administration can lead to a significant loss of the dose due to spillage and drainage.

✔ Intranasal administration of some drugs produce blood concentrations similar to when the drug is intravenously administered.

✔ Inhalation dosage forms deliver drugs to the lungs. MDI aerosols, dry powder inhalers, and nebulizers are common devices used to administer drugs through this route.

✔ Dermal formulations vary from gels and lotions to aerosols, ointments, and pastes. Transdermal patches are also common dosage forms.

✔ Vaginal dosage forms (e.g., suppositories, tablets, solutions) are most often used for local effect. However, long term systemic effects can be achieved with IUDs.

SELF TEST

MATCH THE TERMS: I   *the answer key begins on page 511*

1. alveolar sacs (alveoli) ____

2. aqueous ____

3. biocompatibility ____

4. buccal ____

5. buffer system ____

6. colloids ____

7. conjunctiva ____

8. contraceptive ____

9. depot ____

10. diluent ____

11. disintegration ____

12. dissolution ____

13. emulsions ____

14. hemorrhoid ____

15. hydrates ____

16. injectability ____

17. inspiration ____

18. intrauterine device (IUD) ____

19. lacrimal canalicula ____

20. lacrimal gland ____

21. local effect ____

22. nasal cavity ____

23. nasal inhaler ____

24. nasal mucosa ____

a. absorbs water.

b. ingredients in a formulation designed to control the pH.

c. mixture of two non-miscible liquids where one is dispersed throughout the other as tiny droplets.

d. water based.

e. when drug activity is at the site of administration.

f. pouch between the teeth and cheek in the mouth.

g. painful swollen veins in the anal/rectal area, generally caused by strained bowel movements from hard stools.

h. a solvent that dissolves a freeze-dried powder or dilutes a solution.

i. the ease of flow when a suspension is injected into a patient.

j. the area in the muscle where the formulation is injected during an intramuscular injection.

k. particles up to a hundred times smaller than those in suspensions that are, however, also suspended in a solution.

l. not irritating; does not promote infection or abscess.

m. the gland that produces tears for the eye.

n. the tear ducts.

o. the eyelid lining.

p. the small sacs of specialized tissue that transfer oxygen out of inspired air into the blood and carbon dioxide out of the blood and into the air for exhalation.

q. breathing in.

r. an intrauterine contraceptive device that is placed in the uterus for a prolonged period of time.

s. device or formulation designed to prevent pregnancy.

t. the cavity behind the nose and above the roof of the mouth that filters air and moves mucous and inhaled contaminants outward and away from the lungs.

u. a device which contains a drug that is vaporized by inhalation.

v. the cellular lining of the nose.

w. the breaking apart of a tablet into smaller pieces.

x. when the smaller pieces of a disintegrated tablet dissolve in solution.

REVIEW

MATCH THE TERMS: II   *the answer key begins on page 511*

1. necrosis ____

2. ophthalmic ____

3. percutaneous absorption ____

4. pH ____

5. sterile ____

6. stratum corneum ____

7. sublingual ____

8. syringeability ____

9. systemic effect ____

10. transcorneal transport ____

11. viscosity ____

12. water soluble ____

13. wheal ____

a. a condition which is free of all microorganisms.

b. the absorption of drugs through the skin, often for a systemic effect.

c. related to the eye.

d. a measure of a liquid's thickness or resistance to flow.

e. under the tongue.

f. when a drug is introduced into the circulatory system and carried to the site of activity.

g. measures the acidity or the opposite (alkalinity) of a substance.

h. the ease with which a suspension can be drawn from a container into a syringe.

i. a raised blister-like area on the skin caused by an intradermal injection.

j. drug transfer into the eye.

k. the outermost cell layer of the epidermis.

l. the property of a substance being able to dissolve in water.

m. increase in cell death.

CHOOSE THE BEST ANSWER   *the answer key begins on page 511*

1. Which route of administration is not an enteral route?
   a. rectal
   b. inhalation
   c. buccal
   d. sublingual

2. Which of the following routes is least likely to give a systemic effect?
   a. oral
   b. sublingual
   c. rectal
   d. intradermal

3. Within the alimentary tract, pHs of 5–7 are typically found in the
   a. stomach.
   b. large intestine.
   c. small intestine.
   d. mouth.

4. A dissolution step would not be necessary for drug absorption from a/an
   a. capsule.
   b. intramuscular suspension.
   c. intravenous solution.
   d. suppository.

5. Modified release tablets might be called
   a. extended release.
   b. prolonged action.
   c. long acting.
   d. all of the above.

6. Nonaqueous solutions often contain glycerin, alcohol, and
   a. polyethylene glycol.
   b. polyvinyl alcohol.
   c. propylene glycol.
   d. chloroform.

7. A gel
   a. is two non-mixable components and an emulsifier.
   b. is a network of interlacing particles.
   c. has undissolved drug in a solvent.
   d. is a saturated solution of sucrose.

8. The best known example of a drug given by sublingual administration is
   a. nifedipine.
   b. nitroglycerin.
   c. digoxin.
   d. diltiazem.

9. Which parenteral route of administration would typically use the longest needle with the smallest gauge?
   a. intravenous
   b. intramuscular
   c. subcutaneous
   d. intradermal

10. Which intravenous dosage form requires the technician to consider syringeability and injectability?
    a. emulsions
    b. gels
    c. solutions
    d. suspensions

11. Which will not be caused by particulate material in an intravenous injection?
    a. air emboli
    b. thrombus
    c. phlebitis
    d. blood clots

12. Which is not used to administer a drug by parenteral route?
    a. syringe
    b. elastomeric pump
    c. infusion pump
    d. none of the above

13. _____ injections are administered into the top layer of the skin at a slight angle using short needles.
    a. Intraarterial
    b. Transcorneal
    c. Subcutaneous
    d. Intradermal

14. A raised blister-like area on the skin caused from an intradermal injection is called a
    a. thrombus.
    b. pachyderma.
    c. wheal.
    d. phlebitis.

Match questions 15–18 with the following key:
    a. deltoid
    b. 0.1 ml
    c. 20 seconds
    d. implants

15. Intravenous administration _____

16. Intramuscular administration _____

17. Intradermal administration _____

18. Subcutaneous administration _____

REVIEW

19. Which ophthalmic formulation will maintain the drug in contact with the eye the longest?
    a. solution
    b. suspension
    c. gel
    d. ointment

20. When administering ophthalmic drops, why is instilling two drops at a time not recommended?
    a. The eye only holds about 10 microliters.
    b. The second drop will be lost due to spillage.
    c. The average drop size is 50 microliters.
    d. The second drop will cause corneal abrasion.

21. What percent of an administered ophthalmic solution is actually delivered to the eye?
    a. 5%
    b. 20%
    c. 50%
    d. 75%

22. When administering a nasal spray,
    a. lay on the bed with the head hanging over the edge.
    b. keep both nostrils open.
    c. breathe through the nostril while spraying the solution.
    d. exhale immediately.

23. A drug is administered by inhalation using a metered dose inhaler (MDI) aerosol. Which pathway will the drug follow?
    a. mouth, trachea, alveoli, bronchioles
    b. mouth, bronchioles, trachea, alveoli
    c. mouth, trachea, bronchioles, alveoli
    d. bronchioles, alveoli, nasal cavity, trachea

24. Which device would be used to administer a volatile drug intranasally?
    a. nasal solution as a drop
    b. nasal inhaler
    c. plastic squeeze bottle
    d. nasal MDI aerosol

25. A spacer with an MDI aerosol will
    a. help coordinate actuation and inspiration.
    b. increase expiration.
    c. act as a nebulization chamber.
    d. also fit on dry powder inhalers.

26. Which layer of skin contains the stratum corneum?
    a. dermis
    b. muscle
    c. epidermis
    d. subcutaneous

27. Which dermal formulation is a base with drug incorporated into it?
    a. ointment
    b. cream
    c. gel
    d. lotion

28. Plasters are generally used with the _____ route of administration.
    a. dermal
    b. rectal
    c. intranasal
    d. vaginal

29. The primary reason to use a vaginal applicator is to
    a. prevent a "mess" during application.
    b. prevent patients from using oral tablets by the route.
    c. place the formulation high in the vaginal tract.
    d. enable patients to retrieve the formulation if needed.

PARENTERALS: STERILE FORMULATIONS

LEARNING OBJECTIVES

At the completion of study, the student will:

➥ describe the differences between LVP and SVP solutions, and explain the purpose of common specialty parenteral solutions.

➥ explain the importance of using laminar flow hoods and aseptic techniques in compounding parenteral solutions.

➥ describe the use of administration sets and positive pressure pumps to administer parenteral solutions to patients.

➥ list and explain the factors that affect incompatibilities in parenteral solutions.

➥ discuss the purposes of the following aspects of a quality assurance program: inspection of compounded products, disposal of drugs and supplies, environmental quality assessment, and infection control.

➥ compare and contrast the units of measurement that are unique to parenteral solutions.

CHAPTER OUTLINE

PARENTERALS: STERILE FORMULATIONS

There are special requirements for how parenteral products are made, packaged, and how they are administered.

Most parenteral formulations are required to be sterile, meaning that the formulation is free from bacteria and other microorganisms. Sterility is not a relative term: the formulation is either sterile or nonsterile. This applies to the injectable formulations given by the intravenous, intramuscular, subcutaneous, and intradermal routes of administration. Dosage forms used for ophthalmic (e.g., intraocular), intranasal, and inhalation administration are also required to be sterile. Only dermal and vaginal formulations are not required to be sterile.

Sterility is required because these formulations have rapid access to the circulatory system and can cause a patient the greatest harm if an infection develops.

In addition to being a sterile dosage form, many parenteral formulations must also be free from particulate material, pyrogen-free, isotonic, and at physiological pH.

These requirements are met by the manufacturer of a sterile parenteral dosage form.

They produce sterile formulations that are ready for immediate use. However, it is not practical for a manufacturer to supply all of the many different sterile dosage forms used in a pharmacy practice. Many manufacturers' formulations are modified in the pharmacy by technicians, under the authorization of a pharmacist. These modified formulations must still be sterile, pyrogen-free, etc.

This chapter will highlight how many types of sterile solution formulations are manipulated in a pharmacy setting.

These manipulations generally occur in a laminar flow hood or biological safety cabinet, and require that the operator use **aseptic techniques.** The most common sterile solutions manipulated can be classified as large volume parenterals (LVP), small volume parenterals (SVP), total parenteral nutrition (TPN) solutions, dialysis solutions, and irrigation solutions.

SPECIAL PRECAUTIONS

There are a number of special considerations and precautions that must be taken with parenteral dosage forms.

✔ **Solutions must be sterile—i.e., free from bacteria and other microorganisms.**

Techniques that maintain sterile conditions and prevent contamination must be followed. These are called **aseptic techniques.**

✔ **Solutions must be free of all visible particulate material.**

Examples of such contaminants are glass, rubber cores from vial closures, cloth or cotton fibers, metal, and plastic. Undissolved particles of an active drug will be present in intravenous suspensions, but no contaminants should be present.

✔ **Solutions must be pyrogen-free.**

Intravenous solutions can cause pyretic (fever) reactions if they contain pyrogens. **Pyrogens** are chemicals that are produced by microorganisms. They are soluble in water and are not removed by sterilizing or filtering the solution.

✔ **The solution must be stable for its intended use.**

Most admixtures are prepared hours in advance of when they are to be administered. So the stability of a particular drug in a particular intravenous solution must be considered in the admixture preparation. This information is generally available in a number of reference sources.

✔ **The pH of an intravenous solution should not vary significantly from physiological pH, about 7.4.**

Sometimes, other factors may be more important, such as when acidic or alkaline solutions are needed to increase drug solubility or used as a therapeutic treatment themselves.

✔ **Intravenous solutions should be formulated to have an osmotic pressure similar to that of blood.**

Osmotic pressure is the characteristic of a solution determined by the number of dissolved particles in it. Osmolarity is a unit of measure of osmotic pressure and is expressed in terms of osmoles (Osmol) or milliosmoles (mOsmol) per liter.

Blood has an osmolarity of approximately 300 mOsmol per liter. Both 0.9% sodium chloride solution and 5% dextrose solution have a similar osmolarity. When a solution has an osmolarity equivalent to that of blood, it is called **isotonic.**

Intravenous solutions that have greater osmolarity than blood are called **hypertonic**, and those with lower osmolarity, **hypotonic.** Both hypertonic and hypotonic solutions may cause damage to red blood cells, pain, and tissue irritation. However, it is at times necessary to administer such solutions. In these cases, the solutions are usually given slowly through large, free flowing veins to minimize the reactions.

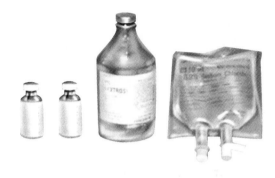

Which parenteral?

Besides meaning any route of administration other than enteral, "parenteral" is commonly used to describe dosage forms administered through syringes or administration sets. It is also used to describe the various bottles, vials, and bags used in preparing and delivering solutions for intravenous administration. It is possible to say that parenterals are prepared and parenterally administered at parenteral sites. As a result, extreme care must be taken when using the word "parenteral" so that the intended meaning is clear to all.

ABCD *aseptic techniques* techniques or methods that maintain the sterile condition of products.

pyrogens chemicals produced by microorganisms that can cause pyretic (fever) reactions in patients.

osmotic pressure a characteristic of a solution determined by the number of dissolved particles in it.

isotonic when a solution has an osmolarity equivalent to that of blood.

hypertonic when a solution has a greater osmolarity than that of blood.

hypotonic when a solution has a lesser osmolarity than that of blood.

LVP SOLUTIONS

Large volume parenteral (LVP) solutions are intravenous solutions packaged in containers holding 100 ml or more.

Common uses of LVP solutions without additives include correction of electrolyte and fluid balance disturbances, nutrition, and vehicles for administering other drugs. The most common sizes are 100, 250, 500, and 1,000 ml. There are three types of containers: glass bottle with an air vent tube, glass bottle without an air vent tube, and plastic bags. The top of the LVP solution container is hung on an administration pole. At the other end of the container are two ports of about the same length. One is the administration set port, and the other is the medication port. Graduation marks to indicate the volume of solution in the container are on its front. They are marked at 25 ml to 100 ml intervals depending on the overall size of the container.

The administration set port has a plastic cover on it to maintain the sterility of the bag.

The cover is easily removed. Solution will not drip out of the bag through this port because of a plastic diaphragm inside the port. When the spike of the administration set is inserted into the port, the diaphragm is punctured, and the solution will flow out of the bag into the administration set. This inner diaphragm cannot be resealed once punctured.

The medication port is covered by a protective rubber tip.

Drugs are added to the LVP solution through this port using a needle and syringe. There is an inner plastic diaphragm about one half inch inside the port, just like the administration set port. This inner diaphragm is also not self-sealing when punctured by a needle, but the protective rubber tip prevents solutions from leaking from the bag once the diaphragm is punctured.

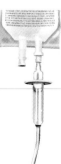

an LVP administration port

REGULATORY REQUIREMENTS FOR PARENTERALS

The United States Pharmacopeia (USP) and the Food and Drug Administration (FDA) provide regulations and guidelines for the manufacture, compounding, dispensing, and distribution of drug products in the United States.

In 2009, a chapter of USP (<797>) titled, "Pharmaceutical Compounding—Sterile Preparations" established requirements for the aseptic preparation of sterile dosage forms. The standards apply to health care institutions, pharmacies, physician practice facilities, and other facilities in which **compounded sterile preparations (CSPs)** are prepared, stored, and dispensed.

A CSP was defined as follows:

➡ Preparations prepared according to the manufacturer's labeled instructions and other manipulations when manufacturing sterile products that expose the original contents to potential contamination.

➡ Preparations containing nonsterile ingredients or employing nonsterile components and devices that must be sterilized before administration.

➡ Biologics, diagnostics, drugs, nutrients, and radiopharmaceuticals that possess either of the above two characteristics, and which include, but are not limited to, baths and soaks for live organs and tissues, implants, inhalations, injections, powders for injection, irrigations, metered sprays, and ophthalmic and otic preparations.

Plastic bags have advantages not found with glass bottles.

They do not break. They weigh less. They take up less storage space, and they take up much less disposal space. The plastic bag system is not vented to outside air. It collapses as the solution is administered, so a vacuum is not created inside.

Some drugs and solutions may not be used with plastic because they interact with it.

In these cases, glass IV bottles are used. They are packaged with a vacuum, sealed by a solid rubber closure, and the closure is held in place by an aluminum band. Graduation marks are along the sides of the bottle and are usually spaced every 25 ml to 50 ml. The solution bottle is hung on an administration pole in an inverted position using the aluminum or plastic band on the bottom of the bottle. Nitroglycerin and amiodarone are examples of dosage solutions dispensed in glass bottles.

Solutions flow from the glass containers to the patient through a special administration set.

For solutions to flow out of a glass container, air must be able to enter the container to relieve the vacuum as the solution leaves. Some bottles have air tubes built into the rubber closure for this. Some bottles do not, in which case a special administration set with a filtered airway in the spike must be used.

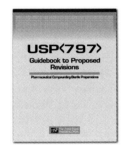

The intent of Chapter <797> is to "prevent harm and fatality that could result from microbial contamination (nonsterility), excessive bacterial endotoxins, large content errors in the strength of correct ingredients, and incorrect ingredients in compounded sterile products (CSPs)."

Chapter <797> provides guidelines for the development and implementation of essential policies and procedures for the safe preparation of CSPs. It states that policies and procedures developed by pharmacies must provide for: cleaner facilities (compared to nonsterile compounding); air quality evaluation and maintenance; and specific training and testing of personnel in aseptic manipulation, sterilization, and solution stability principles and practices.

The level of involvement of the pharmacy technician in developing and implementing these procedures will vary from institution to institution and practice to practice. However, all personnel who prepare CSPs must understand these fundamental practices and precautions.

Common LVP Solutions

Many intravenous solutions are commercially available. Four common solutions used either as LVP solutions or as the primary part of an admixture solution are:

➡ sodium chloride solution;
➡ dextrose solution;
➡ Ringer's solution;
➡ Lactated Ringer's solution.

Various combinations of different strengths of sodium chloride and dextrose solutions are also available, e.g., 5% dextrose and 0.45% sodium chloride, or 5% dextrose and 0.225% sodium chloride.

 compounded sterile preparation (CSP) a compounded sterile parenteral dosage form that will be parenterally administered.

SVP SOLUTIONS

Small volume parenteral (SVP) solutions are packaged products that are either directly administered to a patient or added to another parenteral formulation.

When a drug is added to a parenteral solution, the drug is referred to as the **additive**, and the final mixture is referred to as the **admixture**. SVP solutions are supplied in prefilled syringes, ampules, glass or plastic vials sealed with a rubber closure, or plastic minibags. Powdered drugs are supplied in vials that must be reconstituted (dissolved in a suitable solvent) before being added to the intravenous solution.

Ampules are elongated sealed glass containers with a neck that must be snapped off.

Most ampules are weakened around the base of the neck for easy breaking. These will have a colored band around the base of the neck. Some ampules, however, must first be scored and weakened with a file or the top may shatter. Once an ampule is opened, it becomes an open-system container.

Minibags are made of the same plastic materials as LVPs and contain the same types of solutions found in LVPs.

Minibags are just smaller in size since they contain only 50–100 ml of solution.

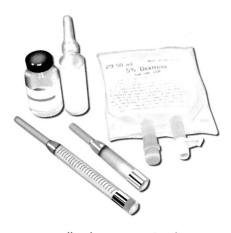

small volume parenterals

additive a drug that is added to a parenteral solution.

admixture the resulting solution when a drug is added to a parenteral solution.

ADDING SVPs TO LVPs

Generally the LVP solution is used as a continuous infusion because of its large volume and slow infusion rate. SVP solutions can be introduced into the on-going LVP infusion by injecting the SVP into the medication port of the container or the volume control chamber of the administration set. However, most often the SVP is put into a minibag and used as a piggyback on the LVP.

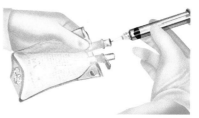

Using a Needle and Syringe to Add a SVP to a LVP:

1. Assemble the needle and syringe.

2. If the drug in the SVP is in powder form, reconstitute it with the recommended diluent.

3. Swab the SVP and medication port of the LVP with an alcohol swab.

4. Draw the necessary volume of drug solution into the syringe from the SVP.

5. Insert the needle into the medication port and through the inner diaphragm. The medication port should be fully extended to minimize the chance of going through the side of the port.

6. Inject the SVP solution into the LVP.

7. Remove the needle from the LVP.

8. Shake and inspect the admixture.

Note: This procedure will be done in a laminar flow hood.

READY-TO-MIX SYSTEMS

Ready-to-mix systems consist of a specially designed minibag with an adapter for attaching a drug vial. The admixing takes place just prior to administration. The major advantages of ready-to-mix systems include a significant reduction in waste and lower potential for medication error because the drug vial remains attached to the minibag and can be re-checked if necessary. However, the systems do cost more, and there is the potential that the system will not be properly activated so that the patient receives only the diluent or a partial dose.

Some ready-to-mix systems are: Add-Vantage®; Add-a-Vial®; Mini-Bag Plus®; and CRIS® Controlled Release Infusion System.

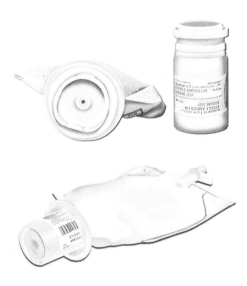

the Add-Vantage® system before and after mixing

Drugs and other additives can be packaged in glass or plastic vials.

The drugs or other additives may be either in liquid form or as **lyophilized** (freeze dried) powders. Powders must be reconstituted with a suitable solvent (**diluent**) before use. Vials have a rubber stopper through which a needle is inserted to withdraw or add to the contents. Before withdrawing solution from a vial, an equal volume of air is usually drawn up in the syringe and injected into the vial. This pressurizes the vial and helps in withdrawing solution from the vial. Some medications are packaged under pressure or can produce gas (and pressure) upon reconstitution. In such cases, air is not injected into the vial before withdrawing the solution.

Vials may be prepared for single or multidose use.

Single dose vials do not contain preservatives and should be discarded after one use. Multidose vials contain a preservative to inhibit bacterial contamination once the vial has been used. Also, the rubber closure will reseal on a multidose vial. These vials can be used for a number of doses of variable volume.

There are two varieties of prefilled syringes.

One type, a cartridge type package, is a single syringe and needle unit which is to be placed in a special holder before use. Once the syringe and needle unit is used, it is discarded but the holder can be used again with a new unit. Another type of prefilled syringe consists of a glass tube closed at both ends with rubber stoppers. The prefilled tube is placed into a specially designed syringe that has a needle attached to it. After using this type of prefilled syringe, all of the pieces are discarded.

 ready-to-mix a specially designed minibag where a drug is put into the SVP just prior to administration.

lyophilized freeze-dried.

diluent a solvent that dissolves a lyophilized powder or dilutes a solution.

SPECIAL SOLUTIONS

TOTAL PARENTERAL NUTRITION SOLUTIONS

Total parenteral nutrition (TPN) solutions are complex admixtures used to provide nutritional support to patients who are unable to take in adequate nutrients through their digestive tract. These admixtures are composed of dextrose, fat, protein, electrolytes, vitamins, and trace elements. They are hypertonic solutions.

Base parenteral nutrition solutions are available in 2,000 and 3,000 ml sizes. The base solution consists of:

➡ an amino acid solution (for protein);
➡ a dextrose solution (for carbohydrate calories).

These solutions, sometimes referred to as macronutrients, make up most of the volume of a parenteral nutrition solution. Several electrolytes, trace elements, and multiple vitamins (together referred to as micronutrients) may be added to the base solution to meet individual patient requirements. Common electrolyte additives include sodium chloride (or acetate), potassium chloride (or acetate), calcium gluconate, magnesium sulfate, and sodium (or potassium) phosphate. Multiple vitamin preparations containing both water soluble and fat soluble vitamins are usually added on a daily basis. A trace element product containing zinc, copper, manganese, selenium, and chromium may be added.

Intravenous fat (lipid) emulsion can be added as a source of essential fatty acids and a concentrated source of calories. Fat provides nine calories per gram, compared to 3.4 calories per gram provided by dextrose. Intravenous fat emulsion may be admixed into the total parenteral nutrition solution or piggybacked into the administration line. When intravenous fat emulsion is admixed with a TPN solution, the resulting solution is referred to as a **total nutrient admixture (TNA)**.

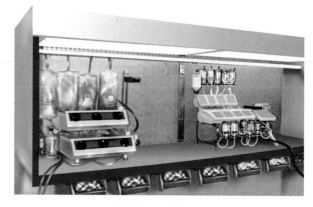

TPN Preparation Systems

Due to the complexity and time needed to prepare TPN solutions, pharmacies use high-speed compounders, automixers, or micromixers. These machines can deliver from two to ten different components safely, accurately, and quickly.

TPN Administration

TPN solutions are generally (though not always) administered via the subclavian vein under the collar bone over 8 to 24 hours. Slow administration using this vein minimizes the adverse effects that may occur with such a hypertonic solution. The subclavian vein is large and close to the heart, so the solution is diluted rapidly by the large volume of blood in the heart.

To assure their accurate delivery, nutrition solutions are almost always administered with an intravenous infusion pump. Parenteral nutrition solutions are commonly administered through an in-line filter in the administration set positioned as close to the patient as possible. However, intravenous fat emulsion, either alone or as part of a TNA solution, can be administered through an in-line filter only if it has a pore size of 1.2 micron or larger. An alternative is to piggyback the intravenous fat emulsion into the administration set below the in-line filter.

total parenteral nutrition (TPN) solution complex solutions with two base solutions (amino acids and dextrose) and additional micro-nutrients.

total nutrient admixture (TNA) solution a TPN solution that contains intravenous fat emulsion.

peritoneal dialysis solution a solution placed in and emptied from the peritoneal cavity to remove toxic substances.

irrigation solution large volume splash solutions used during surgical or urologic procedures to bathe and moisten body tissues.

DIALYSIS SOLUTIONS

Dialysis refers to the passage of small particles through membranes. This is caused by **osmosis,** the action in which a drug in a solution of a higher concentration will move through a permeable membrane (one that can be penetrated) to a solution of a lower concentration. This principle is the basis for another type of special solution.

Peritoneal dialysis solutions are used by patients who have compromised kidney function. The solution is administered directly into the peritoneal cavity (the cavity between the abdominal lining and the internal organs) to remove toxic substances, excess body waste, and serum electrolytes through osmosis. *These solutions are hypertonic to blood so the water will not move into the circulatory system. But the toxic substances will move into the dialysis solution.*

Peritoneal solutions are administered several times a day. The solution is permitted to flow into the abdominal cavity, and then remains in the cavity for 30 to 90 minutes. It is then drained by a siphon tube into discharge bottles. This procedure is repeated many times a day and may use up to 50 liters of solution. For this reason, peritoneal dialysis solutions are supplied in containers that are 2,000 ml or larger in capacity.

IRRIGATION SOLUTIONS

Irrigation solutions are not administered directly into the venous system but are subject to the same stringent controls as intravenous fluids. They are packaged in containers that are larger than 1,000 ml capacity and are designed to empty rapidly.

Surgical irrigation solutions (splash solutions) are used to:

➡ bathe and moisten body tissues;

➡ moisten dressings;

➡ wash instruments.

They are typically Sodium Chloride for Irrigation or Sterile Water for Irrigation.

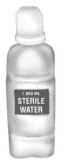

Urological irrigation solutions are used during operations to:

➡ maintain tissue integrity;

➡ remove blood to maintain a clear field of vision.

Glycine 1.5% Irrigation and Sorbitol 3% Irrigation solutions are commonly used because they are non-hemolytic (i.e., do not damage blood cells).

 osmosis the action in which a drug in a higher concentration solution passes through a permeable membrane to a lower concentration solution.

dialysis movement of particles in a solution through permeable membranes.

LAMINAR FLOW HOODS

Microorganisms invisible to the eye are present in dust and particulate matter in natural air and on most surfaces, even those that appear clean.

Unless aseptic techniques are used to prepare parenteral solutions, contamination can easily occur from the environment in which the product is being prepared or from the person preparing it.

The best way to reduce the environmental risk is to use a laminar flow hood which establishes and maintains an ultraclean work area.

Room air is drawn into a laminar hood and passed through a prefilter to remove relatively large contaminants such as dust and lint. The air is then channeled through a high efficiency particulate air (**HEPA**) filter that removes particles larger than 0.5 μm (microns).* The purified air then flows over the work surface at a uniform velocity (i.e., **laminar flow**) of 80–100 ft./min. The constant flow of air from the hood prevents room air from entering the work area and removes contaminants introduced into the work area by material or personnel. However, they do not protect personnel or the environment from the hazards of drug products.

The surfaces of the hood's work area are clean, not sterile.

Therefore, it is necessary to use techniques which maintain the sterility of all sterile items. These are called aseptic techniques. They apply to the technician, the laminar flow hood, and all substances and materials involved in the procedure.

*Laminar flow hoods used in preparing parenteral formulations must be ISO Class 5 (less than 100 particles of 0.5 micron size per cubic foot).

 HEPA filter a high efficiency particulate air filter.

laminar flow continuous movement at a uniform rate in one direction.

horizontal flow hood a laminar flow hood where the air crosses the work area in a horizontal direction.

vertical flow hood a laminar flow hood where the air crosses the work area in a vertical direction.

TYPES OF LAMINAR FLOW HOODS

Laminar flow hoods are designed as either "horizontal" or "vertical" flow hoods.

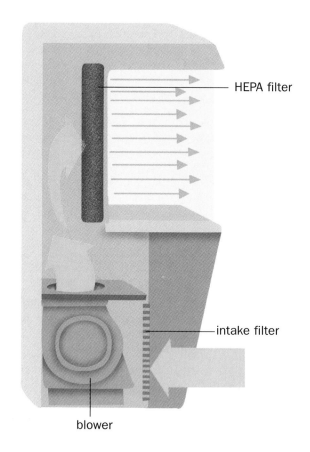

HEPA filter

intake filter

blower

a horizontal flow hood

Horizontal flow hoods take up room air and channel it through the HEPA filter. The air crosses the work area in a horizontal direction and exits the hood. The illustration above shows a design where room air enters the hood through the bottom. Other models have room air entering from the back or top of the hood.

R safety you should know
Laminar flow hoods do not provide a sterile environment. They provide an ultraclean work area.

view from above of a horizontal hood

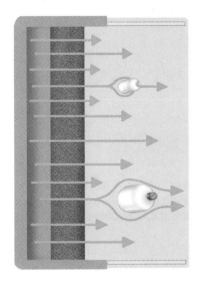

The illustration above shows how air is channeled around objects in the work area of a horizontal hood. Note that there is a "dead" area (sometimes called the "zone of turbulence") in front of the large container. Proper consideration needs to be given to the placement of materials inside the work area because of the air flow pattern. Smaller items should be placed close to the HEPA filter and larger items closer to the opening of the hood.

Hand movements should also be considered so that they do not disturb the air flow pattern. For example, moving the hands between the HEPA filter and the materials placed on the hood will disrupt or block the air flow, which will decrease the efficiency of the hood in that area. This can happen with an act as simple as wrapping the hand around an item. It is best to approach materials from the opening side of the hood, and avoid the tendency to grasp the item with the full hand.

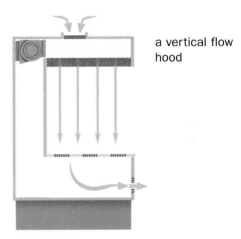

a vertical flow hood

Vertical flow hoods have the filtered air enter at top of the work area, and move downward. Some models have the air move downward all the way through the work area before it is returned to the room air.

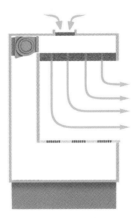

Other models of vertical flow hoods have the air move downward initially but then turn inside the work area and exit from the hood through the opening of the front of the hood.

When working in a vertical laminar flow hood, moving the hands over the items placed on the hood will block the air flow, decreasing the hood's efficiency in that area.

BIOLOGICAL SAFETY CABINETS

Biological safety cabinets are designed differently than laminar flow hoods.

They take air into the cabinet through the work surface vents and recirculate it through a HEPA filter located in the top of the cabinet. The air is channeled so that a major portion is recirculated back into the cabinet, and a minor portion is passed through another HEPA filter before being exhausted into the room. Once the air is filtered, it is directed downward toward the work surface, just as with a vertical laminar flow hood. However, as the air approaches the work surface, it is pulled through vents at the front, back, and sides of the work surface and again recirculated back into the cabinet.

There are two types of biological safety cabinets.

A Class 2, type A, which was just described, represents the minimum recommended environment for preparing chemotherapy agents. Class 2, type B biological safety cabinets have greater intake air flow velocities and are vented outside the building rather than back into the room.

Either type of biological safety cabinet should be used when preparing chemotherapy drugs.

Biological safety cabinets protect both personnel and the environment from contamination. Laminar flow hoods should not be used to prepare chemotherapy agents because they blow air across the work surface toward the operator and into the work environment.

Institutions will have policies and procedures for personnel working with cytotoxic and hazardous drugs.

In addition to working in a biological safety cabinets, these policies will cover areas such as personnel training in the identification, containment, collection, segregation, and disposal of these agents. The procedures should also describe the use of equipment, protective clothing to be worn, and procedures to be followed in case of exposure.

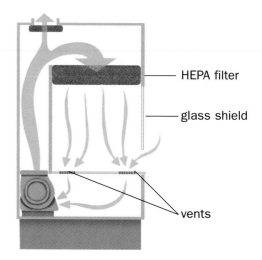

This is a Class 2, type A biological safety cabinet. These safety cabinets protect both personnel and the environment from contamination.

Common Chemotherapy Drugs

Route	Drug(s)
Oral	Capecitabine
Intravenous	Doxorubicin
Intraarterial (into the arteries)	Floxuridine
	Fluorouracil
	Mitomycin-C
	Cisplatin
	Streptomycin
Intralesional (directly into a tumor)	Vinblastine
	Vincristine
Intraperitoneal (into the cavity surrounding the abdominal organs)	Paclitaxel
	Mitoxantrone
	Carboplatin
	Alpha interferon
Intrathecal (into the spinal fluid)	Methotrexate
	Cytarabine

R **safety you should know**
Biological safety cabinets protect both personnel and the environment from contamination.

CLEAN ROOMS

L aminar flow hoods and biological safety cabinets are required to be housed in an area that is isolated from the main traffic in a pharmacy. These areas are commonly referred to as "clean rooms." Originally, clean room facilities varied significantly between pharmacies, but the USP/NF <797> regulations have brought mandatory requirements for such facilities.

USP/NF <797> regulations state that clean room facilities must be in a designated area of the pharmacy where traffic is very limited and air flow is unrestricted.

Further, only designated personnel should enter the space, and only for the purpose of aseptic preparations. The room should be large enough to accommodate all the necessary equipment such as the laminar air flow hoods (or safety cabinets) needed for aseptic compounding, and provide for the proper storage of drugs and supplies. There should be an additional room adjacent to the clean room (the anteroom) where gowning and hand washing take place.

The regulations also state that clean rooms must have air flow properties where the air quality, temperature, and humidity are tightly regulated in order to greatly reduce the risk of cross-contamination.

The air in a clean room must be repeatedly filtered to remove dust particles, particulates, and other impurities. The clean room usually has only one door, which should remain closed when not in use. It should have positive pressure, which means that when the door is open, the air will flow out of the clean room.

Sterile products must be prepared in a clean room with an ISO Class 7 environment.

ISO Class 7 means that any air flow unit used in the clean room is capable of producing an environment containing no more than 10,000 airborne particles of a size 0.5 micron or larger per cubic foot of air.

PREPARING FLOW HOODS OR SAFETY CABINETS FOR USE

Turning on Hoods or Cabinets

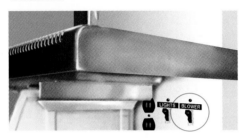

✔ Turn the hood or cabinet on and let it operate for at least 30 minutes before use in order to produce an ultraclean environment. Maintain a designated "clean" area around the hood.

Cleaning Hoods or Cabinets

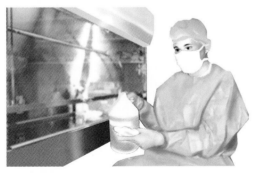

✔ Clean the inside of the hood with a suitable disinfectant. First clean the metal pole used to hang the containers.
✔ Then the sides of the hood are cleaned using up and down motions moving from the back of the hood toward the front.
✔ Then the bottom of the hood is cleaned using side-to-side motions moving from the back of the hood toward the front.
✔ If using a spray bottle to dispense the disinfectant, be sure not to spray the HEPA filter.

ASEPTIC TECHNIQUES IN HOODS AND CABINETS

Personnel involved with admixing parenteral solutions must use good aseptic techniques.

Aseptic techniques are the sum total of methods and manipulations required to minimize the contamination of sterile products. Contamination can be from microorganisms and/or particulate material. Working in a laminar flow hood does not, by itself, guarantee a sterile formulation.

Positioning of material and aseptically working inside hoods and cabinets requires training, practice, and attention to details.

Following are some general aseptic techniques for working in a laminar flow hood or biological safety cabinet:

✔ Never sneeze, cough, or talk directly into a hood.

✔ Close doors or windows. Breezes can disrupt the air flow enough to contaminate the work area.

✔ Perform all work at least 6 inches inside the hood to derive the benefits of the laminar air flow. Laminar flow air begins to mix with outside air near the edge of the hood.

✔ Maintain a direct, open path between the HEPA filter and the area inside the hood.

✔ Place nonsterile objects, such as solution containers or your hands, downstream from sterile ones. Particles blown off these objects can contaminate anything downstream from them.

✔ Do not put large objects at the back of the work area next to the filter. They will disrupt air flow.

The guidelines on these pages must also be followed, along with any facility and manufacturer guidelines that apply.

R̸ safety you should know
Sterile supplies often have instructions for use as well as expiration dates. Always follow such instructions along with any facility or manufacturer instructions.

Clothing and Barriers

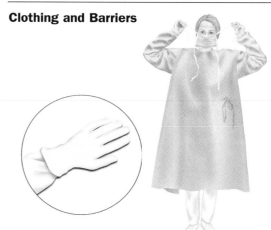

✔ Wear clean lint-free garments or barrier clothing, including gowns, hair covers, and a mask.

✔ Wear sterile gloves.

✔ Follow facility or manufacturer guidelines for putting on and removing barrier clothing. Unless barriers are put on properly, they can easily become contaminated.

Collect Supplies

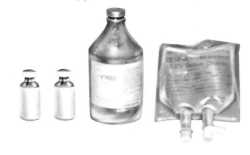

✔ Assemble all necessary supplies checking each for expiration dates and particulate material.

✔ Plastic solution containers should be squeezed to check for leaks.

✔ Use only pre-sterilized needles, syringes, and filters. Check the protective covering of each to verify they are intact.

✔ Remove dust coverings before placing supplies in the hood.

Wash Hands

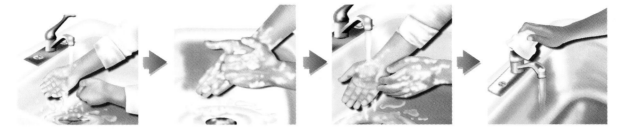

✔ Remove all jewelry.

✔ Stand far enough away from the sink so clothing does not come in contact with it.

✔ Turn on water. Wet hands and forearms thoroughly. Keep hands pointed downward.

✔ Scrub hands vigorously with an antibacterial soap.

✔ Work soap under fingernails by rubbing them against the palm of the other hand.

✔ Interlace the fingers and scrub the spaces between the fingers.

✔ Wash wrists and arms up to the elbows.

✔ Thoroughly rinse the soap from hands and arms.

✔ Dry hands and forearms thoroughly using a nonshedding paper towel.

✔ Use a dry paper towel to turn off the water faucet.

✔ After hands are washed, avoid touching clothes, face, hair, or any other potentially contaminated object in the area.

Position Supplies in Hood

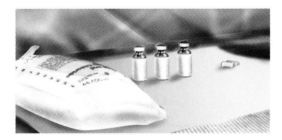

✔ Place supplies in the hood with smaller supplies closer to the HEPA filter and larger supplies further away from the filter.

✔ Space supplies to maximize laminar flow.

✔ Plan for the work area to be at least three inches from the back of the hood, and six inches inside the front of the hood.

Sterilize Puncture Surfaces

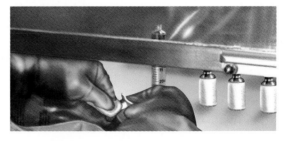

✔ Swab all surfaces that require entry (puncture) with an alcohol wipe. Avoid excess alcohol or lint that might be carried into the solution.

✔ Use a new alcohol wipe with each surface.

WORKING WITH VIALS

There are two types of parenteral vials that are used in making admixtures.

One contains the drug already in the solution. The other contains a powder that must be dissolved in a diluent to make a solution. In either case, a needle will be used to penetrate the closure in the vial.

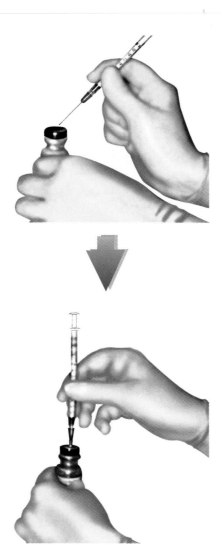

PREVENTING CORING

There is the potential of **coring** when pushing a needle through the rubber stopper of a vial or medication port.

As the needle penetrates the stopper, it can cut small pieces from the stopper which can fall into the vial. To prevent coring, follow these steps:

✔ Place the vial on a flat surface and position the needle point on the surface of the rubber closure so that the bevel is facing upward and the needle is at about a 45 to 60 degree angle to the closure surface.

✔ Put downward pressure on the needle while gradually bringing the needle up to an upright position. Just before penetration is complete, the needle should be at a vertical (90 degree) angle.

 coring when a needle damages the rubber closure of a parenteral container causing fragments of the closure to fall into the container and contaminate its contents.

VIALS CONTAINING SOLUTIONS

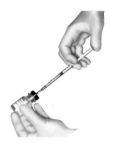 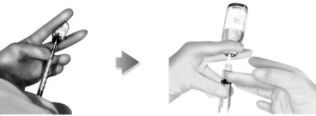

✔ Draw into the syringe a volume of air equal to the volume of solution to be withdrawn from the vial.

✔ Penetrate the vial without coring and inject the air. This will pressurize the vial and help in withdrawing the solution.

✔ Turn the vial upside down. Using one hand to hold the vial and the barrel of the syringe, pull back on the plunger with the other hand to fill the syringe. Fill the syringe with a slight excess of solution.

✔ Tap the syringe to allow air bubbles to come to the top of the syringe. Press the plunger to push air and excess solution into the vial.

✔ Transfer the solution into the final container, again minimizing coring.

VIALS CONTAINING LYOPHILIZED POWDER

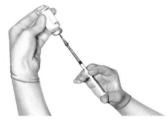 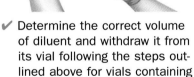 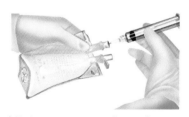

✔ Determine the correct volume of diluent and withdraw it from its vial following the steps outlined above for vials containing solutions.

✔ Transfer the diluent into the vial containing powder.

✔ Once the diluent is added, remove a volume of air into the syringe that is slightly more than the volume of diluent added. This will create a slight negative pressure in the vial and lowers the chance that aerosol droplets will be sprayed when the needle is withdrawn.

✔ After withdrawing the needle, swirl the vial until the drug is dissolved.

✔ Using a new needle and syringe, use the steps outlined above for vials containing solutions to withdraw the correct volume of reconstituted drug solution into the syringe.

✔ Transfer the reconstituted solution to the final container, again making sure to minimize coring.

WORKING WITH AMPULES

Ampules are always broken open at the neck.

Ampules have a colored stripe around the neck if they are pre-scored to indicate the neck has been weakened by the manufacturer to facilitate opening. Some ampules are not pre-scored by the manufacturer, and the neck must first be weakened (scored) with a fine file.

TO OPEN AN AMPULE

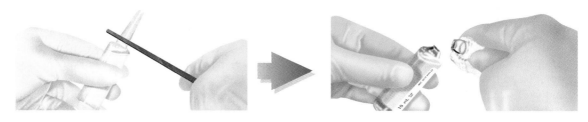

✔ If the ampule is not pre-scored, use a fine file to lightly score the neck at its narrowest point. Do not file all the way through the glass.

✔ Hold the ampule upright and tap the top to settle the solution into the bottom of the ampule.

✔ Swab the neck of the ampule with an alcohol swab.

✔ Wrap a gauze pad around the neck of the ampule. This will help protect fingers if the ampule shatters and will reduce the possibility of splinters becoming airborne.

✔ Grasp the top of the ampule with the thumb and index finger of one hand. Grasp the bottom of the ampule with the other hand.

✔ Quickly snap the ampule moving your hands outward and away. Do not open the ampule toward the HEPA filter or any other sterile supplies in the hood. If the ampule does not snap easily, rotate it slightly and try again.

✔ Inspect the opened ampule for glass particles that may have fallen inside, and use a filter needle if necessary when withdrawing the solution.

 ampules sealed glass containers with an elongated neck that must be snapped off.

TRANSFERRING SOLUTION

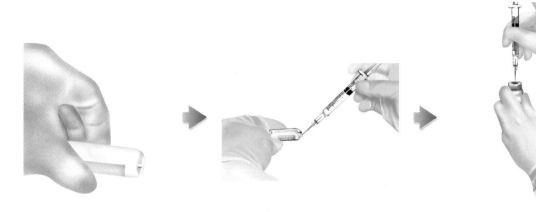

✔ Hold the ampule down at about a 20 degree angle.

✔ Attach a filter needle to a syringe.

✔ Insert the filter needle into the ampule. Avoid touching the opening of the ampule with the needle point.

✔ Position the needle on the shoulder area of the ampule. Place its beveled edge against the side of the ampule to avoid pulling glass particles into the syringe.

✔ Withdraw solution into the syringe but keep needle submerged to avoid drawing air into the syringe.

✔ Withdraw needle from ampule and remove all air bubbles from the syringe.

✔ Exchange the filter needle for a new filter needle or membrane filter and transfer the solution into the final container.

SYRINGES & NEEDLES

Many of the manipulations performed with aseptic techniques require the use of syringes, needles, and filters.

The basic parts of a syringe are the barrel, plunger, and tip. The barrel is a tube that is open at one end and tapers into a hollow tip at the other end. The plunger is a piston-type rod with a slightly cone-shaped stopper that passes inside the barrel of the syringe. The tip of the syringe provides the point of attachment for a needle. The volume of solution inside a syringe is indicated by graduation lines on the barrel. Graduation lines may be in milliliters or fractions of a milliliter, depending on the capacity of the syringe. The larger the capacity, the larger the interval between graduation lines.

There are several common types of syringe tips.

Slip-Tip® tips allow the needle to be held on the syringe by friction. The needle is reasonably secure, but it may slip off if not properly attached or if considerable pressure is used. **Luer-Lok®** tips have a collar with grooves that lock the needle in place. **Eccentric** tips, which are off-center, are used when the needle must be parallel to the plane of injection such as in an intradermal injection. **Oral syringes** have tips larger than a Slip-Tip®. Needles will not fit on oral syringes. Therefore, they are used to administer liquids by routes other than parenteral administration.

Syringes come in sizes ranging from 1 to 60 ml.

As a rule, the correct syringe size is the next size larger than the volume to be measured. For example, a 3 ml syringe should be selected to measure 2.3 ml, or a 5 ml syringe to measure 3.8 ml. In this way, the graduation marks on the syringe will be in the smallest possible increments for the volume measured. Syringes should not be filled to capacity because the plunger can be easily dislodged.

SYRINGES

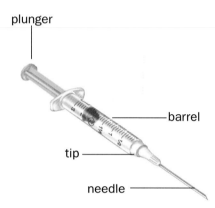

a syringe with graduation marks

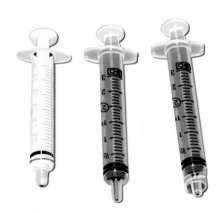

different syringe tips: oral (left); Slip-Tip® (center); and Luer-Lok® (right).

Drawing Liquids into the Syringe

Liquids are drawn into the syringe by pulling back on the plunger. The tip of the syringe must be fully submerged in the liquid to prevent air from being drawn into the syringe. Generally, an excess of solution is drawn into the syringe so that any air bubbles may be expelled by holding the syringe tip up, tapping the syringe until the air bubbles rise into the hub, and depressing the plunger to expel the air. This ensures that the hub will be completely filled with solution and the volume of delivery will be accurate.

Measuring Volume

The volume of solution in a syringe is measured to the edge of the plunger's stopper while the syringe is held upright and all the air has been removed from the syringe.

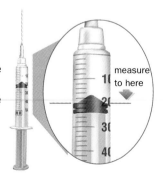

measure to here

Disposable needles should always be used when preparing admixtures as they are presterilized and individually wrapped to maintain sterility.

NEEDLES

Parts

A needle has three parts: the **hub**, the **shaft**, and the **bevel**. The hub is at one end of the needle and is the part that attaches to the syringe. It is designed for quick and easy attachment and removal. The shaft is the long, slender stem of the needle that is angled at one end to form a point called the "bevel." The hollow bore of the needle shaft is known as the **lumen**.

Sizes

Needle sizes are indicated by length and **gauge**. The length of a needle is measured in inches from where the shaft meets the hub to the tip of the bevel. Needle lengths range from 3/8 inch to three and a half inches. Some special use needles are even longer. The gauge of a needle, used to designate the size of the lumen, ranges from 27 (the smallest) to 13 (the largest). *In other words, the higher the gauge number, the smaller the lumen.* The hubs are color-coded for each gauge size.

Needle sizes are chosen based on both the viscosity (thickness) of the parenteral solution and the type of rubber closure in the container. Needles with relatively small lumens can be used for most dosage forms. However, some viscous solutions require needles with larger lumens. One problem is that larger needles are more likely to cause coring. Therefore, small gauge needles are used if the rubber closure can be easily cored, regardless of the solution viscosity.

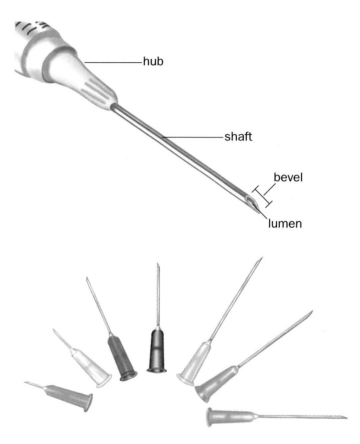

hub

shaft

bevel

lumen

different needle sizes

Slip-Tip®, Luer-Lok®, eccentric, oral different types of syringe tips.

hub the part of the needle that attaches to the syringe.

shaft the stem of the needle that provides the overall length of the needle.

bevel an angled surface at the tip of a needle.

gauge a measurement with needles: the higher the gauge, the smaller the lumen.

lumen the hollow center of a needle.

FILTERS

Filters are used to remove particulate materials or microorganisms from solutions.

They can be attached to the end of a syringe, to the end of an administration set, or they can be part of the needle. They are divided into two basic groups: depth filters and membrane filters. **Depth filters** work by trapping particles as solution moves through twisting channels. A **membrane filter** consists of many small pores of a uniform size that retain particles larger than the pores. Filters have a wide range of pore sizes. Common ones are 0.22, 0.45, 1.2, 5, or 10 microns.

Filters can be found in a variety of packaging.

Membrane filters often are packaged in a round plastic holder that can be attached easily to the end of a syringe. Some filters are attached to administration sets and serve as "final filters," filtering the solution immediately before it enters the patient's vein. Some administration sets have filters that are already built into the set. Filters also can be placed inside of needles; these are called *filter needles*. Double-ended filter needles comprise a simple unit that has a filter between two needles. This allows the transfer of solution directly from one container to another container and eliminates the need for using a syringe to transfer the solution. Filters also are supplied as single units to be used in specialized filtration apparatus.

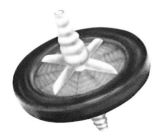

Membrane Filters

A membrane filter similar to the one above is often placed between the syringe and needle before the medication is introduced into a LVP or SVP container. Double-ended filter needles are also used to transfer solutions from a vial directly into a bottle or bag. This eliminates the need of using a syringe.

MEMBRANE FILTERS

Membrane filters are intended to filter a solution only as it is expelled from a syringe. A common scenario would be to transfer a reconstituted powder drug solution into a LVP or SVP following these steps:

1. A needle is attached to the syringe.
2. The reconstituted powder drug solution is pulled into the syringe.
3. Air bubbles are removed from the syringe.
4. The needle is removed from the syringe.
5. A membrane filter is then attached to the syringe.
6. Another needle is placed on the end of the filter.
7. Air is eliminated from the filter chamber by holding the syringe in a vertical position so that the needle is pointing upward. The air in the filter chamber is then expelled by slowly pushing in the plunger. Air must be expelled before the filter becomes wet or the air will not pass through the filter. Do not pull back on the plunger when the membrane filter is being used because the filter may rupture.
8. Once air has been expelled, the needle is introduced into the final LVP or SVP container and pressure is slowly and continuously applied to push the solution through the filter into the container.

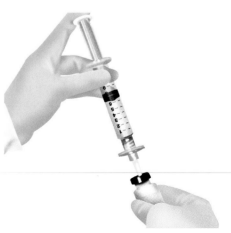

a membrane filter attached to a syringe and needle

DEPTH FILTERS

Depth filters are constructed of randomly oriented fibers or particles (e.g., diatomaceous earth, porcelain, asbestos) that have been pressed, wound, or otherwise bonded together to form a tortuous pathway for solution flow.

The depth filter is rigid enough so the solution may be filtered either as it is pulled into or expelled from the syringe, but not both ways in the same procedure. If a drug solution is to be filtered as it is pulled into a syringe, the following steps are used:

1.   The filter needle is attached to the syringe.

2.   The solution is pulled into the syringe.

3.   The filter needle is removed.

4.   A new needle is attached to the syringe.

5.   The solution is expelled from the syringe.

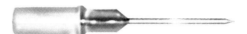

The depth filter is inside the hub of this filter needle.

FINAL FILTERS

A filter that filters a solution immediately before it enters the patient's vein is called a **final filter**. Some administration sets contain final filters as part of the set. Some filters are designed to be attached to administration sets and serve as final filters.

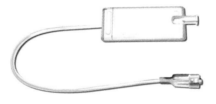

a Pall® final filter

 depth filter a filter that can filter solutions being drawn into or expelled from a syringe, but not both ways in the same procedure.

membrane filter a filter that filters solution as the solution is expelled from the syringe.

final filter a filter placed immediately before a solution enters a patient's vein.

ADMINISTRATION DEVICES

ADMINISTRATION SETS

LVP solutions are usually administered with administration sets.

An administration set is a length of flexible plastic tubing with a spike at one end and a needle adapter at the other. The spike fits into the administration set port of the LVP container. The solution flows from the LVP container through the plastic tubing to the needle adapter at the other end. A needle or catheter can be attached to the needle adapter.

On the tubing, a clamp provides one means of regulating the **flow rate** (the rate at which the solution is to be administered to the patient, generally measured in ml/hour). The clamp may be a roll clamp or a slide clamp.

The flow rate can also be determined by counting the number of drops per minute that enter a drip chamber. A drip chamber is a small reservoir in the plastic tubing near the LVP container. Fluid collects in the drip chamber, and then flows continuously through the remainder of the tubing without mixing with air. Drip chambers may be a regular drip chamber (e.g., 10 drops/ml), or a minidrip chamber (e.g., 60 drops/ml).

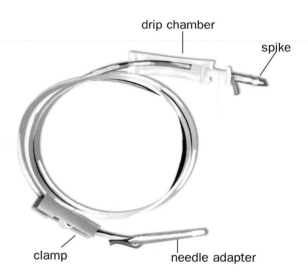

an administration set

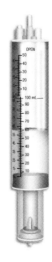

a volume control chamber

A volume control chamber is often used with a clamp to control the flow rate. A volume control chamber is a plastic cylindrical device with graduation marks along the sides for measuring the volume of solution. As the IV solution flows from the LVP container, the chamber is filled to a measured volume. A clamp immediately above the chamber is closed when the desired volume of solution has been added. In this manner, the volume control chamber serves as a minireservoir from which the solution is allowed to flow when a clamp below the chamber on the administration set is opened. It also is a safety precaution that will limit the volume of fluid that may be infused accidentally. These chambers are generally recommended only for pediatric patients.

Source for the administration set and volume control chamber illustrations: Adapted from Figure 2.4 and 2.9 respectively in Hunt, *Training Manual for Intravenous Admixture Personnel, Fifth Edition.* ®Copyright 1995 Baxter Healthcare Corporation.

flow rate the rate (in ml/hour or ml/minute) at which the solution is administered to the patient.

Flashball flexible rubber tubing near the needle adapter on an administration set; used to determine if the needle is properly placed in the veins.

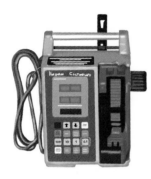

A controller may also be used to regulate the flow rate. Most controllers use a photoelectric sensor to compare the actual gravity flow rate to a programmed (desired) flow rate and relax or constrict the administration set tubing to increase or decrease the flow rate. Combination controllers /pumps provide both the safety of low infusion pressures from the controller part of the device and the availability of a positive pressure pump in the other part of the device. The user selects whether to use the device as a controller or a pump.

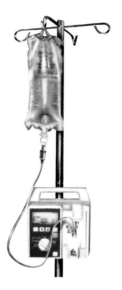

an LVP connected to an administration set with a controller

An administration set can have many variations. The spike may have an air vent built into it. A drip chamber or a volume control chamber may or may not be present. The length of the tubing varies as well as the lumen size (i.e., regular or microbore). There may also be a filter incorporated into the tubing.

Some administration sets have a piece of flexible rubber tubing located near the needle adapter called a **Flashball**. The Flashball can be squeezed before starting the administration to see if the needle is correctly located in the patient's vein. If blood comes up into the Flashball, the needle is properly placed.

IV CATHETERS

An IV catheter is a 1- to 5-inch piece of fine, flexible plastic tubing connected to a plastic hub that is in turn attached to a syringe or to an administration set. The catheter has a needle to allow for insertion but it is pulled out after insertion. IV catheters are sometimes used instead of needles because they are more flexible and therefore can be less irritating to the patient. It is important to remember, however, that the risk of inflammation increases the longer any foreign material is left inserted in a vein.

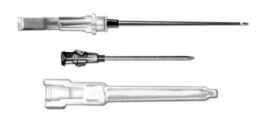

ADMINISTRATION DEVICES (cont'd)

PIGGYBACKS

Intermittent intravenous medications are often administered using **piggybacks**. This involves infusing medications in a small volume of solution at regular intervals, typically thirty to sixty minutes. The intermittent IV solution flows into the patient's vein through the same administration set as the LVP, and at the same time. When the intermittent infusion is not being administered, the LVP infusion continues to keep the vein open.

The LVP solution container and the piggyback solution container are connected at a Y-type connector in the administration set. The minibag container is placed higher than the LVP container so its greater pressure will ensure the minibag solution will enter the administration set. At the appropriate time, the clamp to the piggyback container is opened. The minibag solution is prevented from flowing into the LVP container by a one-way check valve on the LVP container. The two solutions are not mixed together except in the administration set tubing below the Y-connector.

Piggyback containers are usually made of the same material as the plastic LVP bags and hold 50–100 ml of 5% Dextrose Injection or 0.9% Sodium Chloride Injection.

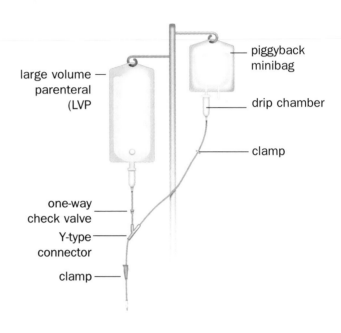

large volume parenteral (LVP

piggyback minibag

drip chamber

clamp

one-way check valve

Y-type connector

clamp

HEPARIN LOCKS

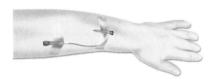

In some instances, a patient may not have a primary LVP solution, yet must receive minibag medications. This is done through a **heparin lock**, which is a short piece of tubing attached to a needle or intravenous catheter. When the tubing is not being used for the minibag, heparin is used to fill the tubing. Heparin prevents blood from clotting in the tube.

piggybacks small volume solutions connected to an LVP.
heparin lock an administration device used when a primary LVP solution is not available.

POSITIVE PRESSURE PUMPS

Positive pressure infusion devices (pumps) generate a pressure that will cause fluid to flow through tubing into the patient's vascular system. These devices overcome minor occlusions and resistance associated with an intravenous system, viscous solutions, and vascular back pressure. Most pumps have operating pressures in the 2–12 pounds per square inch (PSI) range. Pressures around 2 PSI are used to keep the vascular access open (called "keep open"), whereas arterial access requires pressures about 10–12 PSI.

Cassette Pumps

Cassette pumps are often used as ambulatory pumps since many are about the size of a hand, allowing the patient to have freedom of movement.

In this type of pump, a cassette acts as a reservoir and fits into the pump housing. Tubing connects the cassette to the patient. The pump makes the cassette fill and then empty in two separate, sequential cycles to deliver a measured volume of fluid.

Syringe type cassette pumps move a motor-driven plunger into and out of a fluid filled chamber. In a piston-activated diaphragm cassette pump, a flexible diaphragm is mounted near a moving piston. Each inward stroke of the piston compresses the diaphragm, directing solution to the patient. Each outward stroke allows the diaphragm to relax and refills the chamber.

Multiple chamber pumps allow one chamber to refill while the other directs fluid to the patient.

Elastomeric Reservoirs

These are tennis ball sized pumps with a balloon-like reservoir surrounded by a rigid, protective outer shell. The elastic reservoir is filled with a solution which exerts a constant positive pressure forcing the solution through the tubing into the patient. The combination of the pressure and dimensions of the tubing determine the flow rate of the pump.

Syringe Pumps

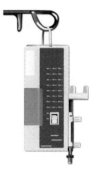

In this type of pump, a syringe attached to a pump expels solution from the syringe by advancing either the plunger or the barrel at a predetermined rate. Syringe pumps are commonly used for infusion of intermittent medications such as antibiotics. They are also used to administer antineoplastic drugs, analgesics, and anesthetics. Because they can deliver solutions at very low and precisely controlled flow rates, they are especially useful for neonatal, infant, and critical care applications where small volumes need to be given over extended periods of time.

Peristaltic Pumps

Peristaltic pumps infuse solutions in "micropulses" produced by a massaging action on the IV tubing. Special infusion sets are used because the tubing has been reinforced with a silastic insert at the point of contact with the peristaltic mechanism. This reinforcement keeps the tubing from stretching and deforming, which would lead to variations in the flow rate. A linear peristaltic pump has finger-like projections that occlude the tubing in a successive manner in a rippling, wave-like motion. Rotary peristaltic pumps compress the tubing against a rotor housing with rollers mounted on it. As the rotor turns, the rollers occlude the tubing and force the fluid to flow toward the patient while drawing new fluid from the IV bag.

PARENTERAL INCOMPATIBILITIES

Not all drugs are compatible with each other: an incompatibility may exist between two or more drugs or between a drug and an IV solution.

The number of unexpected or undesired combinations is relatively low compared with the number of IV admixtures prepared. But incompatibilities can lead to a patient not receiving the full dose of the medication or to an adverse reaction.

Some incompatibilities, such as a color change or hazy appearance, can be seen.

Precipitates form in the solution, or an evolution of gas may even be smelled. For example, variations in color can occur for imipenem-cilastatin or dobutamine. When ceftazidime is reconstituted, carbon dioxide gas is released. The precipitate that forms when paclitaxel is refrigerated dissolves at room temperature. Reading the package insert or checking with the pharmacist can confirm the reason for these changes in appearance.

But other incompatibilities are not indicated by color changes, precipitation, or gas formation.

If two or more drugs react that are incompatible with each other, one drug can cause the degradation of the other drug(s). These types of incompatibilities are confirmed by analytical methods.

Incompatibility Information Resources

The most often used resource for incompatibility information is the manufacturers' package insert. There are also incompatibility charts that list drugs horizontally across the top and vertically down one side. Where the column and row intersect, there is a code relating information about the compatibility or incompatibility of the two drugs. These charts also list specific solutions that should not be used with a drug when making an admixture.

Other sources of information include articles in professional magazines, reference books such as Trissel's *Handbook on Injectable Drugs*, and the *American Hospital Formulary Service, Drug Information*. There is computer software available based on these references.

MINIMIZING INCOMPATIBILITIES

The following guidelines can help minimize incompatibilities.

✔ Use solutions promptly after preparation. This will ensure that the most stable formulation is being administered. Drugs in solutions tend to degrade in a relatively short time. If an admixture is not immediately used, it should be placed in the refrigerator (if appropriate).

✔ Minimize the number of drugs added to a solution at one time. As the number of added drugs increase, so does the likelihood of an incompatibility. It also becomes more difficult to find incompatibility information when more drugs have been added to one solution.

✔ Check incompatibility resources to verify which drugs will produce a very high or very low pH solution. Since many drugs are acidic, their combination with a drug solution that has a very low pH is likely to result in an incompatibility. The same would be true for basic drugs in solutions with very high pH.

✔ Check incompatibility resources closely when one additive is a drug containing calcium, magnesium, or phosphate. These salt forms can precipitate many drugs and each other.

✔ Check incompatibility references closely when an additive drug contains an acetate or lactate. These solutions tend to have increased buffer capacities and are resistant to changes in pH.

SOME CONTRIBUTING FACTORS

Following are some common factors that can affect the compatibility and/or stability of drugs in IV admixtures.

pH

Combining two drugs that require two different pH values for the final solution can cause one or both drugs to either degrade or precipitate.

Light

Some drugs will start to break down and lose their therapeutic effect if exposed to light.

➡ Example: Amphotericin B, cisplatin, and metronidazole must be protected from light to maintain their potency.

Temperature

Storing and maintaining IV solutions at the appropriate temperature are important factors in keeping admixtures stable. Because heat increases the rate of most chemical reactions (including degradation), most drugs are more stable when refrigerated than at room temperature.

➡ Example: Cefazolin IV is stable for only 24 hours at room temperature, but for 96 hours under refrigeration.

However, some drugs should not be refrigerated because a precipitate will form.

Dilution

The concentration of a drug in a solution may be a factor in its compatibility with other drugs. A common problem is mixing electrolytes for parenteral nutrition solutions. Make sure that a drug is properly diluted before combining it with another drug.

➡ Example: Up to 15 mEq of calcium can be added to a liter of solution containing up to 30 mEq of phosphate but higher concentrations of either drug will cause precipitation.

Buffer Capacity

This is the ability of a solution to resist a change in pH when either an acidic or alkaline substance is added. In general, IV solutions do not have high buffer capacities so when a drug with a high buffer capacity is added, the resulting solution will have a pH closest to the drug added.

Time

Many drugs start to degrade shortly after being added to an IV solution. Others may require a longer period of time before degradation is evident.

Filters

Filters, especially final filters, can reduce the concentration of a drug if it becomes trapped by the filter.

➡ Example: An in-line filter can cause up to a 90% reduction in the delivered concentration of nitroglycerin.

Solutions

Some drugs require a specific solution or diluent to be used with them. Choosing the wrong solution can cause the drug to be broken down more quickly or can cause a precipitate to form.

➡ Example: amphotericin B is not compatible with normal saline.

➡ Example: Some drugs such as trastuzumab (Herceptin®) are packaged with a specific diluent for reconstitution.

Chemical Complexation

Complexation occurs when two drugs are combined and a new chemical combination is formed, often reducing the therapeutic effect of one of the drugs.

➡ Example: The combination of tetracycline and calcium reduces the activity of tetracycline.

➡ Example: Cisplatin-AQ should not be used with needles, administration sets, or filters that contain aluminum.

Plastics

Some drugs are incompatible with the plastics in containers or certain administration sets. This is especially true of polyvinyl chloride (PVC) plastics. Plasticizers can be leached out of the plastic bag or from the administration set into the IV solution, or the drug can bind to the plastic material making it unavailable for the therapeutic effect. Albumin is sometimes added to admixtures because it preferentially binds to plastic surfaces.

QUALITY ASSURANCE & INFECTION CONTROL

The USP/NF <797> regulations require that every parenteral compounding facility to have a quality assurance program.

Quality assurance (QA) is a series of activities ensuring that a compounded formulation will be safe, stable, and of the proper identity, strength, purity, and quality. Another goal is to provide for product uniformity since a given formulation may be compounded by different pharmacy technicians at different times.

A major component of a quality assurance program is to have a written environmental quality and infection control plan.

Such plans provide for:

✔ semi-annual testing and certification of ISO classified work areas;

✔ routine monitoring of environmental airborne particulates and microbiologicals;

✔ routine monitoring of operating temperatures and humidity;

✔ maintaining continuous positive pressure and pressure differentials or gradients between clean areas;

✔ continuous HEPA filtered air;

✔ maintaining environmentally zoned areas based on critical activities (i.e., ISO Class 5, 7, or 8);

✔ and limiting access to environmentally controlled areas.

Inspection

 Formulated or admixed solutions should be inspected after compounding. Visual inspection can show two of the six characteristics of parenteral solutions: particulate material and stability. (Lack of stability is indicated by precipitation or crystallization in the solution).

Visual inspection cannot reveal anything about the sterility, pH, osmolarity, presence of pyrogens, or chemical degradation of the drug. Special equipment and skilled personnel are needed to determine these factors. Since sterility cannot be determined visually, good aseptic technique must be used when preparing parenteral solutions.

Final Check

The final check by the pharmacy technician should verify that:

✔ the label is complete and error-free;

✔ the correct base parenteral components (size, strength) have been used;

✔ the correct drug additive (components, strength, quantity) has been added to the base parenteral component;

✔ if an IV solution, the admixture is clear and free from particulate matter. This part of the inspection can be aided by holding the admixture in front of both a black and white background.

✔ the correct beyond-use date is stated.

Hazardous Waste Regulations

The Resource Conservation and Recovery Act (RCRA) regulates handling hazardous waste from its generation to disposal. These regulations apply to drugs and chemicals discarded by pharmacies, hospitals, clinics, and other commercial entities.

Hazardous materials are divided into two lists. "P-list" wastes include epinephrine, nitroglycerin, and physostigmine. "U-list" wastes are toxic, flammable, corrosive, or reactive and include cyclophosphamide. These materials are considered hazardous even in trace amounts of no more than 3% of the capacity of a container.

Hazardous waste must be collected and stored according to specific EPA and Department of Transportation (DOT) requirements. Properly labeled, leak proof, and spill proof containers of non-reactive plastic and sharps containers are required for areas where hazardous waste is generated. Hazardous drug waste may be initially contained in thick, sealable plastic bags before placing in approved containers.

Transport of waste containers from satellite accumulation areas to storage sites must be done by individuals who meet OSHA-mandated hazardous waste training. Hazardous waste must be properly manifested and transported by a federally permitted transporter to a federally permitted storage, treatment, or disposal facility.

Another part of an environmental quality and infection control plan specifies the methods and frequency of cleaning and sanitizing parenteral compounding areas.

This is the responsibility of the pharmacy personnel since these areas are off limits to untrained or unsupervised housekeeping personnel.

Recommended standard operating procedures for cleaning sterile compounding facilities, including all anteroom carts, equipment, work benches, work surfaces, and floors, are to:

✔ clean and sanitize the direct and contiguous compounding area at the beginning of each shift;

✔ clean and sanitize work surfaces in the anteroom daily;

✔ mop floors daily when no aseptic operations are in progress;

✔ empty storage shelving in the anteroom of all supplies and clean and sanitize at least weekly;

✔ clean and sanitize the walls and ceilings in the work space at least monthly.

---

sharps needles, jagged glass or metal objects, or any items that might puncture or cut the skin.

Sharps Disposal

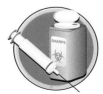

Once a parenteral solution has been prepared and inspected, any used syringes, bottles, vials, or other supplies should be disposed of properly in a container labeled **sharps**. A sharp is any object that might puncture or cut the skin of anyone who handles them. Sharps containers should be easily identified, leak proof, puncture proof, and be able to be sealed permanently.

Following are procedures for preparing materials for disposal into a sharps container:

✔ Excess solutions should be returned to their original vial, an empty vial, or some other closed container before disposal.

✔ Needles must be left on syringes to prevent possible injuries.

✔ To prevent aerosolization of any remaining solution, needles should not be clipped.

✔ Used needles should never be recapped. They should be discarded as an intact unit, along with IV catheters or other sharp objects.

✔ Sharps containers should be disposed of when three-quarters full or at least daily.

UNITS OF MEASUREMENT

There are different ways to express the concentration of a drug in a parenteral solution.

Each method of expressing the concentration is related to a particular property of the solution. The common concentrations and their units are listed on these pages.

MOLARITY

Molarity is an expression of the number of moles of a drug in a volume of solution. A mole is the number of grams numerically equal to the **molecular weight** of the drug. The molecular weight is the sum of the atomic weights of all the atoms that make up the drug molecule. Potassium chloride (KCl) has a molecular weight of 74.6. So, one mole of potassium chloride is 74.6 grams.

Molarity concentrations are expressed as mole/liter (written as mol/L, or M). A 1M solution of potassium chloride contains 74.6 grams of the drug in 1,000 ml (1 liter) of solution.

Some molarity concentrations are expressed as millimoles per liter (written as mM/L). A millimole is one-thousandth of a mole.

Salt Forms

Drugs come in different salt forms for a variety of reasons, and the salt form and **"waters of hydration"** must be factored into determining the molecular weight of a drug. For example, chloride is available as the sodium salt, the potassium salt, and the calcium salt.

Waters of hydration are water molecules that can attach to drug molecules. Calcium chloride ($CaCl_2$) exists in three different forms, **anhydrous** (no waters), dihydrate (2 associated waters), and hexahydrate (six waters of hydration). *The dihydrate form is the one used in making parenteral solutions.*

OSMOLES

Another expression for an amount of drug is the osmole (Osmol). An osmole is equal to the molecular weight of the drug divided by the number of **ions** formed when a drug dissolves in solution.

$$\text{osmole} = \frac{\text{molecular weight}}{\text{\# of ions}}$$

For example, potassium chloride forms two ions when it dissolves in solutions. Therefore, 1 Osmol of potassium chloride would be its molecular weight (74.6 grams) divided by two: 37.3 grams. Anhydrous calcium chloride forms three ions when it dissolves in solution: one calcium ion and two chloride ions. 1 Osmol would be its molecular weight (111.0 grams) divided by three: 37.0 grams.

Most drug solution concentrations are expressed as Osmol/liter (written as Osmol/L). Some concentrations are expressed as mOsmol/L. A milliosmol is one-thousandth of an osmole.

 molecular weight the sum of the atomic weights of a molecule.

waters of hydration water molecules that attach to drug molecules.

anhydrous without water molecules.

ions molecular particles that carry electric charges.

equivalent weight a drug's molecular weight divided by its valence, a common measure of electrolyte concentration.

valence the number of positive or negative charges on an ion.

EQUIVALENTS

Another expression for an amount of drug is the **equivalent weight (Eq)**. It is used to describe concentrations of electrolytes such as potassium chloride, sodium chloride, sodium acetate, etc.

When an electrolyte dissolves in solution, it divides into ions, particles which carry electric charges that can be positive or negative. The number of positive *or* negative charges (but not both added together) is called the **valence** of the ions. It indicates the ions' ability to combine with other atoms or molecules.

An equivalent weight is equal to the molecular weight of the drug divided by the valence of the ions that form when the drug is dissolved.

$$\text{equivalent weight} \; = \; \frac{\text{molecular weight}}{\text{valence}}$$

Equivalent concentrations are expressed as an equivalent weight per liter (written as Eq/L). Equivalent concentrations are also expressed as milliequivalents per liter (written as mEq/L). A milliequivalent is one-thousandth of an equivalent weight.

EXAMPLE

Potassium chloride (KCl) splits into one potassium ion (K^+) and one chloride ion (Cl^-).

➥ KCl's valence is 1 since there is either one positive charge on the potassium ion or one negative charge on the chloride ion.

➥ The equivalent weight of KCL is 74.6 grams divided by one: 74.6 grams.

EXAMPLE

Anhydrous calcium chloride ($CaCl_2$, 111.0 grams) splits into one calcium ion having two positive charges (++) and two chloride ions, each having one negative charge (-).

➥ Its valence is 2.

➥ The equivalent weight of $CaCl_2$ is 111.0 grams divided by two: 55.5 grams.

PERCENTAGE WEIGHT PER VOLUME

Percentage concentrations refer to the drug's weight per 100 ml if the drug is a solid, or the drug's volume per 100 ml if the drug is a liquid.

$$\text{solid: } \% \; = \; \frac{\text{weight (gm)}}{\text{100 ml}}$$

$$\text{liquid: } \% \; = \; \frac{\text{volume (ml)}}{\text{100 ml}}$$

For example, a 5% dextrose solution contains 5 grams of dextrose (a solid) in 100 ml of solution. A 5% acetic acid solution (common household vinegar) contains 5 ml of acetic acid (a liquid) per 100 ml of solution.

Percentage concentrations are applied to other formulations besides parenteral solutions. A 10% zinc oxide ointment would have 10 grams of zinc oxide (a solid) in 100 grams of ointment.

INTERNATIONAL UNITS

Because the potency and purity of drugs from biological sources vary depending on the source, they are measured by units of activity rather than by weight. Units may be abbreviated as IU, or U, and are expressed for example as 2,000 U, 1,000,000 U, etc. However, most institutions do not recommend the "IU" or "U" abbreviation as it can be mis-interpreted. It is suggested that international units be spelled out.

Drugs commonly measured in international units include penicillin, insulin, heparin, and some vitamins.

REVIEW

KEY CONCEPTS

PARENTERALS: STERILE FORMULATIONS

✔ Parenteral solutions must be sterile, free of all visible particulate material, pyrogen-free, stable for their intended use, have a pH around 7.4, and in most (but not all) cases isotonic.

LVP SOLUTIONS

✔ Large volume parenterals (LVP) are 100 ml or more and come in plastic bags or glass bottles.

✔ USP/NF <797> is the federal set of procedures and guidelines for making parenteral formulations.

SVP SOLUTIONS

✔ When a drug is added to a parenteral solution, the drug is referred to as the additive, and the final mixture is referred to as the admixture.

SPECIAL SOLUTIONS

✔ Parenteral nutrition solutions are complex admixtures composed of dextrose, fat, protein, electrolytes, vitamins, and trace elements used to meet patient nutritional needs.

LAMINAR FLOW HOODS

✔ A laminar flow hood establishes and maintains an ultraclean work area for preparing admixtures.

BIOLOGICAL SAFETY CABINETS AND CLEAN ROOMS

✔ Chemotherapy agents are to be made in a biological safety cabinet, not a laminar flow hood.

✔ Clean rooms are isolated rooms that house air flow hoods such as laminar flow hoods and biological safety cabinets.

ASEPTIC TECHNIQUES FOR HOODS AND CABINETS

✔ Aseptic techniques maintain the sterility of all sterile items and are used in preparing admixtures.

WORKING WITH VIALS

✔ There is the potential of coring the rubber stopper of a vial.

WORKING WITH AMPULES

✔ Ampules may be pre-scored by the manufacturer or need to be scored with a file.

SYRINGES AND NEEDLES

✔ Syringes come in sizes ranging from 1 to 60 ml.

✔ Needle sizes are indicated by length and gauge. Large needle lumens may be needed for highly viscous solutions but are more likely to cause coring.

FILTERS

✔ Syringe filters are often used to remove particulate materials from solutions, and sometimes to remove microorganisms.

ADMINISTRATION DEVICES

✔ LVP solutions are usually administered with an administration set. In addition to the basic components of flexible plastic tubing, spikes, clamps, and needle adapters, administration sets can have many other features such as drip chambers, clamps, or Flashballs.

✔ Parenteral administration devices use either gravity or a pump to push the solution into the patient.

PARENTERAL INCOMPATIBILITIES

✔ An incompatibility can exist between the drugs in an admixture or between a drug and the base IV solution.

QUALITY ASSURANCE & INFECTION CONTROL

✔ A significant part of preparing parenteral admixtures is to have and follow an environmental quality and infection control plan.

✔ Every admixture should be inspected to make sure the medication order, label, and added components are correct and in agreement with each other.

✔ Drugs and supplies used in making parenteral admixtures should be disposed of properly. This may involve using a sharps container, or following procedures prescribed by the EPA and local landfill requirements.

UNITS OF MEASUREMENT

✔ Equivalent (Eq/L) or milliequivalent (mEq/L) concentrations are commonly used to describe concentrations of electrolytes in parenteral solutions.

✔ Percentage concentrations refer to the drug's weight per 100 ml if the drug is a solid, or the drug's volume per 100 ml if the drug is a liquid.

SELF TEST

MATCH THE TERMS: I   *the answer key begins on page 511*

1. additive _____

2. admixture _____

3. ampules _____

4. anhydrous _____

5. aseptic techniques _____

6. bevel _____

7. compounded sterile preparation (CSP) _____

8. coring _____

9. depth filter _____

10. dialysis _____

11. diluent _____

12. equivalent weight _____

13. final filter _____

14. Flashball _____

15. flow rate _____

16. gauge _____

17. HEPA filter _____

18. heparin lock _____

a. sealed glass containers with an elongated neck.

b. a filter placed immediately before a solution enters a patient's vein.

c. a high efficiency particulate air filter.

d. a solvent that dissolves a lyophilized powder or dilutes a solution.

e. a needle measurement.

f. an angled surface, at the tip of a needle.

g. movement of particles in a solution through permeable membranes.

h. methods that maintain sterility of sterile products.

i. the resulting solution when a drug is added to a parenteral solution.

j. a compounded sterile parenteral dosage form that will be parenterally administered.

k. the rate (in ml/hour or ml/minute) at which the solution is administered to the patient.

l. an injection device used when a primary LVP solution is not available.

m. a drug that is added to a parenteral solution.

n. without water molecules.

o. when a needle damages the rubber closure of a parenteral container causing fragments to fall into the container.

p. a filter that can filter solutions being drawn into or out of a syringe, but not both ways in the same procedure.

q. a drug's molecular weight divided by its valence, a common measure of electrolyte concentration.

r. flexible rubber tubing near the needle adapter of an administration set used to determine if the needle is properly placed in the vein.

REVIEW

the answer key begins on page 511

MATCH THE TERMS: II

1. horizontal flow hood _____

2. hub _____

3. hypertonic _____

4. hypotonic _____

5. ions _____

6. irrigation solution _____

7. isotonic _____

8. laminar flow _____

9. lumen _____

10. lyophilized _____

11. membrane filter _____

12. molecular weight _____

13. osmosis _____

14. osmotic pressure _____

15. peritoneal dialysis solution _____

16. piggybacks _____

17. pyrogens _____

18. ready-to-mix _____

19. shaft _____

20. sharps _____

21. Slip-Tip®, Luer-Lok®, eccentric, oral _____

22. total nutrient admixture (TNA) solution _____

23. total parenteral nutrition (TPN) solution _____

a. chemicals produced by microorganisms that can cause fever reactions in patients.

b. molecular particles that carry electric charges.

c. when a solution has an osmolarity equivalent to that of blood.

d. when a solution has a lesser osmolarity than that of blood.

e. when a solution has a greater osmolarity than that of blood.

f. freeze dried.

g. complex solutions with two base solutions (amino acids and dextrose) and additional micro-nutrients.

h. a TPN solution that contains intravenous fat emulsion.

i. the action in which a drug in a higher concentration solution passes through a permeable membrane to a lower concentration solution.

j. a solution placed in and emptied from the peritoneal cavity to remove toxic substances.

k. large volume splash solutions used during surgical or urologic procedures to bathe and moisten body tissues.

l. continuous movement at a uniform rate in one direction.

m. different types of syringe tips.

n. the part of the needle that attaches to the syringe.

o. the stem of the needle that provides the overall length of the needle.

p. the hollow center of a needle.

q. a filter that filters solution as the solution is expelled from the syringe.

r. a characteristic of a solution determined by the number of dissolved particles in it.

s. any object that can puncture or cut the skin of anyone who handles them.

t. small volume solutions connected to an LVP.

u. the sum of the atomic weights of a molecule.

v. water molecules that attach to drug molecules.

w. the number of positive or negative charges on an ion.

x. a specially designed minibag where a drug is put into the SVP fluid just prior to administration.

24. valence _____

25. vertical flow hood _____

26. waters of hydration _____

y. a laminar flow hood where the air crosses the work area in a horizontal direction.

z. a laminar flow hood where the air crosses the work area in a vertical direction.

CHOOSE THE BEST ANSWER

the answer key begins on page 511

1. Which parenteral solution is not required to be sterile?
   a. subcutaneous injection
   b. vaginal
   c. intranasal
   d. inhalation

2. Pyrogens
   a. grow in parenteral solutions.
   b. are not water soluble.
   c. produce fever.
   d. can be removed by filtration.

3. The purpose of USP/NF <797> is to prevent harm and fatality to patients that can result from
   a. nonsterile formulations.
   b. excessive bacterial endotoxins.
   c. large errors in the strength of correct ingredients.
   d. all of the above

4. Add-a-Vial®, Add-Vantage® system, and the Mini-Bag Plus® system are examples of
   a. prefilled syringe systems.
   b. multiple dose glass vial systems.
   c. ready-to-mix systems.
   d. dry powder for constitution systems.

5. Multidose vials
   a. can be reused within 48 hours if refrigerated.
   b. can be reused within 24 hours if refrigerated.
   c. do not contain preservatives.
   d. contain preservatives.

6. Irrigation solutions are administered
   a. through a filter needle.
   b. through a special administration set.
   c. orally.
   d. by pouring them out of the bottle.

7. In horizontal laminar flow hoods, air blows
   a. down toward the work area.
   b. away from the operator.
   c. toward the operator.
   d. up toward the HEPA filter.

8. With laminar flow, the air moves in _____ direction(s).
   a. four
   b. three
   c. two
   d. one

9. If a laminar flow hood is turned off between aseptic processing sessions, how long should it run before it is used again?
   a. does not matter
   b. at least 15 minutes
   c. at least 30 minutes
   d. it should never be turned off

10. Which is not a correct statement regarding clean rooms?
    a. Must be a designated area of the pharmacy.
    b. Must have restricted air flow.
    c. Must accommodate most of the equipment for aseptic compounding.
    d. Must have proper storage of supplies.

REVIEW

11. Which must be used to create and maintain a sterile environment?
    a. ISO Class 5 laminar flow hood
    b. aseptic technique
    c. positive pressure clean room
    d. none of the above

12. Aseptic techniques are methods used to maintain
    a. pH.
    b. sterility of sterile products.
    c. osmotic pressure.
    d. pyrogens.

13. When using the laminar flow hood, a technician should work inside the hood at least
    a. two inches.
    b. four inches.
    c. six inches.
    d. eight inches.

14. Why is air generally injected into a vial before a volume of solution is removed?
    a. Keeps the drug dissolved in the solution.
    b. Provides a negative pressure in the vial so the solution will not spray when the needle is removed.
    c. Helps withdraw the solution by pressurizing the vial.
    d. Prevents the vial closure from coring.

15. When opening an ampule, snap the ampule neck
    a. toward the HEPA filter.
    b. away from the HEPA filter but toward sterile supplies that have been swabbed with an alcohol pad.
    c. toward the HEPA filter but away from sterile supplies that have not been swabbed with an alcohol pad.
    d. away from the HEPA filter or any other sterile supplies.

16. You are to use 2.4 ml of diluent to reconstitute a vial of medication. What size of syringe should be used?
    a. 20 ml
    b. 10 ml
    c. 5 ml
    d. 3 ml

17. Which part of an administration set is used to set the flow rate?
    a. spike
    b. volume control chamber
    c. Flashball
    d. needle adapter

18. Peristaltic, cassette, and elastomeric pumps are examples of
    a. automixers.
    b. positive pressure pumps.
    c. controllers.
    d. administration sets.

19. Incompatibilities between a drug and a base IV fluid are evident when _____ is observed.
    a. a precipitate
    b. gas evolution
    c. a color change
    d. all of the above

20. Visual inspection of parenteral solutions can show the presence of _____ and _____.
    a. particle contamination, precipitation
    b. pH, precipitation
    c. chemical degradation of a drug, osmolarity
    d. pyrogens, precipitation

21. Which concentration term used with parenteral solutions does not use the drug's molecular weight to determine its value?
    a. molarity
    b. osmoles
    c. equivalents
    d. percentage weight per volume

9

COMPOUNDING

COMPOUNDING

Extemporaneous compounding is the on-demand preparation of a drug product according to a physician's prescription to meet the unique needs of an individual patient.

Compounding has always been a component of Pharmacy. There is an art involved in using raw ingredients to formulate a drug product that meets the special needs of particular patients. It requires specialized knowledge of the physical and chemical properties of drugs and their vehicles. It also requires proper training and skill. This chapter will focus on the terminology, equipment, and basic principles of extemporaneous compounding.

There are various aspects of compounding.

It can mean the preparation of suspensions, dermatologicals, and suppositories; the conversion of one dosage form into another; the preparation of select dosage forms from bulk chemicals; the preparation of intravenous admixtures, parenteral nutrition solutions, and pediatric dosage forms from adult dosage forms; the preparation of radioactive isotopes; or the preparation of cassettes, syringes, and other devices for administering drugs in the home.

The demand for pharmaceutical compounding has grown substantially.

Reasons for this include the growth of home health care, the unavailability of certain drug products, orphan drugs, veterinary compounding, and biotechnology derived drug products. Newly evolving dosage forms and therapies also suggest that compounding will become more common in pharmacy practice.

Technicians, under pharmacist supervision, are increasingly involved in compounding.

Specific responsibilities will vary from environment to environment. Therefore, it is necessary to know and understand the specific responsibilities and requirements that apply to your job.

SPECIAL NEEDS

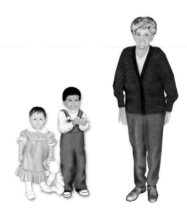

Compounding is done for many special reasons, including:

- ➡ Pediatric patients requiring diluted adult strengths of drugs;

- ➡ patients needing an oral solution or suspension of a product that is only available in another form;

- ➡ patients with sensitivity to dyes, preservatives, or flavoring agents found in commercial formulations;

- ➡ dermatological formulations with fortified (strengthened) or diluted concentrations of commercially available products;

- ➡ specialized dosages for therapeutic drug monitoring;

- ➡ care for hospice patients in pain management;

- ➡ compounding for animals.

Chapter <795> regulations from USP/NF pertaining to the nonsterile compounding of formulations.

Chapter <797> regulations from USP/NF pertaining to the sterile compounding of formulations.

COMPOUNDING AND MANUFACTURING

There are many guidelines published by federal and state agencies that pertain to compounding. These guidelines address topics ranging from the definition of compounding to specifications for compounding equipment and personal training. The USP has defined compounding and manufacturing as follows:

Compounding is "the preparation, mixing, assembling, packaging, or labeling of a drug or device in accordance with a licensed practitioner's prescription under an initiative based on the practitioner /patient/pharmacist/compounder relationship in the course of professional practice."

Manufacturing is "the production, propagation, conversion, or processing of a drug or device, either directly or indirectly, by extraction of the drug from substances of natural origin or by means of chemical or biological synthesis.

Manufacturing also includes (1) any packaging or repackaging of the substance(s) or labeling or relabeling of containers for the promotion and marketing of such drugs or devices; (2) any preparation of a drug or device that is given or sold for resale by pharmacies, practitioners, or other persons; (3) the distribution of inordinate amounts of compounded preparations or the copying of commercially available drug products; and (4) the preparation of any quantity of a drug product without a licensed prescriber/patient/pharmacist/compounder relationship."

Compounding is the result of a practitioner's prescription order based on the practitioner-patient-pharmacist relationship.

Compounding is regulated by the State Boards of Pharmacy and the U.S. Pharmacopeia.

The USP has the federal authority to set standards pertaining to pharmacy compounding. This authority was established in the 1906 Pure Food and Drugs Act. Many state boards of pharmacy accept USP standards as their standards, but some states have made their own regulations.

In the last several years, the USP has been extremely active in setting standards for compounding.

Expert committees have been created and charged with the responsibility of developing standards for compounding nonsterile and sterile products. Standards on various topics are grouped into "chapters" and published annually in the resource book called the USP/NF. Chapters are assigned numbers that detail their legal enforceability. Those chapters numbered below 1000 are legally enforceable by the FDA. Those above 1000 can be considered guidelines.

In 2000, *Chapter <795>*, Pharmaceutical Compounding—Nonsterile Preparations, was published, making these standards enforceable.

Chapter <797>, Pharmaceutical Compounding—Sterile Preparations, became official in 2004. The USP/NF has over 60 chapters that pertain to compounding such as Containers <661>; Good Compounding Practices <1075>; Pharmaceutical Stability <1150>; and Pharmaceutical Dosage Forms <1151>.

Overall, the USP/NF provides a broad base of regulations and guidelines to direct the practice of compounding.

Another significant inclusion in the USP/NF is monographs of the most commonly compounded preparations used in practice. These "official" formulations have the advantage of USP/NF's testing, quality assurance, and beyond-use date assignment. Therefore, when a formulation is compounded as described in a monograph, the stability can be assumed to be identical to that stated in the monograph, and the beyond-use date assignment given in the monograph can be applied to the compounded formulation. The USP/NF has published over 150 monographs.

COMPOUNDING REGULATIONS

Regulations on Compounding in a Pharmacy

The USP establishes standards of quality, strength, purity, packaging, and labeling for medications. Currently, the USP provides standards for more than 3,700 prescription and non-prescription drugs, nutritional and dietary supplements, and medical devices. It also provides additional standards for personnel, facilities, and record keeping. Summaries of significant parts of these standards are given here. The technician should consult the USP/NF for further information and additional regulations.

Personnel

The standards give the responsibility and authority for the management of the compounding area to the pharmacist. They outline the duties of the pharmacist and the pharmacist's responsibilities for other personnel in the compounding area. These standards also list the qualifications a pharmacist must have to compound and recommends further training and continuing education responsibilities.

Facilities and Equipment

The standards go into great detail about the physical design and maintenance of the compounding area. They specify that the compounding area, either nonsterile or sterile, should be a designated area away from the "routine dispensing and counseling functions and high traffic areas" of the pharmacy. The standards also recommend compounding equipment that should be in the compounding area.

Ingredient Standards

Raw chemicals are supplied in many levels of purity. The table below summarizes some of the different purity classifications applied to chemicals (from least pure to most pure). It is desired that USP or NF grade be the "lowest" grade of purity used in compounding; if that grade is not available, then a "higher" grade of purity can be used if deemed acceptable by the pharmacist.

Quality Assurance and Quality Control

QA is a program of activities used to assure that the procedures used in compounding a product lead to products that comply with specifications and standards. QC is a set of testing procedures that determine the quality of the compounded formulation.

Grade of Chemical	Description
Technical (commercial)	Commercial or industrial quality, generally of indeterminate quality
CP (chemically pure)	More refined than technical grade, but still of unknown quality; only partial analytical information available
USP/NF	Meets standards set by the USP/NF
FCC	Meets specifications of Food Chemical Codex
ACS reagent	High purity; meets specifications of the Reagent Chemicals Committee of the American Chemical Society
AR (analytical reagent)	Very high purity
HPLC	Very high purity; used in high pressure chromatography
Spectroscopic grade	Very high purity
Primary standard	Highest purity; used in standard solutions for analytical purposes

formulation record formulas and procedures (i.e., recipes) for what should happen when a formulation is compounded.

compounding record a record of what actually happened when the formulation was compounded.

Packaging and Storage

The pharmacist is responsible for the appropriate packaging of compounded formulations. The appropriate container will depend on the physical and chemical properties of the compounded formulation and its intended use. Packaging materials should not chemically react with any drug or ingredient in the formulation. Other packaging considerations include its strength, visibility, moisture protection, ease of use, and cost.

The pharmacist is also responsible for the storage of all ingredients, drugs, supplies, and formulations in the compounding area. Materials used in compounding should be stored according to the manufacturers' labeling or USP/NF requirements. Materials should be marked with the date of receipt and the date the container is opened, and the materials should be rotated to use the oldest stock first. Materials should not be used beyond their expiration date. Materials that specify storage temperatures use the definitions listed in the table below.

Documentation and Record Keeping

Documentation and record keeping provide information that is directly applicable to the formulation being compounded. They provide a basis for professional judgement and for legal liability. They also provide for consistency when formulations are compounded over and over again. And if there is a problem in the formulation, they provide a mechanism to systematically review procedures and ingredients.

The guidelines recommend that four sets of records be kept in the compounding area:

➥ a **formulation record** (compounding formulas and procedures, a master sheet, a "recipe")—what should happen when the formulation is compounded;

➥ a **compounding record**—what actually happened when the formulation was compounded;

➥ standard operating procedures (SOPs) for equipment maintenance, equipment calibration, handling and disposal of supplies, etc.;

➥ ingredients records with certificates of purity and MSDSs (Material Safety Data Sheets).

Note: Sample document templates for a formulation record, a compounding record, and standard operating procedures are in Chapter Nine of *The Pharmacy Technician Workbook and Certification Review, Fourth Edition* that accompanies this text.

Storage Temperature Definitions

Freezer	-20°C to -10°C
Protect from Freezing	Store above 0°C
Cold	Any temperature not exceeding 8°C
Refrigerator	Between 2°C and 8°C
Cool	Between 8°C and 15°C
Room Temperature	Temperature in the work area
Controlled Room Temperature	Thermostatically controlled at 20°C to 25°C
Warm	Between 30°C and 40°C
Excessive Heat	Any temperature above 40°C

COMPOUNDING CONSIDERATIONS

Compounding considerations are "questions to ask" before, during, and after the compounding process. For example, there must be an initial decision if it is necessary to compound the prescription. Then there are numerous factors to consider as the prescription is compounded, and finally there are records and checks that must be completed after the compounding is completed. Below is a summary of these considerations. The pharmacy technician will be involved in each of these considerations.

Whether to Compound

➡ Is there a commercial product already available?

➡ If yes, are the commercial product's ingredients different from the prescription so that the product cannot be used?

➡ If no, the pharmacist should determine what is the purpose of the prescription. Can the purpose be achieved without having to compound a product?

Before Beginning the Compounding Process

➡ Is the pharmacy personnel qualified to prepare this prescription?

➡ Are the proper equipment and supplies available?

➡ Can the drug and ingredient identity, quality, and purity be assured?

➡ Is there literature information about the formulation to help determine an appropriate beyond-use date?

➡ What basic quality control measures will be used to assure the prescription is compounded correctly?

➡ Does the patient have the necessary skills to use and store the prescription?

As the Prescription is Being Compounded

➡ Read and interpret the prescription.

➡ Determine a preliminary compounding procedure.

➡ Collect and prepare the required ingredients, drugs, supplies, equipment, and clothing.

➡ Package the formulation in an appropriate container and affix appropriate labels.

➡ Perform quality control procedures.

After Compounding

➡ Recheck all work.

➡ If the compounded formulation is new to the pharmacy, keep a sample or make a second batch to assess its stability or appearance over the expected time of therapy.

➡ Document the compounding process.

➡ Deliver the product to the patient with appropriate consultation.

➡ Return ingredients, supplies, etc., to their proper locations. Perform required equipment maintenance.

 stability the chemical and physical integrity of the dosage form, and when appropriate, its ability to withstand microbiological contaminations.

STABILITY & BEYOND-USE DATES

Stability is defined as "the extent to which a dosage form retains, within specified limits, and throughout its period of storage and use (i.e., its shelf-life), the same properties and characteristics that it possessed at the time of its manufacture."

A beyond-use date is different than an expiration date. Expiration dates are required on commercially manufactured products and are determined after extensive study of the product's stability. Most expiration dates are in the order of "years." Beyond-use dates are used for compounded preparations only and are generally in the order of "days" or "months."

Assigning a Beyond-Use Date

It is not possible to use a manufacturer's expiration date and "extrapolate" or "estimate" a beyond-use date for a compounded formulation. The compounded formulation probably will not be identical to the manufactured product. It may have a different drug concentration, use different diluents, be a different fill volume, and packaged in a different container type.

When assigning a beyond-use date, follow these procedures.

➥ When possible, beyond-use dates should be in accordance with the manufacturer's approved labeling. This means that the product was formulated according to the manufacturer's directions, or that the formulation contains the same concentration of drug, in the same diluent, in the same packaging, for the same intended period of use, etc. If the formulation is an "official" USP/NF compounded preparation, the beyond-use date and packaging requirements are given in the monograph.

➥ When the above is not possible, use drug-specific and general stability documentation from reference books or primary literature.

➥ Published references often do not evaluate exactly the same formulation, or a study may not have examined the stability for a long enough period of time. In these cases, USP/NF Chapter <795> gives the following maximum recommended beyond-use dates for nonsterile compounded products:

Nonaqueous liquids and solid formulations

➥ If the source of the active drug is a manufactured drug product, the beyond-use date is not later than 25% of the time remaining until the drug product's expiration date, or 6 months, whichever is earlier.

➥ If the source of the active drug is a USP or NF substance, the beyond-use date is not later than 6 months.

Water containing formulations

➥ When prepared from ingredients in solid form, the beyond-use date should be not later than 14 days when stored at cold temperature.

For all other formulations

➥ The beyond-use date is not later than the intended duration of therapy or 30 days, whichever is earlier.

	Risk Level	Room Temperature	Refrigeration	Freezer
USP/NF Chapter <797> gives these maximum beyond-use dates for sterile compounded drug products that are *not* tested for sterility.	Low	48 hours	14 days	45 days
	Medium	30 hours	9 days	45 days
	High	24 hours	3 days	45 days

EQUIPMENT

Each individual compounded prescription can be viewed as a four step process: measure, mix, mold, and package.

Not all steps are needed in every compounded prescription, but they indicate the type of equipment necessary for compounding.

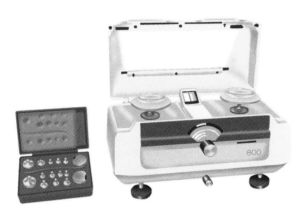

TYPES OF EQUIPMENT

For Measuring

Balance, weights, weighing containers, volumetric glassware (graduates, pipets, flasks, syringes).

For Mixing

Beakers, Erlenmeyer flasks, spatulas, funnels, sieves, mortar and pestle.

For Molding

Hot plates, suppository molds, capsule shells, ointment slabs.

For Packaging

Prescription bottles, capsule vials, suppository boxes, ointment jars.

Class A Prescription Balances

A balance is used to determine the weight of a powder, dosage form, liquid, etc. Most pharmacies have a Class A prescription balance. The Class A balance is a 2 pan torsion type balance that uses both internal and external weights. The balance has a rider which adds the internal weights to the right hand pan. The rider is always **calibrated** in the metric system (grams), though some riders also have calibration marks in the apothecary system (grains).

Sensitivity

Class A balances have a sensitivity requirement of up to 6 mg. The **sensitivity** of a balance is the amount of weight that will move the balance pointer one division mark on the marker plate.

Capacity

Class A balances have a minimum weighable quantity of 120 mg of material with a 5% error. 5% is generally considered an acceptable error in most pharmaceutical processes. Most Class A balances have a maximum weighable quantity of 60 grams, though some will weigh up to 120 grams.

Weights

A proper set of metric weights is essential for prescription compounding. These are usually brass cylindrical weights ranging from 1 gram to 50 grams and fractional weights of 10 mg to 500 mg. Weights should be stored in their box. They must be handled with forceps (not with fingers!) to prevent soiling and erosion of the weights.

Small Quantities

When a prescription calls for less than 120 mg of an ingredient, a precise amount of the drug (greater than 120 mg) is mixed with an inert (inactive) powder so that a portion of the resulting mix weighing at least 120 mg will contain the amount of drug needed. This portion of the mixed powders is called an **aliquot**.

aliquot a portion of a mixture.

calibrate to set, mark, or check the graduations of a measuring device.

sensitivity the amount of weight that will move the balance pointer one division mark on the marker plate.

trituration the process of grinding powders to reduce particle size.

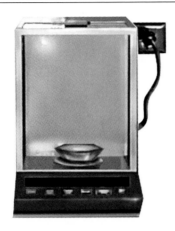

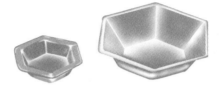

Electronic or Analytical Balance

Another method for weighing quantities smaller than 120 mg with acceptable accuracy is to use either an electronic or analytical balance. Electronic balances come in a variety of sizes and shapes. Most are top-loading balances and have sensitivities around 1 mg. Analytical balances may be found in some pharmacies, but are generally found in research laboratories. They have extremely high sensitivities and are designed to weigh milligram and microgram quantities of materials.

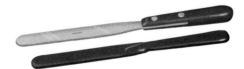

Spatulas

Spatulas are used to transfer solid ingredients. They are also used as the mixing instruments in semisolid dosage forms such as ointments and creams. Spatulas are available in a variety of sizes and are made of stainless steel, hard rubber, or plastic. Stainless steel spatulas can be corroded with certain materials such as iodine and in these cases, the rubber or plastic spatulas should be used. Always clean the spatulas before use.

Weighing Papers or Weighing Boats

Weighing papers or weighing boats should always be placed on the balance pans before any weighing is done. These protect the pans from damage and also provide a convenient way to transfer the weighed material from the balance to another vessel. Weighing papers are made of nonabsorbable glassine paper and weighing boats are made of polystyrene. When using weighing papers, the paper should be diagonally creased from each corner and then flattened and placed on the pans. This ensures a collection trough in the paper. New weighing papers or weighing boats should be used with each new drug weighing to prevent contamination.

Mortars and Pestles

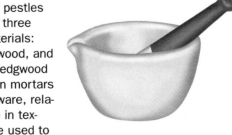

Mortars and pestles are made of three types of materials: glass, wedgwood, and porcelain. Wedgwood and porcelain mortars are earthenware, relatively coarse in texture, and are used to grind crystals and large particles into fine powders. The process of grinding powders to reduce the particle size is called **trituration**. Glass mortars and pestles are preferable for mixing liquids and semisolid dosage forms.

USING A BALANCE

Following are some general rules for using a balance and maintaining it in top condition.

✔ Always use the balance on a level surface and in a draft free area.

✔ Always use weighing papers or weighing boats. These protect the pans from abrasions, eliminate the need for repeated washing, and reduce loss of drug to porous surfaces.

✔ A clean weighing paper or boat should be used for each new ingredient to prevent cross-contamination of components.

✔ The balance must be readjusted after a new weighing paper or boat has been placed on a pan. Weighing papers taken from the same box can vary in weight by as much as 30 mg. Larger weighing boats can vary as much as 200 mg.

✔ Always arrest the balance before adding or removing weight from either pan. Although the balance is noted for its durability, repeated jarring of the balance will ultimately damage the working mechanism of the balance and reduce its accuracy.

✔ Use a spatula to add or remove ingredients from the balance. Do not pour ingredients out of the bottle.

✔ Always clean the balance, close the lid, and arrest the pans before storing the balance between uses.

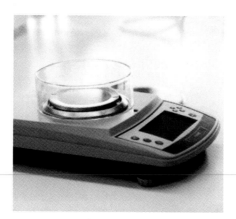

an electronic balance

USING AN ELECTRONIC BALANCE

Electronic balances have digital displays and may have internal calibration capabilities. These may either be top-loading or encased to protect the balance from dust and drafts. To use an electronic balance, follow these guidelines:

✔ Move the balance to a place in the compounding area where it will not have to be moved again during the day.

✔ Turn the leveling feet all the way into the balance and then move them in the same direction until the level bubble is within the black circle of the sight glass. If needed, further adjust one foot to center the bubble.

✔ Turn on the balance.

✔ For the first use of the day, check internal weight calibration.

✔ Remove the top ring of the draft shield (if present) and place the weighing boat in the center of the weighing pan. Replace the draft shield ring. Press TARE key and the balance should read 0.000 g.

✔ Add the ingredients to be weighed through the top ring of the draft shield. If necessary, remove the ring to add or remove some of the ingredient, and then replace the ring before reading the measurement.

✔ Use a lint-free towelette to clean any spills off the weighing boat.

✔ Turn off the balance at the end of the day.

arrest knob the knob on a balance that prevents any movement of the balance pans.

USING A PRESCRIPTION BALANCE

In order to obtain an accurate weight of components on the prescription balance, appropriate techniques must be used. The following steps should always be taken to ensure accuracy:

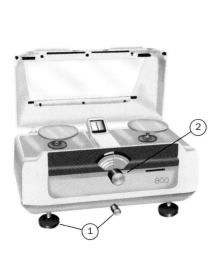

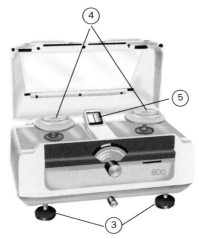

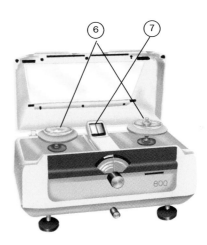

1. Lock the balance by turning the **arrest knob**. *Level the balance front to back* by turning the leveling screw feet all the way into the balance and then moving them the same direction until the 4 sides of the bottom of the balance are equidistant from the bench top. For balances with leveling bubbles, move the leveling screw feet until the bubble is in the middle of the tube.

2. Set the internal weights to zero. This is done by turning the calibrated dial (i.e., rider) to zero.

3. Unlock the balance and *level it left to right* by adjusting the leveling screw feet in opposite directions. To shift the pointer left, rotate the feet inward. To shift the pointer to the right, rotate the feet outward. Continue adjusting the screw feet slowly until the pointer rests at the center of the marker plate.

4. Lock the balance. Place a weighing boat or paper on each weighing pan. (If using weighing papers, fold diagonally and then gently flatten.)

5. Unlock the balance by releasing the arrest knob. If the pointer does not rest at the center of the marker plate, then level the balance from left to right to account for weight differences between the weighing boats or papers.

6. Lock the balance and place the required weights in the boat on the right pan. Place the material to be weighed in the boat on the left pan.

7. Unlock the balance and note the shift of the pointer on the marker plate. If the pointer shifts left, too much of the drug is on the pan and a portion should be removed. If it shifts right, there is too little drug and more should be added. Always arrest the balance when adding or removing material from the left pan.

8. Once you have made an accurate measurement, double check that you have weighed the correct substance (check the label) and that you have used the correct weights (internal and external).

VOLUMETRIC EQUIPMENT

In compounding, liquid drugs, solvents, or additives are measured in volumetric glassware or plasticware.

Volumetric means "measures volume." Common volumetric vessels are pipets, cylindrical and conical graduates, burets, syringes, and volumetric flasks. The volume capacity is etched on the vessel wall, and some devices will have graduation marks to measure partial volume.

Volumetric vessels are either "to deliver" (TD) or "to contain" (TC).

"To deliver" means that the vessel must be completely emptied to dispense the needed volume. Single volume pipets, syringes, droppers and some calibrated pipets are TD vessels. "To contain" means that the vessel does not need to be completely emptied to dispense the needed volume. Volumetric flasks and cylindrical and conical graduated cylinders and some calibrated pipets are TC vessels.

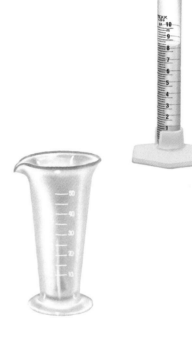

Graduated Cylinders

Graduated cylinders, both cylindrical and cone-shaped, are used for measuring and transferring liquids. Cylindrical graduates are the preferred device because they are more accurate. Graduated cylinders are available in sizes ranging from 5 ml to 4,000 ml. When selecting a graduated cylinder, always choose the smallest one capable of containing the volume to be measured. Avoid measurements of volumes that are below 20 percent of the capacity of the graduated cylinder because the accuracy is unacceptable. For example, a 100 ml graduated cylinder cannot accurately measure volumes below 20 ml. When measuring small volumes, such as 20 ml and less, it is often preferable to use a syringe or pipet.

Volumetric Flasks

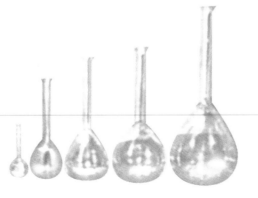

Volumetric flasks have slender necks and wide bulb-like bases. Volumetric flasks are single volume glassware and come in sizes ranging from 5 ml to 4,000 ml. There is a calibration mark etched on the neck of the flask. When the flask is filled to that mark, the flask contains that volume. Volumetric flasks are hard to use if dissolving solids in liquid because of the narrowness of the neck. If solids are to be dissolved in the flask, it is best to partially fill the flask with liquid, dissolve, and then fill the flask with more liquid to the calibration mark.

volumetric measures volume. Volumetric vessels are either TD (to deliver) or TC (to contain).

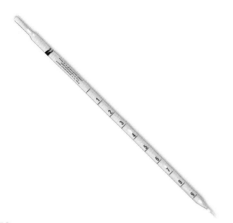

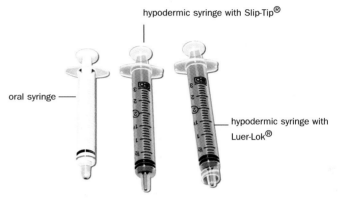

oral syringe

hypodermic syringe with Slip-Tip®

hypodermic syringe with Luer-Lok®

Pipets

Pipets are thin glass tubes recommended for the delivery of all volumes less than 5 ml and required for delivering volumes less than 1 ml (in the absence of an appropriate syringe). A rubber pipet bulb is used to draw liquid into the pipet. There are two basic types of pipets:

➡ The single volume or transfer pipet is the most accurate and simplest to use, but is limited to the measurement of a single fixed volume. They are normally used for the accurate transfer of 1.0, 2.0, 5.0, 10.0, and 25.0 ml of liquid.

➡ The calibrated pipet has several calibration marks from a point near the tip to the capacity of the pipet. It can deliver multiple volumes of liquid with good precision.

➡ A micropipet is a type of pipet with two parts, a hand piece and a disposal tip. The handle section usually has a turn screw that adjusts the volume of liquid drawn into the pipet tip. Each micropipet is calibrated for a range of volumes such as 1–20, 1–100, 1–200 or 1–1000 microliters. When determining which range to use, select the smallest range that will accommodate the volume of liquid to be measured.

Syringes

Syringes come in sizes from 0.5 ml to 60 ml and in a variety of materials and styles. For most compounding tasks involving small volumes, a disposable hypodermic syringe or an oral syringe made of plastic is used. Syringes have graduation marks on the barrel for measuring partial volumes. As when selecting a graduated cylinder, choose the smallest syringe capable of containing the volume to be measured.

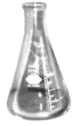 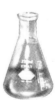

℞ Erlenmeyer flasks (right), beakers, and prescription bottles, regardless of markings, are *not volumetric glassware*, but are simply containers for storing and mixing liquids. The designated volume is only the *approximate* capacity of the vessel.

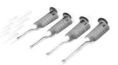

micropipets

LIQUID MEASUREMENT

Selecting a Liquid Measuring Device

✔ *Always use the smallest device (graduated cylinder, pipet, syringe) that will accommodate the desired volume of liquid.* This will minimize the potential for errors of measurement associated with misreading the scale.

✔ Use a calibrated pipet, micropipet, or syringe to measure/deliver volumes less than 1 ml.

✔ Remember that oily and viscous liquids will be difficult to remove from graduated cylinders and pipets, and at best require long drainage time. Consider using a syringe instead, or measuring by weight rather than volume.

✔ Never use prescription bottles, non-volumetric flasks, beakers, or household teaspoons as measurement devices.

✔ Liquids have a **meniscus** when they are poured into containers. The surface of the liquid curves downward toward the center. If the container is very narrow, the meniscus can be quite large. When reading a volume of a liquid against a graduation mark, *hold the measuring device so the meniscus is at eye level and read the mark at the bottom of the meniscus.* Viewing the level from above will create the incorrect impression that there is more volume in the measuring device.

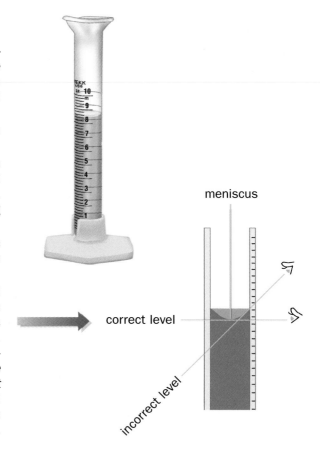

meniscus

correct level

incorrect level

Droppers

Medicine droppers can be used to deliver small doses of liquid medication. But the medicine dropper must first be calibrated because the drop size will vary from dropper to dropper and from liquid to liquid. Personal factors can also contribute to the inaccuracy of droppers. Two individuals dispensing the same liquid from identical droppers may produce drops of different sizes because of variations in the pressure, speed of dropping, and the angle at which the dropper is held.

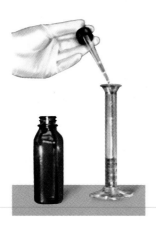

To calibrate a medicine dropper, slowly drop the drug formulation into a small cylindrical graduate (10 ml), and count the number of drops needed to add several milliliters (ml) to the graduated cylinder. Calculate the average number of drops per ml. Some commercially produced medications are packaged with a marked dropper which has already been calibrated for that preparation.

Graduated Cylinders

Cylindrical graduates are more accurate than conical ones. The following steps will help maximize accuracy when using either a cylindrical or conical graduate.

1. Either place the graduated cylinder on a flat surface that will allow you to view it at eye level or hold the graduated cylinder by the base with the left hand (for a right-handed person) and elevated so that the desired mark is at eye level.

2. Hold the solution container with the right hand and pour the liquid to be measured into the center of the graduated cylinder. This will minimize the liquid adhering to the wall of the graduated cylinder (especially viscous liquids).

3. As the surface of the liquid approaches the desired mark, decrease the pouring rate or use a dropper or pipet to bring the level to final volume. The final volume should be determined by aligning the bottom of the meniscus with the desired graduation mark.

4. Transfer the liquid from the graduated cylinder to the appropriate vessel or container, allowing about 15 seconds for aqueous and hydroalcoholic liquids to drain. Approximately 60 seconds (or more) will be required for more viscous liquids such as syrups, glycerin, propylene glycol, and mineral oil.

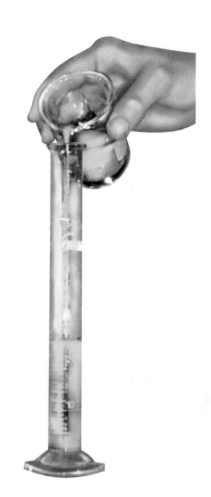

Special Precautions When Using Graduated Cylinders

✔ While graduated cylinders are volumetric devices, they are not mixing devices. They should not be used as a container for dissolving solids in liquids. A solution should first be prepared in a beaker or flask, and then placed in the graduated cylinder for final volume adjustments.

✔ Do not assume that the final volume of a prescription will be the sum of the individual volumes of ingredients. This is particularly important with the admixture of aqueous and nonaqueous solutions such as alcohol and water. When these solutions are mixed, the total volume is less than the sum of the two volumes.

 meniscus the curved surface of a column of liquid.

LIQUID MEASUREMENT
(cont'd)

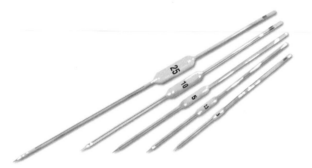

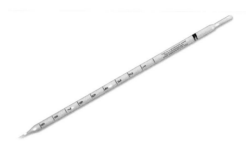

Single Volume Pipets

Single volume pipets have only one graduation mark, and that is the indicated volume of the pipet (e.g., 5 ml, 10 ml, etc.). As a result, the pipet is filled, and then emptied. There is no partial filling done with a single volume pipet. The steps in using a single volume pipet are:

1. Using a rubber bulb for suction, draw the liquid into the pipet until it is above the graduation mark.

2. Remove the pipet from the solution.

3. Wipe the end of the pipet with a tissue or Kimwipe®.

4. While holding the pipet in a vertical position, release the pressure inside the bulb and allow the liquid to flow into a waste beaker until the bottom of the meniscus coincides with the graduation mark. Droplets which remain suspended from the tip of the pipet can be removed by touching the pipet to the inside of the waste beaker.

5. Allow the pipet to drain for 30 seconds (or up to 3 minutes for viscous liquids) while touching the tip of the pipet to the inner side of the receiving vessel.

Calibrated Pipets

The calibrated pipet is filled and emptied the same way as a single volume pipet. However, it has multiple graduation marks that allow partial volumes to be transferred by noting the meniscus level before and after delivery. For example, you can deliver 1.50 ml of a liquid by filling the pipet to 8.50 ml and then allowing it to drain until the meniscus reaches 7.00 ml. A second delivery could be made by allowing the meniscus to reach 5.50 ml. The final graduation of the pipet is usually some distance above the pipet tip so that delivery is performed from graduation to graduation and not from graduation to tip as with the single volume pipet.

From a practical standpoint, *the calibrated pipet is the preferred pipet for compounding.* Just about any prescription requiring small volumes can be compounded with just three basic sizes of pipets: a 1 ml pipet subdivided in 1/100 ml graduations, a 2 ml pipet subdivided in 1/10 ml graduations, and a 5 ml pipet subdivided in 1/10 ml graduations.

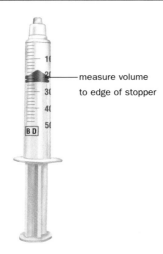

 measure volume
to edge of stopper

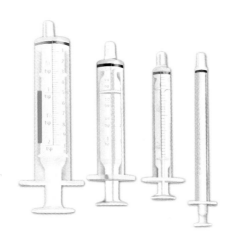

Syringes

Syringes come in a variety of sizes ranging from 0.5 ml (calibrated in 0.01 ml graduations) to 60 ml (calibrated in 2 ml graduations). Syringes may be used to deliver a wide range of liquid volumes with a high degree of accuracy. Measurements made with syringes are more accurate and precise than those made with cylindrical graduates. They are especially useful for measuring and delivering viscous liquids. Besides being easy to use, plastic disposable syringes are unbreakable and economical. Like graduated cylinders and pipets, select a syringe that equals or barely exceeds the volume to be measured.

Liquids are pulled into the syringe by pulling back on the plunger. The tip of the syringe must be fully submerged in the liquid to prevent drawing air into the syringe. Generally, an excess of solution is drawn into the syringe so that any air bubbles may be expelled by holding the syringe tip up, tapping the syringe until the air bubbles rise into the hub, and depressing the plunger to expel the air. This ensures that the hub will be completely filled with solution and the volume of delivery will be accurate.

Oral Syringes

Oral syringes are available for accurately administering liquid medication to the patient. They are especially useful when administering non-standard doses. Oral syringes have tips that are larger than tips on hypodermic syringes so needles cannot be placed on these syringes. After the dose is drawn into the syringe, a cap is placed on the tip to prevent leakage and prevent contamination.

Oral syringes can be used with a device called an Adapt-a-Cap®. Adapt-a-Caps® do not work with hypodermic syringes (i.e., Slip-Tip® or Luer-Lok®). The cap portion of the Adapt-a-Cap® screws onto the bottle containing the liquid, and the oral syringe is fitted into the other side of the cap. When the bottle is inverted, liquid can be withdrawn by pulling back on the syringe plunger. When the required volume has been withdrawn, the bottle is righted, and the syringe is removed from the Adapt-a-Cap®. There are different size caps to fit on bottles with different size openings.

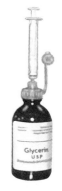

MIXING SOLIDS AND SEMISOLIDS

Mixing Powders

When mixing two powders of unequal quantity, a technique called **geometric dilution** is used. The smaller amount of powder is diluted in steps by additions of the larger amount of powder. If the two powders are just mixed together without this technique, a homogenous (fully and evenly combined) mixture will not result.

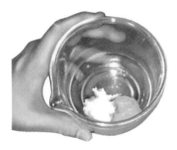 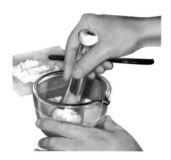 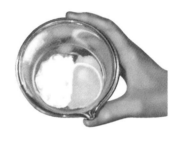

The smaller amount of powder is first triturated with an approximate equal portion of the larger amount of powder in a mortar. This first triturate is then mixed with an approximate equal portion of the larger amount of powder, and these are again triturated in the mortar. This dilution process is continued until all of the two powders have been mixed in the mortar.

Spatulation mixes powders using a spatula. The mixing can be done in a mortar, on an ointment slab, or in a plastic bag.

This method is used when mixing eutectic powders. Eutectic powders partially liquefy when they are brought together. First, the powders are mixed with a "carrier" powder (i.e., magnesium oxide, calcium carbonate, starch, lactose) and then blended by spatulation. Some eutectic compounds are aspirin, salicylic acid, camphor, benzocaine, and lidocaine.

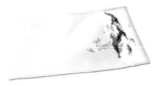

When powders are triturated together in a mortar with a pestle, the overall size of the particles is reduced. With spatulation, there is no particle size reduction so the powders must be of fine particle size and of uniform size before the process begins. There is also no pressure applied to the mixture when it is blended so the resulting blend is light and "fluffy."

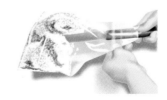

geometric dilution a technique for mixing two powders of unequal quantity.

spatulation mixing powders with a spatula.

levigation triturating a powder drug with a solvent in which it is insoluble to reduce its particle size.

Ointment Slabs

Some ointments and creams are prepared on ointment slabs which are porcelain or ground glass plates, often square or rectangular, that provide a hard nonabsorbable surface for mixing compounds. Spatulas are used to mix the ingredients of the formulation. Many times drugs are **levigated** prior to being incorporated into an ointment to reduce the grittiness of the final formulation.

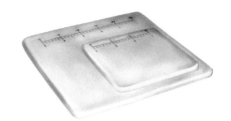

Levigation

Levigation is a technique used to reduce the particle size of a powder drug by triturating it with a solvent in which the drug is insoluble.

This is generally done before the drug is incorporated into a formulation such as a suspension, ointment, or suppository base.

For example, hydrocortisone (used in ointments) is levigated with glycerin before being incorporated into an ointment base. This reduces the size of the hydrocortisone particles so the resulting ointment will be smooth, not gritty.

Levigation can be done with a mortar and pestle or on an ointment slab.

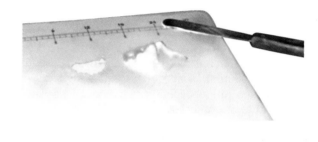

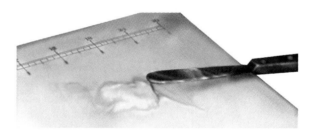

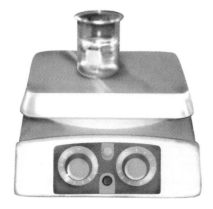

Hot Plates

Sometimes solids are mixed by melting them together in a beaker on a hot plate. The hot plate needs to be a special low temperature (25°C to 120°C) hot plate, and not a standard laboratory type hot plate; those hot plates heat at 125°C to 150°C at their lowest setting. If a low temperature hot plate is not available, a water bath or steam bath will suffice. Most solids and semisolids used in pharmaceutical compounding will completely melt by 70°C. The melt is removed from the hot plate and allowed to cool to room temperature with constant stirring using a stirring rod, spatula, or magnetic stirring bar. Forced cooling in cold water, ice water, or ice will change the consistency and texture of the final product.

SELECT DOSAGE FORMS

Aqueous Solutions

Solutions are probably the most commonly compounded products. Solutions are clear (but not necessarily colorless) liquids in which the drug is completely dissolved. The simplest compounded solution is the addition of a drug in liquid form to a liquid base solution called a "vehicle." This involves the careful measurement of the drug using graduated cylinders or syringes, and then diluting the drug to the final volume with the liquid vehicle. The resulting mixture should be thoroughly shaken or stirred to ensure adequate mixing. Purified water is the most common liquid used in pharmaceutical solutions, but combinations of ethanol, glycerin, propylene glycol, or a variety of syrups may be used, depending on the product requirements.

When solids are to be dissolved in solution, they must be carefully weighed using a prescription balance. Most solids dissolve easily in a solvent. However, some may need to be triturated first to reduce the particle size and increase the dissolution rate. Others require that the solvent be heated (but not overheated, since some drugs decompose at higher temperatures). Some drugs require vigorous shaking, stirring, or **sonication** (the application of sound waves using sonic mixing equipment) to affect dissolution.

The solubility of the drug must be known before attempting to dissolve it in a solution. If a drug is not soluble in a vehicle, then no amount of mixing will help.

The solubility of a drug in a solvent may be described in a variety of ways. References generally express the solubility in terms of the volume of solvent required to dissolve one gram of the drug. A small distinction, but an important one, needs to be made about these solubility values. The solubilities are given as grams of solute per milliliter of solvent, not per milliliter of final solution. If the concentration is going to be close to the solubility, this distinction may be relevant. Solubilities may also be expressed in more subjective terms such as those given in the table below from the USP/NF.

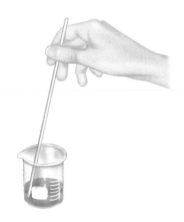

Most solutions require thorough shaking or stirring for adequate mixing.

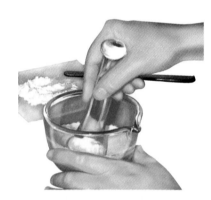

Some solids need to be triturated before mixing in a solution.

Descriptive Terms	Parts of Solvent Needed for 1 Part Solute
Very soluble	< 1
Freely soluble	1–10
Soluble	10–30
Sparingly soluble	30–100
Slightly soluble	100–1,000
Very slightly soluble	1,000–10,000
Practically insoluble or insoluble	> 10,000

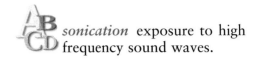

Syrups

A syrup is a concentrated or nearly saturated solution of sucrose in water. Syrups containing flavoring agents are known as flavoring syrups (e.g., Cherry Syrup, Acacia Syrup, etc.); medicinal syrups are those which contain drugs (e.g., Guaifenesin Syrup).

When a reduction in calories or sucrose properties is desired, syrups can be prepared from sugars other than sucrose (e.g., glucose, fructose), non-sugar polyols (e.g., sorbitol, glycerin, propylene glycol, mannitol), or other non-nutritive artificial sweeteners (e.g., aspartame, saccharin). Non-nutritive sweeteners do not produce the same viscosity as with sugars and polyols, so viscosity enhancers such as methylcellulose are added. Polyols, though less sweet than sucrose, produce good viscosity and have some preservative and solvent qualities. A 70% sorbitol solution is a commercially available syrup vehicle.

Syrups are primarily made by two methods, with or without heat. Using heat is a faster method, but it cannot be used with heat sensitive ingredients. When using heat, the temperature must be carefully controlled to avoid overheating sucrose and making the syrup darker in color and more likely to ferment. When making syrups without heat, stirring or shaking generally provides the energy to produce the solution. In this case, a mixing vessel that is about twice as large as the final volume of the product is needed to provide room for adequate mixing.

Nonaqueous Solutions

Nonaqueous solutions are those that contain solvents other than water, either alone or in addition to water. There are several types of nonaqueous solutions:

- elixir
- tincture
- spirit
- fluid extracts
- glycerates
- collodions
- liniments
- oleaginous solutions

Elixirs, collodions, and oleaginous solutions are the most commonly compounded nonaqueous solutions. Elixirs are clear, sweetened, hydroalcoholic liquids intended for oral use. Oleaginous solutions (e.g., corn oil, peanut oil, mineral oil) can be used for oral, topical, or parenteral administration. Collodions are limited to topical application. Because elixirs are hydroalcoholic solutions, they can be used to dissolve either alcohol soluble or water soluble drugs. Collodions and oleaginous solutions would be suitable for more lipophilic (i.e., oil loving) ingredients.

When compounding these formulations, separately dissolve the alcohol soluble ingredients in the alcohol (or oleaginous) portion and the water soluble ingredients in the water portion. Then add the aqueous solution to the alcohol solution, stirring constantly. This will keep the alcohol concentration as high as possible so that the final solution does not become turbid.

water soluble ingredients   alcohol soluble ingredients

pouring water soluble ingredients into alcohol soluble ingredients

SELECT DOSAGE FORMS
(cont'd)

Suspensions

The term suspension refers to a two phase system consisting of a finely divided solid dispersed in a liquid. The smallest particle size that can be suspended is approximately 0.1 micrometer. The primary concern in formulating suspensions is that they tend to settle over time, so the dose is unevenly dispersed in the liquid. A well-formulated suspension remains dispersed or settles very slowly, and can be redispersed easily with shaking. The settling properties of a suspension are controlled by (1) the addition of **flocculating agents** to enhance particle "dispersibility" and (2) the addition of **thickening agents** to reduce the settling (sedimentation rate) of the suspension.

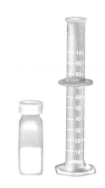

➡ Flocculating agents are electrolytes which carry an electrical charge. The flocculating agent imparts the electrical charge onto the suspended particle; since all of the particles will have the same charge, there is a slight repulsion between the particles as they settle. What results are clusters of particles or floccules which are loosely associated with each other and may be easily redispersed by shaking.

➡ Thickening agents are added to suspensions to thicken the suspending medium, thereby reducing the sedimentation rate of the floccules. Typical thickening agents include carboxymethylcellulose, methylcellulose, bentonite, and tragacanth.

To begin compounding a suspension, the solid drug to be suspended is levigated in a mortar with a pestle. This will reduce the drug's particle size. Common levigating agents are mineral oil or glycerin. Then, a portion of the vehicle is added to the mortar, and mixed with the levigated drug until a uniform mixture results. This mixture is then put into the final container or a volumetric measuring device. The mortar and pestle are rinsed with portions of the remaining vehicle, and each rinsing is added to the final container or volumetric measuring device until the final volume is reached. Suspensions should be dispensed in containers that contain enough air space for adequate shaking. The bottle should contain the auxiliary label "Shake well."

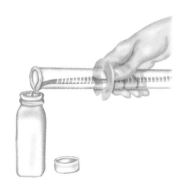

mixing

Some commercially available suspensions require reconstitution with water before they are dispensed. Water is added to the package container and shaken to form the suspension.

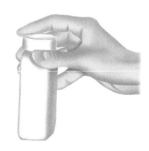

shaking

 flocculating agent electrolytes used in the preparation of suspensions to form particles that can be easily redispersed.

thickening agent an ingredient used in the preparation of suspensions to increase the viscosity of the liquid.

 Thickening agents are often referred to as viscosity enhancers or suspending agents.

Flavoring

The human tongue contains about 10,000 taste buds which distinguish salty, bitter, sour, and sweet tastes. The "flavor" experience is a complex combination of taste, smell, texture, appearance, and temperature. Most patients want:

➡ immediate flavor recognition;
➡ rapid full flavor development;
➡ acceptable mouth feel;
➡ short "after-taste";
➡ and no undesirable sensations.

Discovering the flavoring agent best suited to masking an unpleasant drug taste is often an empirical matter. It will also be patient dependent. For the basic tastes, several flavors have been found to work well.

Sweeteners

Some desired properties of sweeteners include colorless, odorless, solubility in water at the concentrations needed for sweetening, pleasant tasting with no "after-taste," and stable over a wide pH range. Simple Syrup, 70% sorbitol solution, sodium saccharin (0.05%), nutrasweet (0.1%), and dextrose have many of these properties.

When increasing the sweetness of a formulation that contains both a sweetening agent and a flavoring agent, increase the sweetener concentration first. All flavoring agents are bitter and need sweetening to make them more pleasing to the taste. If a desirable sweetness cannot be found by changing the sweetener concentration, then experiment with increasing the flavoring agent concentration.

Coloring

Coloring agents are not required in every formulation; they are contraindicated in all sterile solutions. However, clear, water-like oral solutions may be perceived to be inert or lack potency. Dark colors such as dark purple, navy, black, and brown may also be rejected because they are often associated with poisons. More pleasant, fruity colors are generally preferred and should be coordinated with flavors and scents (i.e., yellow with lemon, red with cherry). Flesh-toned colors may be added to topical preparations so the product is less visible on the skin.

From a practical standpoint, the pharmacy technician may consider food colorings sold in grocery stores to be safe and appropriate to use. These are red, blue, yellow, or green aqueous solutions and are ideally suited to coloring aqueous solutions. Blends may be used to produce nearly any color.

Taste	Flavor
Salty	Cinnamon, raspberry, orange, butterscotch
Sweet	Fruit, berry, vanilla
Bitter	Cocoa, chocolate, mint, cherry, walnut
Sour/Acid	Fruit, citrus, cherry
Oily	Wintergreen, peppermint, lemon, anise
Metallic	Mint, marshmallow

Sweetener	Sweetness Compared to Sucrose (Approx.)
Sorbitol	0.5–0.7
Mannitol	0.7
Saccharin	500
Sodium Saccharin	300
Aspartame	180
Stevia	200

SELECT DOSAGE FORMS (cont'd)

Emulsions

An emulsion is an unstable system consisting of at least two **immiscible** liquids, one of which is dispersed in the form of small droplets throughout the other, and a stabilizing agent. The dispersed liquid is known as the internal or discontinuous phase, whereas the liquid serving as the dispersion medium is known as the external or continuous phase.

When oils, petroleum hydrocarbons, and/or waxes are the dispersed phase, and water or an aqueous solution is the continuous phase, the system is called an **oil-in-water (o/w) emulsion**. An o/w emulsion is generally formed if the aqueous phase makes up greater than 45% of the total weight, and a **hydrophilic emulsifier** is used.

When water or aqueous solutions are dispersed in an oleaginous (oil based) medium, the system is known as a **water-in-oil (w/o) emulsion**. W/O emulsions are generally formed if the aqueous phase constitutes less than 45% of the total weight and an **lipophilic emulsifier** is used.

Emulsifiers

Emulsions will separate into two distinct phases or layers over time. Some separation can be overcome with shaking. However, some separations result in emulsions that "break" and these cannot be redispersed. Emulsions are stabilized by adding an emulsifier or emulsifying agents. Emulsifiers provide a protective barrier around the dispersed droplets. Some commonly used emulsifying agents include tragacanth, sodium lauryl sulfate, sodium dioctyl sulfosuccinate, and polymers known as the Spans® and Tweens®.

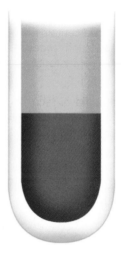

emulsion before mixing

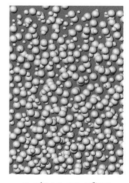

a close-up after mixing

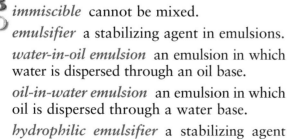

immiscible cannot be mixed.

emulsifier a stabilizing agent in emulsions.

water-in-oil emulsion an emulsion in which water is dispersed through an oil base.

oil-in-water emulsion an emulsion in which oil is dispersed through a water base.

hydrophilic emulsifier a stabilizing agent for water-based dispersion mediums.

lipophilic emulsifier a stabilizing agent for oil based dispersion mediums.

 Stabilizing agents used in emulsions are called emulsifiers, surfactants, or surface active agents.

Methods for Preparing Emulsions: Continental (Dry Gum), Wet Gum, and Beaker

There are various methods used to make emulsions. Each requires that energy be put into the system in the form of either shaking, heat, or the action of a mortar and pestle.

The Continental method is one method for preparing emulsions. This is sometimes referred to as the Dry Gum method. In this method, the initial or **primary emulsion** is formed from oil, water, and a "gum" type emulsifier which is usually acacia. The primary emulsion is formed from 4 parts oil, 2 parts water, and 1 part emulsifier. The 4 parts oil and 1 part emulsifier represent their total amounts for the final product. In a dry wedgwood or porcelain mortar, the 1 part gum is triturated with the 4 parts oil until the powder is thoroughly levigated. Then the 2 parts water are added, and the mixture is vigorously and continually triturated until the primary emulsion is formed (usually 1–2 minutes). It appears as creamy white and produces a "cracking" sound as it is triturated. Additional ingredients are incorporated after the primary emulsion is formed, and the product is then brought to the final volume with the external phase vehicle.

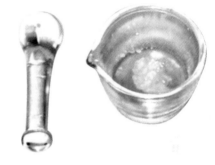

gum and water in preparation for the Wet Gum method

In the Wet Gum method, the primary emulsion is formed by triturating the 1 part gum with 2 parts water to form a **mucilage,** and then slowly adding the 4 parts oil, in portions, with trituration after each addition. After all the oil is added, the mixture is triturated for several minutes to form the primary emulsion. Then other ingredients may be added as in the Continental method.

Some emulsions will have a consistency of a lotion or a cream (i.e., a semisolid). The method of choice in making these types of emulsions is the beaker method. The ingredients of the formulation are divided into water soluble and oil soluble components. All oil soluble components are dissolved in one beaker and all water soluble components are dissolved in a separate beaker. Both phases are then heated to approximately 70°C using a low temperature hot plate or steam bath. The two beakers are removed from the heat, and the internal phase is slowly added to the external phase with continual stirring. The product is allowed to cool to room temperature but is constantly stirred with a stirring rod, spatula, or magnetic stirring bar.

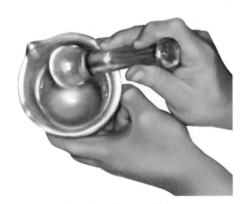

forming the mucilage

primary emulsion the initial emulsion to which ingredients are added to create the final product.

mucilage a wet, slimy liquid formed as an initial step in the wet gum method.

SELECT DOSAGE FORMS (cont'd)

Ointments

Ointments are used for many different purposes, e.g., as protectants, antiseptics, emollients, antipruritics, kerotolytics, and astringents.

One major type of compounded ointment is a simple mixture of an active drug in an ointment base. There are five types of ointment bases ranging from oleaginous to water **miscible**. A particular ointment base is chosen for its fundamental properties, or for its potential to serve as a drug delivery vehicle.

If the base ointment base is to be a drug delivery vehicle, the primary consideration will be its ability to release drug. Oleaginous (oil based) bases generally release substances slowly and unpredictably, since water cannot penetrate them well enough to dissolve the drug and allow for diffusion out of the ointment. Water miscible or aqueous bases tend to release drugs more rapidly.

These types of ointments are generally compounded on an ointment slab. In the simple case of combining two ointments or a drug and an ointment, each component is carefully weighed and placed on an ointment slab. The ingredients are combined by geometric dilution using two spatulas to mix the ointment. One spatula will be used to continually remove ointment from the other spatula. Using a spatula, the ointment is transferred into an ointment jar just big enough for the final volume. When filling the ointment jar, use the spatula to bleed out air pockets. Wipe any excess material from the outside of the jar, including the cap screw threads.

Drugs in powder or crystal form, such as salicylic acid, precipitated sulfur, or hydrocortisone need to be triturated or levigated in a mortar with a pestle before incorporating them into an ointment base. This will prevent a gritty texture in the final product. Another technique to reduce particle size is to dissolve the drug in a very small amount of solvent and then let the solvent evaporate.

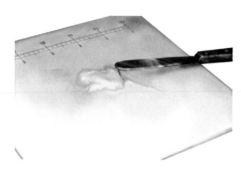

Ointments are generally compounded on an ointment slab.

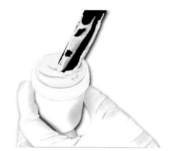

transferring ointment into an ointment jar

Properties of Ointment Bases

Property	Oleaginous Bases	Absorption Bases	Water/Oil Emulsion Bases	Oil/Water Emulsion Bases	Water Miscible Bases
Water Content	anhydrous	anhydrous	hydrous	hydrous	hydrous
Spreadability	difficult	difficult	moderate to easy	easy	moderate to easy
Washability	nonwashable	nonwashable	non- or poorly washable	washable	washable
Greasiness	greasy	greasy	greasy	nongreasy	nongreasy
Occlusiveness	yes	yes	sometimes	no	no
Examples	White Petrolatum, White Ointment	Hydrophilic Petrolatum, Aquaphor®	Hydrous Lanolin, Eucerin®, Nivea®	Hydrophilic Ointment	PEG Ointment

miscible capable of being mixed together.

Another major type of compounded ointment is one where the base is formed as part of the compounding process. The general scenario is to heat oleaginous type ingredients in one beaker and aqueous type ingredients in another beaker, and then combine the two phases and let the mixture congeal.

Following are some suggestions for compounding an ointment base:

➥ When heat is used to melt ingredients, use a water bath or special low temperature hot plate. Most ingredients used in ointment bases will liquefy around 70°C. Some common substances used in base formulations and their melting points are given in the table below.

➥ It is helpful to heat the aqueous phase a few degrees higher than the oil phase prior to mixing. The aqueous phase tends to cool faster than the oil phase. However, use the lowest temperature possible and keep the time of heating as short as possible. This will minimize the quantity of water lost through evaporation.

➥ When melting a number of ingredients, melt the ingredient with the highest melting point first. Then gradually reduce the heat to melt the ingredient with the next highest melting point. Continue this process until all ingredients have been added. This will ensure that the ingredients were exposed to the lowest possible temperature and thus enhance the stability of the final product.

➥ The cooling step in an ointment's preparation is an important part of the compounding process.

✔ Do not accelerate the cooling process by putting the melt in water or ice. This can significantly change the consistency of the final product.

✔ If adding volatile ingredients such as oils, flavors, or drugs, add them when the product is cool. The melt will still be fluid enough for adequate mixing but not hot enough to evaporate the ingredient.

✔ Ointments should be cooled until just a few degrees above solidification before they are poured into tubes or jars. This will minimize "layering" of the ointment in the packaging container.

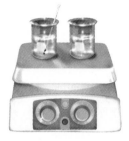

beakers, hot plate, thermometer

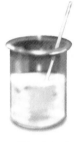

beaker after pouring the two phases together and allowing them to congeal with continuous stirring

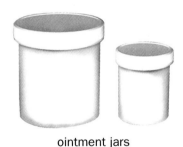

ointment jars

Ingredient	Melting Point (°C)	Ingredient	Melting Point (°C)
Carnauba wax	81–86	Stearic acid	69–70
Cetyl alcohol	45–50	Stearyl alcohol	55–60
Cetyl esters wax	43–47	White wax (Beeswax)	62–65
Cholesterol	147–150	PEG 1500	44–48
Cocoa butter	30–35	PEG 3350	54–58
Glyceryl monostearate	55	PEG 6000	58–63

SELECT DOSAGE FORMS (cont'd)

Suppositories

There are three classes of suppository bases defined by their composition and physical properties:

➡ Oleaginous bases

➡ Water soluble or miscible bases

➡ Hydrophilic bases

Oleaginous Bases

A well-known oleaginous base is cocoa butter (Theobroma Oil) USP. At room temperature, cocoa butter is a solid, but at body temperature, it melts to a bland, non-irritating oil. Cocoa butter is no longer the base of choice because preparing suppositories with it is difficult, and the suppositories require refrigeration. Synthetic triglycerides can be used that do not have the formulation difficulties of cocoa butter, but they are more expensive. There are also newer bases composed of mixtures of fatty acids that do not have the formulation problems or the expense (e.g., FattiBase®, Witepsol®).

Water Soluble or Miscible Bases

Water soluble or miscible bases contain glycerinated gelatin or polyethylene glycol (PEG) polymers. Glycerinated gelatin is a useful suppository base, particularly for vaginal suppositories. Glycerinated gelatin suppositories are gelatinous solids that tend to dissolve slowly to provide prolonged release of active ingredients. Polyethylene glycol (PEGs) polymers are chemically stable, non-irritating, miscible with water and mucous secretions, and can be formulated by molding or compression in a wide range of hardnesses and melting points. Like glycerinated gelatin, they do not melt at body temperature, but dissolve slowly to provide a prolonged release of drugs.

Polyethylene glycols are available in various molecular weight ranges. Those of 200, 400, or 600 molecular weight are liquids. Those with molecular weights over 1,000 are solids. Certain PEGs may be used individually as suppository bases but, more commonly, formulas call for combinations of two or more molecular weights mixed in various proportions to give a desired hardness or dissolution time. Since PEGs suppositories dissolve in body fluids and need not be formulated to melt at body temperature, they can be formulated with much higher melting points and can be safely stored at room temperature.

Hydrophilic Bases

Hydrophilic bases are mixtures of oleaginous and water miscible bases. They generally contain a small percentage of cholesterol or lanolin to assist in water absorption.

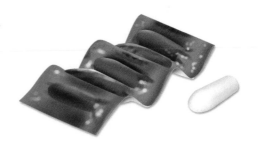

Some PEG Formulations

Molecular Weight	Percent
PEG 300	60%
PEG 8000	40%
PEG 300	48%
PEG 6000	52%
PEG 1000	95%
PEG 3350	5%
PEG 1000	75%
PEG 3350	25%
PEG 300	10%
PEG 1540	65%
PEG 3350	25%
PEG 8000	50%
PEG 1540	30%
PEG 400	20%
PEG 3350	60%
PEG 1000	30%
PEG 400	10%

compression molding a method of making suppositories in which the ingredients are compressed in a mold.

fusion molding a suppository preparation method in which the active ingredients are dispersed or dissolved in a melted suppository base.

Molding Methods

Suppositories are usually prepared by **compression molding** or **fusion molding.** Compression molding is a method of preparing suppositories by mixing the suppository base and the drug ingredients and forcing the mixture into a special compression mold.

Fusion molding is a method in which the drug is dispersed or dissolved in a melted suppository base. The fusion method can be used with all types of suppositories and must be used with most of them. In this method, the suppository base is melted on a low temperature hot plate, and the drug is dissolved or dispersed in the melted base. The mixture is then removed from the heat, and poured into a suppository mold, over filling each cavity. The mixture is allowed to congeal (harden), and the excess material is removed from the top of the mold.

Suppository Molds

There are many types of suppository molds: metal (aluminum or steel) molds, plastic molds, or rubber molds. The metal molds come in a variety of cavity sizes, from six to one hundred. The two halves of the mold are held together with screws. When the suppository mixture has congealed, the excess mass on top of the suppository mold can be removed with a hot spatula or knife scraped flat across the surface of the mold. The screws on the mold are loosened, and the mold is separated. Never open a mold by prying it apart with a knife or spatula. This will damage the matching mold faces which have been accurately machined to give a tight seal. The suppositories are removed from the mold, generally wrapped in foil paper, and put in a suppository box.

Plastic suppository molds come in long strips and can be torn into any number of cavities. When the suppository has hardened in the cavity, the plastic mold is heat sealed, torn into individual suppository cavities, and put in a suppository box. Rubber molds come in long strips but cannot be separated into individual cavities. Suppositories are allowed to remain in the mold (i.e, unwrapped), and the entire mold is put in the dispensing box.

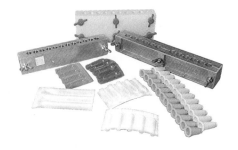

types of suppository molds

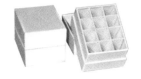

a suppository box

Polyethylene glycol polymers (PEGs) are used in a wide variety of formulations. Low molecular weight PEGs (<1,000) are liquids and impart a softer texture to the formulation. High molecular weight PEGs (>1,000) are solids and add stiffness to the formulation.

SELECT DOSAGE FORMS
(cont'd)

Capsules

Hard gelatin capsules consist of a body and a cap which fits firmly over the body of the capsule. For human use, eight sizes of capsules are available. If the capsule is to be filled with a liquid then the volume of the capsule needs to be known. As a guide, the table below provides capsule sizes and their relative liquid fill capacities.

The total amount of a non-liquid formulation that can be placed in a capsule varies according to the bulk density of the formulation. Several methods have been devised to help select the appropriate size capsule for a particular powder formulation. One method is to compare the density of the formulation being compounded to the density of a known drug: Similar amounts of powder with similar densities will fit in the same size capsule. For example, if a formulation has a density similar to aspirin and 300 mg are needed for each dose, then a #1 capsule would be needed based on the information in the right-hand table below. In general, the smallest capsule that will contain the formulation is used since patients often have difficulty swallowing large capsules.

When filling a small number of capsules, the **"punch" method** is used. The ingredients are triturated to the same particle size and then mixed by geometric dilution. Since some powder will be lost in the punching process, calculate for the preparation of at least two extra capsules. The powder is placed on an ointment slab and smoothed with a spatula to a height approximately half the length of the capsule body. The body of the capsule is held vertically and the open end is repeatedly pushed or "punched" into the powder until the capsule is filled. The cap is then replaced to close the capsule. Each filled capsule is weighed using an empty capsule as a counterweight. Powder is added or removed until the correct weight has been placed in the capsule.

Capsule filling machines are available for filling 100 or 300 capsules at a time. The machines come with a capsule loader which correctly aligns all of the capsules in the machine base. The powder is poured onto the base plate and special spreaders and combs are used to fill the individual capsules. All of the caps are simultaneously returned to the capsule bodies, and the batch is complete. When using a capsule filling machine, it takes practice to ensure that each capsule has the same amount of drug. There is a tendency to overfill the capsules in the center, and underfill the capsules around the edges.

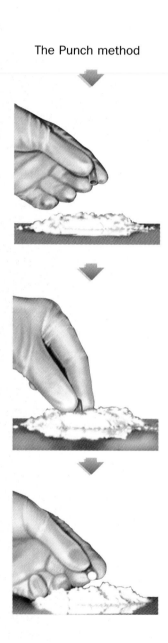

The Punch method

Capsule Size	Liquid Volume (ml)	Capsule Size	Liquid Volume (ml)
000	1.37	2	0.37
00	0.95	3	0.30
0	0.68	4	0.20
1	0.50	5	0.13

punch method a method for filling capsules by repeatedly pushing or "punching" the capsule into an amount of drug powder.

finger cots protective coverings for fingers.

Other Tips for Compounding Capsules:

➡ It is a good practice to remove the exact number of empty capsules needed from the capsule box before compounding begins. This will avoid preparing the wrong number of capsules and will prevent the contamination of other empty capsules with drug particles that cling to hands.

➡ The simplest method to keep a capsule free of moisture during compounding is to use the cap of one capsule as a holder for other capsule bodies during the filling operation. This avoids the capsules coming into contact with the fingers. Another way of protecting the capsules is to wear **finger cots** or rubber gloves.

➡ To remove traces of drug from the outside of the filled capsules, roll them between the folds of clean towel or shake in a towel that has been gathered into the form of a bag.

➡ Liquids that do not dissolve gelatin, e.g., alcohol and fixed oils, may be dispensed in capsules. By calibrated dropper or pipet, the correct volume of liquid is delivered into the empty capsule body. None of the liquid should touch the outside of the body and the size of the capsule should be chosen so that the liquid does not completely fill the body. The capsule is sealed by moistening the lower portion of the inside of the cap with warm water using a camel's hair brush. The moistened cap is placed on the body and given a half turn. The capsules should be placed on an absorbent paper and inspected for leakage.

➡ Capsules will absorb moisture and soften in high humidity. In a dry atmosphere, they become brittle and crack. To protect capsules from the extremes of humidity, dispense them in plastic or glass vials, and store in a cool, dry place. A piece of cotton may be added in the top of the vial to keep the capsules from rattling.

➡ Tablets and smaller capsules can be placed inside capsules. This can be a real convenience to a patient that has many tablets or capsules to take per day.

Capsule Size	Mg of Lactose	Mg of Aspirin
000	1250	975
00	850	650
0	600	490
1	460	335
2	350	260
3	280	195
4	210	130
5	140	65

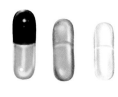

REVIEW

KEY CONCEPTS

COMPOUNDING

✔ Extemporaneous compounding is the on-demand preparation of a drug product according to a physician's prescription, to meet the unique needs of an individual patient.

✔ Compounding is regulated by State Boards of Pharmacy and the U.S. Pharmacopeia. Most states have accepted the USP standards for pharmacy compounding, but some states have their own regulations.

COMPOUNDING REGULATIONS

✔ The pharmacist has the responsibility and authority to manage the compounding area.

✔ Ingredients of USP/NF purity or better are to be used when compounding formulations.

✔ A compounding record and formulation record are required for each compounded formulation.

COMPOUNDING CONSIDERATIONS

✔ There are four areas of considerations when compounding: 1) whether or not to compound; 2) before compounding; 3) during compounding; 4) after compounding.

STABILITY AND BEYOND-USE DATES

✔ Beyond-use dates are required on compounded formulations.

EQUIPMENT

✔ Class A prescription balances can weigh as little as 120 mg of material with a 5% error.

✔ When weighing an amount of ingredient that is less than 120 mg, an aliquot or electronic balance can be used.

USING A BALANCE

✔ Class A prescription balances and electronic balances need to be leveled before any ingredient is weighed.

✔ Weighing papers or weighing boats should always be placed on the balance pans before weighing ingredients.

VOLUMETRIC EQUIPMENT

✔ Liquid drugs, solvents, or additives are measured in volumetric glassware or plasticware such as graduated cylinders, syringes, and pipets.

✔ Erlenmeyer flasks, beakers, and prescription bottles, regardless of markings, are not volumetric glassware.

LIQUID MEASUREMENT

✔ Always use the smallest device that will accommodate the desired volume of liquid.

✔ When reading a volume of a liquid against a graduation mark, hold the graduated cylinder so the meniscus is at eye level and read the mark at the bottom of the meniscus.

MIXING SOLIDS AND SEMISOLIDS

✔ Trituration is the fine grinding of a powder. Levigation is the trituration of a powder drug with a solvent in which the drug is insoluble. Both techniques reduce the drug's particle size.

SELECT DOSAGE FORMS

✔ Aqueous solutions are clear liquids (but not necessarily colorless) made most commonly with purified water but which may also contain ethanol, glycerin, or propylene glycol.

✔ Nonaqueous solutions include elixirs, tinctures, spirits, liniments, and oleaginous solutions.

- ✔ Suspensions are a two phase system consisting of a finely divided solid dispersed in a liquid.
- ✔ The "flavor" experience is a complex combination of taste, smell, texture, appearance, and temperature.
- ✔ An emulsion is an unstable system consisting of at least two immiscible (unmixable) liquids, one that is dispersed as small droplets throughout the other, and a stabilizing agent.
- ✔ There are two major methods of compounding ointments: 1) incorporating a drug into an ointment base and 2) forming the base as a part of the compounding process.
- ✔ There are three classes of suppository bases defined by their composition and physical properties: oleaginous bases, water soluble or miscible bases, and hydrophilic bases.
- ✔ When preparing capsules, the smallest capsule capable of containing the final formulation is used since patients often have difficulty swallowing large capsules.

SELF TEST

MATCH THE TERMS: I   *the answer key begins on page 511*

1. aliquot ____
2. arrest knob ____
3. beyond-use date ____
4. calibrate ____
5. Chapter <795> ____
6. Chapter <797> ____
7. compounding record ____
8. compression molding ____
9. emulsifier ____
10. finger cots ____
11. flocculating agent ____
12. formulation record ____
13. fusion molding ____

a. regulations from USP/NF pertaining to the nonsterile compounding of formulations.
b. the knob on a balance that prevents any movement of the balance pans.
c. a date assigned to compounded prescription telling the patient when the formulation should no longer be taken.
d. regulations from USP/NF pertaining to the sterile compounding of formulations.
e. electrolytes used in the preparation of suspensions.
f. formulas and procedures (i.e., recipes) for what should happen when a formulation is compounded.
g. a record of what actually happened when the formulation was compounded.
h. a portion of a mixture.
i. to set, mark, or check the graduations of a measuring device.
j. a stabilizing agent in emulsions.
k. a method of making suppositories in which the ingredients are compressed in a mold.
l. a suppository preparation method in which the active ingredients are dispersed or dissolved in a melted base.
m. protective coverings for fingers.

REVIEW

MATCH THE TERMS: II   *the answer key begins on page 511*

1. geometric dilution ____

2. hydrophilic emulsifier ____

3. immiscible ____

4. levigation ____

5. lipophilic emulsifier ____

6. meniscus ____

7. miscible ____

8. mucilage ____

9. oil-in-water emulsion ____

10. primary emulsion ____

11. punch method ____

12. sensitivity ____

13. sonication ____

14. spatulation ____

15. stability ____

16. thickening agent ____

17. trituration ____

18. volumetric ____

19. water-in-oil emulsion ____

a. a technique for mixing two powders of unequal quantity.

b. wet, slimy liquid formed as an initial step in the wet gum method.

c. capable of being mixed together.

d. the curved surface of a volume of liquid.

e. the chemical and physical integrity of the dosage form, and when appropriate, its ability to withstand microbiological contaminations.

f. the amount of weight that will move the balance pointer one division mark on the marker plate.

g. measures volume; either TD (to deliver) or TC (to contain).

h. mixing powders with a spatula.

i. exposure to high frequency sound waves.

j. an ingredient used in the preparation of suspensions to increase the viscosity of the liquid.

k. an emulsion in which water is dispersed through an oil base.

l. an emulsion in which oil is dispersed through a water base.

m. the initial emulsion to which ingredients are added to create the final product.

n. the fine grinding of a powder.

o. a method for filling capsules.

p. triturating a powder drug with a solvent in which it is insoluble to reduce its particle size.

q. cannot be mixed.

r. a stabilizing agent for water based dispersion mediums.

s. a stabilizing agent for oil based dispersion mediums.

CHOOSE THE BEST ANSWER *the answer key begins on page 511*

1. _____ is the on-demand preparation of a drug product according to a physician's prescription.
   a. IVPB
   b. Extemporaneous compounding
   c. Trituration
   d. Spatulation

2. Chapter <795> of the USP/NF deals with
   a. compounding sterile products.
   b. compounding nonsterile products.
   c. official compounded formulations and their beyond-use dates.
   d. containers used to package compounded formulations.

3. Which record will document how a compounded formula was actually prepared?
   a. formulation record
   b. compounding record
   c. standard operating procedure
   d. material safety data sheet

4. In assigning a beyond-use date to a compounded prescription,
   a. the manufacturer's beyond-use date should be used as a last resort.
   b. available scientific literature should be used as a last resort.
   c. the expiration date is used.
   d. the USP/NF recommended beyond-use date should be used as a last resort.

5. The sensitivity requirement of a Class A prescription balance is
   a. 6 micrograms.
   b. 60 micrograms.
   c. 60 milligrams.
   d. 6 milligrams.

6. Aliquots can be used with a Class A prescription balance when a prescription calls for less than _____ of an ingredient.
   a. 120 gm
   b. 500 gm
   c. 500 mg
   d. 120 mg

7. Which type of mortar and pestle is recommended for mixing liquids and semisolids?
   a. wedgwood
   b. porcelain
   c. glass
   d. earthenware

8. When weighing a powder on a Class A prescription balance,
   a. pour the powder into the pan on the left side of the balance.
   b. always use the largest weigh boat possible.
   c. keep the balance unarrested.
   d. use a clean weigh boat with each new powder.

9. Which type of glassware is "TC" (i.e., "to contain")?
   a. Erlenmeyer flasks
   b. single volume pipet
   c. beaker
   d. volumetric flask

10. Which piece of equipment must be "tared" before its use?
   a. electronic balance
   b. Class A prescription balance
   c. pipets
   d. electronic mortar and pestle

11. A 100 ml graduated cylinder cannot accurately measure volumes less than
   a. 20 ml.
   b. 50 ml.
   c. 30 ml.
   d. 40 ml.

REVIEW

12. If a 5 ml liquid volume needs to be measured, a _____ should be used.
    a. 10 ml oral syringe
    b. 100 ml cylindrical graduate
    c. 100 microliter micropipet
    d. 25 ml Erlenmeyer flask

13. Viscous liquids such as glycerin or propylene glycol will require approximately _____ to transfer out of a single volume pipet.
    a. 3 minutes
    b. 5 minutes
    c. 10 minutes
    d 15 minutes

14. Which type of syringe is used to administer a dose of liquid medication to a patient?
    a. hypodermic with Luer-Lok®
    b. oral syringe
    c. hypodermic with Slip-Tip®
    d. Adapt-a-Cap®

15. _____ is the technique used to mix two powders of unequal quantity.
    a. Volumetric dilution
    b. Volumetric emulsification
    c. Geometric emulsification
    d. Geometric dilution

16. The fine grinding of a powder is called
    a. melting.
    b. trituration.
    c. levigation.
    d. suspension.

17. Solutions contain
    a. molecular size particles.
    b. particles greater than 0.1 micrometer.
    c. oil, water, and emulsifiers.
    d. hydrated micromolecules that restrict solvent flow.

18. The USP/NF gives "Relative Terms of Solubility." If a drug is soluble, how many parts of solvent are required for one part of drug?
    a. 1–10
    b. 10–30
    c. 30–100
    d. 100–1,000

19. Elixirs, tinctures, and liniments are examples of
    a. syrups.
    b. aqueous solutions.
    c. nonaqueous solutions.
    d. gels.

20. Which characteristic marks a good suspension?
    a. settles quickly and redisperses slowly
    b. settles quickly and redisperses quickly
    c. settles slowly and redisperses slowly
    d. settles slowly and redisperses quickly

21. An aqueous solution of water soluble ingredients is added to an alcoholic solution of alcohol soluble ingredients and the resulting solution turns cloudy or "milky." What is happening?
    a. The alcoholic components are coming out of the solution.
    b. The aqueous components are coming out of the solution.
    c. Nothing; the cloudiness will go away when the solution is stirred.
    d. The small amount of water in the alcohol is separating out.

22. If you need to compound a formulation containing a water-based vehicle and an active drug that is an oil, the appropriate dosage form would be a/an
    a. solution.
    b. elixir.
    c. emulsion.
    d. gel.

10

BASIC BIOPHARMACEUTICS

LEARNING OBJECTIVES

At the completion of study, the student will:

➥ explain how a drug produces a pharmacological effect.

➥ explain why a blood concentration–time profile is an accepted method of indirectly determining the concentration of a drug at the site of action.

➥ identify the influence of the ADME processes on a blood concentration–time curve.

➥ identify and explain the influence of three factors on the processes of absorption, distribution, metabolism, and excretion.

➥ define bioequivalency, and explain how the FDA uses this information.

➥ explain how to determine a drug's half-life.

HOW DRUGS WORK

Drugs produce either desired or undesired effects in the body.

Once they are in the blood, drugs are circulated throughout the body. The properties of both the drug and the body influence where the drug will go, and what concentration it will have at each place. The place where a drug causes an effect to occur is called the **site of action**. Some of the effects caused by the drug are desired effects, and some are undesired. *The objective of drug therapy is to deliver the right drug, in the right concentration, to the right site of action, and at the right time to produce the desired effect.*

When most drugs produce an effect, they are interacting at a molecular level with cellular material or structure.

The cellular material directly involved in the action of the drug is called a **receptor.** The receptor is often described as a lock into which the drug molecule fits as a key, and only those drugs able to interact with the receptors in a particular site of action can produce effects at that site. This is why specific cells only respond to certain drugs, even though their receptors are exposed to any drug molecules that are present in the body. This is also why drugs are **selective** in their action, that is, they only act on specific targeted receptors and tissues.

Receptors are located on the surfaces of cell membranes and inside cells.

There are many different types of receptors, each type having a different influence on the body's processes. Most receptors can be found throughout the body, though some occur in only a few places.

site of action the location where an administered drug produces an effect.

receptor the cellular material located at the site of action that interacts with the drug.

selective (action) the characteristic of a drug that makes its action specific to certain receptors and tissues.

DRUG ACTION AT THE SITE OF ACTION

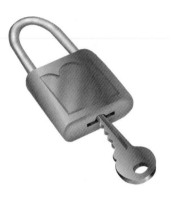

Like a lock and key, only certain drugs are able to interact with certain receptors.

Types of Action

When drugs interact with the site of action, they can:

➡ act through physical action, as with the protective effects of ointments upon topical application;

➡ react chemically, as with antacids that reduce excess gastric acidity;

➡ modify the metabolic activity of pathogens, as with antibiotics;

➡ change the osmolarity of blood and draw water out of tissues and into the blood;

➡ incorporate into cellular material to interfere with normal cell function;

➡ join with other chemicals to form a complex that is more easily excreted;

➡ modify the biochemical or metabolic process of the body's cells or enzyme systems.

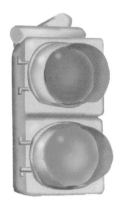

antagonists
block action

agonists activate
receivers

Other Drug Actions

➡ Some drugs work by changing the ability of ions to move into or out of cells. For example, sodium or calcium ion channels can open and allow movement of the ions into nerve cells, stimulating their function. With potassium channels, the opposite can happen. The channels can open and allow the movement of potassium ions out of nerve cells, obstructing their function.

➡ Some drugs modify the creation, release, or control of nerve cell hormones that regulate different physiological processes.

℞ The objective of drug therapy is to deliver the right drug, in the right concentration, to the right site of action, and at the right time to produce the desired effect.

When drug molecules bind with a receptor, they can cause a reaction that stimulates or inhibits cellular functions.

The pharmacological effects of these interactions are termed agonism or antagonism. **Agonists** are drugs that activate receptors and produce a response that may either accelerate or slow normal cellular processes, depending on the type of receptor involved. For example, epinephrine-like drugs act on the heart to increase the heart rate, and acetylcholine-like drugs act on the heart to slow the heart rate. Both are agonists. **Antagonists** are drugs that bind to receptors but do not activate them. They block the receptors' action by preventing other drugs or substances from interacting with them.

The number of receptors available to interact with a drug will directly influence the effect.

A minimum number of receptors have to be occupied by drug molecules to produce an effect. If there are too few drug molecules to occupy the necessary number of receptors, there will be little or no effect. In this case, increasing the dosage will increase the effect. However, once all the receptors are occupied, increasing the dosage will not increase the effect.

Receptors can be changed by drug use.

For example, extended stimulation of cells with an agonist can reduce the number or sensitivity of the receptors, and the effect of the drug is reduced. Extended inhibition of cell functions with an antagonist can increase the number or sensitivity of receptors. If the antagonist is stopped abruptly, the cells can have an extreme reaction to an agonist. To avoid such withdrawal symptoms, some drugs must be gradually discontinued.

 agonists drugs that activate receptors to accelerate or slow normal cellular function.

antagonists drugs that bind with receptors but do not activate them. They block receptor action by preventing other drugs or substances from activating them.

CONCENTRATION & EFFECT

It is difficult to measure the amount of a drug at the site of action and therefore to predict an effect based upon that measurement.

One problem is that many factors influence a drug's movement from the site of administration to the site of action (absorption, elimination, membrane permeability, etc.). It can also be physically impossible to measure the drug at the site of action either because of its unknown location or small size.

One way to monitor the amount of a drug in the body and its effect at the site of action is to use a dose-response curve.

Using a dose-response curve, you would expect a certain effect for any given dose. However, when a series of drug doses is given to a number of people, the results show that some people respond to low doses but others require larger doses for an equal response to be produced. This is due to human variability: different people have different characteristics that affect how a drug product behaves in them. Some differences are due to the product itself, but most come from how the drug is transported from the site of administration to the site of action, and how it interacts with the receptor. For these reasons, dose-response curves are not ideal for relating the amount of drug in the body to its effect.

A better way to relate the amount of a drug in the body to its effect is to determine drug concentrations in the body's fluids.

Of the body's fluids, blood is generally used because of its rapid equilibrium between the site of administration and the site of action. As a result, knowing a drug's concentration in the blood can be directly related to its effect and this is the most common way to analyze the potential effect of a drug.

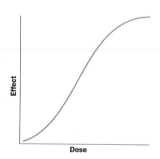

An expected dose-response curve shows that a response increases as the dose is increased.

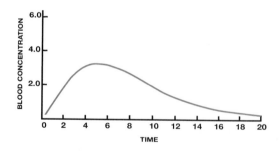

Blood Concentration–Time Profiles

Blood concentration–time profiles have these applications:

➥ Manufacturers use the data to evaluate their drug products.

➥ Pharmacy professionals use them to visualize the consequences of incorrectly compounding a formulation or of using the wrong route of administration.

➥ Researchers and clinicians use them to measure human variability in drug product performance (e.g., influence of age, gender, nationality, or disease).

➥ Physicians and pharmacists use them to monitor the drug therapy of patients.

ABCD *biopharmaceutics* the study of the factors associated with drug products and physiological processes, and the resulting systemic concentrations of drugs.

minimum effective concentration (MEC) the blood concentration needed for a drug to produce a response.

onset of action the time MEC is reached and the response occurs.

therapeutic window a drug's blood concentration range between its MEC and MTC.

A Sample Profile

The illustration on the right shows a typical blood concentration–time profile for a drug given orally. The blood concentration begins at zero at the time the drug is administered (before it has been absorbed into the blood). With time, the drug leaves the formulation and enters the blood, causing concentrations to rise. To produce an effect, the concentrations must achieve a **minimum effective concentration (MEC).** This is when there is enough drug at the site of action to produce a response. The time this occurs is called the **onset of action.** With most drugs, when blood concentrations increase, so does the intensity of the effect, since *blood concentrations reflect the concentrations at the site of action that produce the response.*

Some drugs have an upper blood concentration limit beyond which there are undesired or toxic effects. This limit is called the **minimum toxic concentration (MTC).** The range between the minimum effective concentration and the minimum toxic concentration is called the **therapeutic window.** *When concentrations are in this range, most patients receive the maximum benefit from their drug therapy with a minimum of risk.*

The last part of the curve shows the blood concentrations declining as absorption is complete and elimination is proceeding. The time between the onset of action and the time when the minimum effective concentration is reached by the declining blood concentrations is called the **duration of action.** The duration of action is the time the drug should produce the desired effect.

A n advantage of using blood concentrations as a measure of the "drug amount in the body" is that blood can be repeatedly sampled. When sampling covers several hours or more, a blood concentration–time profile can be developed. Plasma or serum concentrations can be used instead of blood concentrations, and the same type of profile will result.

For many drugs, changes in the blood concentration–time profile reflect changes in concentration at the site of action and therefore changes in effect.

These drugs are typically "monitored" by determining the blood concentration "peak" and "trough" at the beginning and end of a dosing interval. Drugs usually monitored include vancomycin, phenytoin, gentamycin, digoxin, and valproic acid.

There are exceptions to the blood concentration–time profile reflecting the site of action concentration.

The concentration of some drugs at the site of action produces an action hours or days later after the drug is given. Other drugs show no relationship between blood concentrations and concentrations in the site of action. Still others don't depend on blood concentrations to produce an effect.

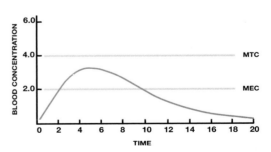

A blood concentration–time profile

minimum toxic concentration (MTC) the upper limit of the therapeutic window. Drug concentrations above the MTC increase the risk of undesired effects.

duration of action the time drug concentration is above the MEC.

ADME PROCESSES & DIFFUSION

Blood concentrations are the result of four simultaneously occurring processes: absorption, distribution, metabolism, and excretion. These four processes are referred to as the ADME processes, but may also be called **disposition**. Metabolism and excretion combined are called **elimination**.

The transfer of drug into the blood from an administered drug product is called absorption.

When a drug product is first administered, absorption is the primary process. Distribution, metabolism, and excretion will also occur, but the amount of drug available for them is much less than the amount of drug available for absorption. So these processes have little effect. As more of the drug is absorbed into the blood, it is available to undergo these other processes and their roles increase.

A drug's distribution will be affected by physiological functions and its own properties.

Though blood may deliver the drug to body tissue, if the drug cannot penetrate to the tissue's membranes, it will not interact with the receptors. The opposite situation can also occur. A drug may be able to penetrate to the tissue's membranes, but if there is not enough blood flow to the tissue, little of the drug will be available. Distribution is also influenced by drug binding to proteins in the blood or in tissues.

The ADME processes are all illustrated by blood concentration–time curves.

Concentrations rise during absorption, but as absorption nears completion, metabolism and elimination become the primary processes, and they cause the blood concentration to decline.

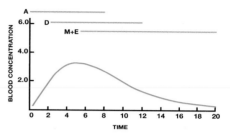

In the first part of a blood concentration–time curve, absorption is the primary process and concentrations rise. As absorption nears completion, metabolism and excretion become the primary processes, causing the concentration to decline. Distribution occurs throughout. The blue lines show the parts of the profile most influenced by the various ADME processes.

Half-life

Half-life is the amount of time it takes for the blood concentration of a drug to decline to *one-half* an initial value. For example, if at 6 hours a drug's blood concentration was 30 mcg/ml, and at 15 hours it was 15 mcg/ml, then the half-life would be 9 hours (15 hours minus 6 hours). To estimate how long it takes to essentially remove the drug from the body via the process of elimination, five times the half-life is used. So, in the preceding example, that would be 5 x the half-life of 9 hours, or 45 hours.

 Even though the ADME processes occur simultaneously, they are studied separately to understand the critical factors responsible for each process.

 disposition a term sometimes used to refer to all of the ADME processes together.

elimination the processes of metabolism and excretion.

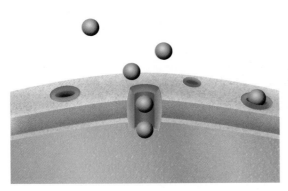

A diagram showing drug molecules penetrating a cell membrane.

Ionization and Unionization

Because they are weak organic acids and bases, most drugs will dissociate (come apart) and associate (attach to other chemicals) in solutions. When acids dissociate, they become ionized. When bases dissociate, they become unionized.

Unionized drugs penetrate biological membranes more easily than ionized drugs for these reasons:

➥ unionized drugs are more lipid-soluble;

➥ charges on biological membranes bind or repel ionized drug;

➥ ionized drugs associate with water molecules, creating larger particles with reduced penetrating capability.

passive diffusion the movement of drugs from an area of higher concentration to lower concentration.

lipoidal fat-like substance.

hydrophobic water repelling; cannot associate with water.

hydrophilic capable of associating with or absorbing water.

active transport the movement of drugs from an area of lower concentration to an area of higher concentration. Cellular energy is required.

Besides the four ADME processes, a critical factor of drug concentration and effect is how drugs move through biological membranes.

Before an effective concentration of a drug can reach its site of action, it must overcome many barriers, most of which are biological membranes.

Biological membranes are complex structures composed of lipids (fats) and proteins.

They are generally classified in three types: those made up of *several layers of cells,* such as the skin; those made up of *a single layer of cells,* as in the intestinal lining; and those of *less than one cell* in thickness, as in the membrane of a single cell.

Most drugs penetrate biological membranes by passive diffusion.

Drugs in the body's fluids will generally move from an area of higher concentration to an area of lower concentration until the concentrations in each area are balanced, or in a state of equilibrium. This process is called **passive diffusion**. It is the most common way a drug penetrates biological membranes and is a primary factor in the distribution process. This movement from higher to lower concentration causes most orally administered drugs to move from the intestine to the blood and from the blood to the site of action.

Drug concentration is not the only factor influencing diffusion.

Membranes are **lipoidal** (fat-like), and drugs that are more lipid (fat) soluble will penetrate them better than those that are not. These drugs are called **hydrophobic drugs.** They hate or repel water and are attracted to fats. **Hydrophilic drugs** (drugs attracted to water) can also penetrate membranes. However, it is thought that they move through water-filled passages called aqueous pores which allow water (and any drug contained in it) to move through the membrane.

In addition to passive diffusion, some drugs may be carried across membranes by *specialized transport mechanisms*.

This type of **active transport** (as opposed to passive diffusion) is thought to explain how certain substances that do not penetrate membranes by passive diffusion nevertheless succeed in entering a cell.

ABSORPTION

Once a drug is released from its dosage formulation, the process that transfers it into the blood is called *absorption.*

Absorption occurs to some extent with any route of administration. For example, even a drug in an intravenous suspension or emulsion must first be released from the dosage form to be absorbed into the blood. However, since many drugs are given orally, this page will look at the ADME processes from the perspective of oral administration.

One of the primary factors affecting oral drug absorption is the *gastric emptying time.*

This is the time a drug will stay in the stomach before it is emptied into the small intestine. Since stomach acid can degrade many drugs and since most absorption occurs in the intestine, gastric emptying time can significantly affect a drug's action. If a drug remains in the stomach too long, it can be degraded or destroyed, and its effect decreased. Gastric emptying time can be affected by various conditions, including the amount and type of food in the stomach, the presence of other drugs, the person's body position, and their emotional condition. Some factors increase the gastric emptying time, but most slow it.

Once a drug leaves the stomach, its rate of movement through the intestines affects its absorption.

Slower than normal intestinal movement can lead to increased drug absorption because the drug is in contact with the intestinal membrane longer. Faster than normal intestinal movement can produce the opposite result since the drug moves through the intestinal tract too rapidly to be fully absorbed.

Bile salts and enzymes from the intestinal tract also affect absorption.

Bile salts improve the absorption of certain hydrophobic drugs. Enzymes added to the intestinal tract's contents from pancreatic secretions destroy certain drugs and consequently decrease their absorption. Enzymes are also present in the intestinal wall and can destroy drugs as they pass from the gut into the blood, decreasing their absorption.

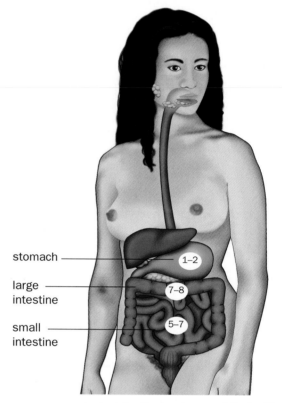

stomach

large intestine

small intestine

gastrointestinal organs and their pH

Most drugs are given orally and absorbed into the blood from the small intestine. The small intestine's large surface area benefits drug absorption. However, there are many conditions in the stomach that can affect absorption positively or negatively before the drug even reaches the small intestine. Once in the intestines, there are many additional factors that can affect a drug's absorption.

R Rapidly administered intravenous solutions (i.e., bolus) do not have an absorption site.

ABCD *absorption* the movement of a drug from the dosage formulation to the blood.

gastric emptying time the time a drug will stay in the stomach before it is emptied into the small intestine.

DISTRIBUTION

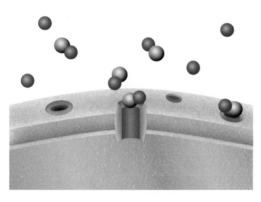

Protein Binding

Many drugs bind to proteins in blood plasma to form a complex that is too large to penetrate biological membranes. So the drug remains inactive.

Protein binding can be considered a type of drug storage or "depot" within the body. Some drugs bind extensively to proteins in fat and muscle, and are gradually released as the blood concentration of the drug falls. These drugs remain in the body a long time, and therefore have a long duration of action.

Selective Action

Though drugs are widely distributed throughout the body once they reach the bloodstream, they will have action that is selective to certain tissues or organs. This is due both to the specific nature of the receptor in the tissue and the various factors that affect the distribution of the drug (e.g., blood flow) to the tissue. This is why drugs can be targeted for specific therapeutic effects.

However, since most receptors can be found in multiple tissues throughout the body, most drugs have multiple effects. This is why a drug may be used for different therapies. For example, terbutaline is used for bronchodilation but it will also delay labor in pregnant women. It is also one reason drugs have side effects.

Distribution involves the movement of a drug within the body once the drug has reached the blood.

Blood carries the drug throughout the body and to its sites of action, as well as to the organs responsible for the metabolism and excretion of the drug.

The blood flow rates to certain organs have a significant effect on distribution.

Drugs are rapidly distributed to organs having high blood flow rates such as the heart, liver, and kidneys. Distribution to areas such as muscle, fat, and skin is usually slower because they have lower blood flow rates.

The permeability of tissue membranes to a drug is also important.

Most tissue membranes are easily penetrated by most drugs. Small drug molecules (those having a low molecular weight) and drugs that are hydrophobic will generally diffuse through tissue membranes with ease. Some tissue membranes have specialized transport mechanisms that assist penetration. A few tissue membranes are highly selective in allowing drug penetration. The blood-brain barrier, for example, limits drug access to the brain and the cerebral spinal fluid.

Protein binding can also affect distribution.

Many drugs will "bind" to proteins in blood plasma, forming a **complex**. The large size of such complexes prevents the bound drug from entering its sites of action, metabolism, and excretion—essentially making the drug inactive. Only free or "unbound" drug can move through tissue membranes and cellular openings. Another drug with a stronger binding capacity can displace a weaker bound drug from a protein, making the weakly bound drug "unbound" and available for pharmacological activity. This has been the basis for a well-known drug interaction between aspirin and coumadin.

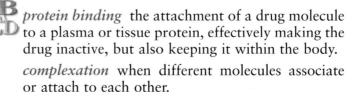

protein binding the attachment of a drug molecule to a plasma or tissue protein, effectively making the drug inactive, but also keeping it within the body.

complexation when different molecules associate or attach to each other.

METABOLISM

Drug metabolism refers to the body's process of transforming drugs.

The transformed drug is called a **metabolite.** Most metabolites are inactive molecules that are excreted. However, the metabolites of some drugs are active, and they will produce effects in the patient until they are further metabolized or excreted.

The primary site of drug metabolism in the body is the liver.

Enzymes are complex proteins that catalyze chemical reactions. The enzymes found in the liver interact with drugs and transform them into metabolites.

In response to the chronic administration of certain drugs, the liver will increase its enzyme activity.

This is called **enzyme induction,** and it results in greater metabolism of a drug. As a result, larger doses of the drug must be administered to produce the same therapeutic effects. Some drugs decrease enzyme activity, a process called **enzyme inhibition.** In this case, smaller doses of the drug will be needed to avoid toxicity from drug accumulation.

The liver may secrete drugs or their metabolites into bile that is stored in the gallbladder.

The gallbladder empties the bile (and any drugs or metabolites in it) into the intestine in response to food entering the intestinal tract. Any drugs or metabolites contained in the bile may be reabsorbed or simply eliminated within the feces. If the drugs or metabolites are reabsorbed back into the blood circulation, this is called **enterohepatic cycling.**

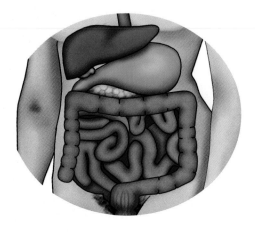

First-Pass Metabolism

With oral administration, once a drug is absorbed from the gastrointestinal tract, it is immediately delivered to the liver. It will then be transferred into the general systemic circulation.

However, before it reaches the circulatory system, the drug can be substantially degraded or destroyed by the liver's enzymes. This is called **"first-pass metabolism"** and is an important factor with orally administered drugs. Because of it, certain drugs must be administered by other routes. Any route of administration other than the oral route either partially or completely bypasses first-pass metabolism.

metabolite the substance resulting from the body's transformation of an administered drug.

enzyme a complex protein that catalyzes chemical reactions.

enzyme induction the increase in hepatic enzyme activity that results in greater metabolism of drugs.

enzyme inhibition the decrease in hepatic enzyme activity that results in reduced metabolism of drugs.

enterohepatic cycling the transfer of drugs and their metabolites from the liver to the bile in the gallbladder, then into the intestine, and then back into circulation.

first-pass metabolism the substantial degradation of an orally administered drug caused by enzyme metabolism in the liver before the drug reaches the systemic circulation.

EXCRETION

Most drugs and their metabolites are excreted in the urine by the kidneys.

Some orally administered drugs are not easily absorbed from the gastrointestinal tract and as a result are significantly excreted in the feces. Excretion can also occur through the bile (if entero-hepatic cycling does not occur) and certain drugs are removed through the lungs in the expired breath.

The kidneys filter the blood and remove waste materials (including drugs and metabolites) from it.

As blood flows through a kidney, some of the plasma water is filtered from it into the **nephron** (the functional unit of the kidney) tubule in a process called **glomerular filtration**. This filtered plasma water may contain waste materials and drugs from other parts of the body. As the water moves along the tubule, additional waste substances and drugs can be secreted into the fluid. Some drugs can be reabsorbed back into the blood during a process called urinary reabsorption. After glomerular filtration, renal secretion, and urinary reabsorption are completed, the remaining fluid is excreted from the body as urine.

The rate of urinary excretion is much faster than that of fecal excretion.

Drugs that will be excreted through the feces generally take a day or two to be excreted, whereas drugs may be excreted through the urine within hours of administration.

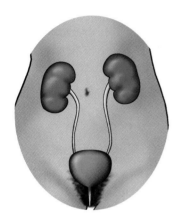

Factors Affecting Urinary Excretion

➡ If the kidney's process of excretion becomes impaired, excretion will be reduced and some drugs will accumulate in the blood. In such cases, the dosage of these drugs must be decreased or the dosing interval lengthened. Drugs such as vancomycin and gentamicin are monitored for this reason.

➡ Some drugs affect the excretion of others. In such cases, the affected drug will accumulate in the blood, and its dosage must be decreased or the dosing interval lengthened.

➡ The pH of the urine can affect the reabsorption of some drugs. A high pH can increase excretion of weak acids such as salicylates and phenobarbital. However, a high pH will decrease the excretion (i.e., increase reabsorption) of weak bases.

➡ The amount of drug excreted in urine is the amount filtered + the amount secreted - the amount reabsorbed.

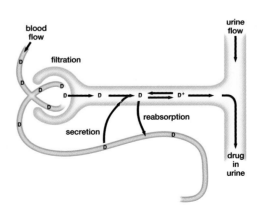

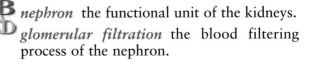

A B C D *nephron* the functional unit of the kidneys.
glomerular filtration the blood filtering process of the nephron.

BIOEQUIVALENCE

The amount of a drug that is delivered to the site of action and the rate at which it becomes available is called the *bioavailability* of the drug.

By FDA definition, bioavailability is measured by determining *the relative amount of an administered dose of a drug that reaches the general systemic circulation and the rate at which this occurs.* As a result, it can be measured using a blood concentration–time profile. Bioavailability is often determined by comparing blood concentration-time profiles from a product to that of an intravenous solution (called absolute bioavailability). Relative bioavailability is determined by comparing blood concentration-time profiles of a product to any other product that is not an intravenous solution.

Comparing the bioavailability of one dosage form to another determines their *bioequivalency.*

The FDA requires drug manufacturers to perform bioequivalency studies on their products before they are approved for marketing. In such studies, the bioavailability of the active ingredient in a test formulation is compared to that in a standard formulation (many times the innovator's product). Bioequivalency studies are also used to compare bioavailability between different dosage forms (tablets, capsules, etc.), different manufacturers, and different production lots.

Bioequivalency can be graphically illustrated by placing the blood concentration–time profiles of the standard and test formulation on the same plot.

In the illustration below, the same dose is contained in both the standard and test formulations, but the two curves are not superimposed. The standard formulation (blue line) has a faster rate of absorption than the test formulation (red line) but the test formulation has a longer duration of action.

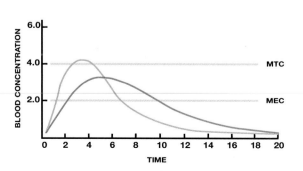

BIOEQUIVALENCE

Bioequivalent Drug Products

Bioequivalent drug products are pharmaceutical equivalents or alternatives which have *essentially* the same rate and extent of absorption when administered in the same dose of the active ingredient under similar conditions.

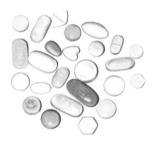

Differences Between Bioavailabilities

Exact bioequivalency between drug products (where blood concentration–time profiles for each product are identical) does not occur, and is not expected. There are simply too many variables that can contribute to differences between products. In tablets, for example, there can be different amounts or types of fillers, binders, lubricants, and other components. The particle size of the active drug itself may be slightly different. The manufacturing process may also produce different results in size, hardness, or other characteristics (especially for different manufacturers, but also for the same manufacturer at different times or different manufacturing facilities). Changes in these or various other factors can affect the bioavailability of a drug. Though there can be differences in the bioavailability of different products, when the differences are not significant the products are bioequivalent.

bioavailability the relative amount of an administered dose that reaches the general circulation and the rate at which this occurs.

bioequivalency the comparison of bioavailability between two dosage forms.

The following terms are used by the FDA to define the type of bioequivalency between drug products:

Pharmaceutical Equivalents

Pharmaceutical equivalents are drug products that contain identical amounts of the same active ingredient in the same dosage form, and are identical in strength, concentration, and route of administration. They do not have to contain the same inactive ingredients, or have the same physical shape, release mechanisms, packaging, or expiration time. Since pharmaceutical equivalents may have different inactive ingredients, different pharmaceutically equivalent products may not be equally suitable for a given patient. One drug formulation may perform differently enough to change the overall effect.

➡ same active ingredient (same salt form)
➡ same amount of active ingredient
➡ same dosage form
➡ inactive ingredients can be different

Pharmaceutical Alternatives

Pharmaceutical alternatives are drug products that contain the identical active ingredient, but not necessarily the same salt form or amount or dosage form. An example is tetracycline hydrochloride 250 mg capsules versus tetracycline phosphate complex 250 mg capsules or quinidine sulfate 200 mg tablets versus quinidine sulfate 200 mg capsules. They do not have to contain the same inactive ingredients, or have the same physical shape, release mechanisms, packaging, or expiration time.

➡ same active ingredient (but different salt form)
➡ amount of active ingredient can be different
➡ dosage form can be different
➡ inactive ingredients can be different

Therapeutic Equivalents

Therapeutic equivalents are pharmaceutical equivalents which produce the same therapeutic effect in patients.

➡ pharmaceutical equivalents that produce the same effects in patients

 The FDA annually publishes *Approved Drug Products With Therapeutic Equivalence Evaluations* (the "Orange Book"). It is available online at www.fda.gov/cder/ob/default.htm. For further discussion, see chapter three of *The Pharmacy Technician Workbook and Certification Review, Fourth Edition.*

 pharmaceutical equivalent drug products that contain identical amounts of the same active ingredient in the same dosage form.

pharmaceutical alternative drug products that contain the same active ingredient, but not necessarily in the same salt form, amount, or dosage form.

therapeutic equivalent pharmaceutical equivalents that produce the same effects in patients.

REVIEW

KEY CONCEPTS

HOW DRUGS WORK

✔ The objective of drug therapy is to deliver the right drug, in the right concentration, to the right site of action, and at the right time to produce the desired effect.

✔ Only those drugs able to interact with the receptors in a particular site of action can produce effects in that site. This is why specific cells respond only to certain drugs.

CONCENTRATION AND EFFECT

✔ To produce an effect, a drug must achieve a minimum effective concentration (MEC). This is when there is enough drug at the site of action to produce a response.

✔ The range between the minimum effective concentration and the minimum toxic concentration is called the therapeutic window. When concentrations are in this range, most patients receive the maximum benefit from their drug therapy with a minimum of risk.

✔ Therapeutic drug monitoring can be useful when the blood concentration of the drug reflects the concentration at the site of action.

ADME PROCESSES AND DIFFUSION

✔ Blood concentrations are the result of four simultaneously occurring processes: absorption, distribution, metabolism, and excretion (the ADME processes).

✔ Besides the four ADME processes, a critical factor of drug concentration and effect is how drugs move through biological membranes. Most drugs penetrate biological membranes by passive diffusion.

ABSORPTION

✔ One of the primary factors affecting oral drug absorption is the gastric emptying time.

DISTRIBUTION

✔ Many drugs bind to proteins in blood plasma to form a complex that is too large to penetrate biological membranes, essentially making the drug inactive.

METABOLISM

✔ Enzymes catalyze the transformation of drugs to metabolites. Most metabolites are inactive molecules that are excreted.

EXCRETION

✔ The kidneys filter blood and remove wastes, drugs, and metabolites from the body.

✔ Urinary excretion = glomerular filtration + renal secretion - urinary reabsorption.

BIOEQUIVALENCE

✔ The amount of a drug that is available to the site of action and the rate at which it becomes available is called the bioavailability of the drug.

✔ Bioequivalent drug products are pharmaceutical equivalents or alternatives which have essentially the same rate and extent of absorption when administered in the same dose of the active ingredient under similar conditions.

✔ Pharmaceutical equivalents are drug products that contain identical amounts of the same active ingredient in the same dosage form, but may contain different inactive ingredients.

✔ Pharmaceutical alternatives are drug products that contain the identical active ingredient, but not necessarily in the same salt form, same amount, or dosage form.

SELF TEST

MATCH THE TERMS: I — *the answer key begins on page 511*

1. absorption ____

2. active transport ____

3. agonists ____

4. antagonists ___

5. bioavailability ____

6. bioequivalency ____

7. biopharmaceutics ____

8. complexation ____

9. disposition ____

10. duration of action ____

11. elimination ____

12. enterohepatic cycling ____

13. enzyme ____

14. enzyme induction ____

15. enzyme inhibition ____

16. first-pass metabolism ____

17. gastric emptying time ____

18. glomerular filtration ____

19. hydrophilic ____

20. hydrophobic ____

21. lipoidal ____

a. the substantial degradation of an orally administered drug caused by enzyme metabolism in the liver before the drug reaches the systemic circulation.

b. the increase in hepatic enzyme activity that results in greater metabolism of drugs.

c. the study of the factors associated with drug products and physiological processes, and the resulting systemic concentrations of drugs.

d. the comparison of bioavailability between two dosage forms.

e. the relative amount of an administered dose that reaches the general circulation and the rate at which this occurs.

f. water repelling; cannot associate with water.

g. capable of associating with or absorbing water.

h. the blood filtering process of the nephron.

i. the time a drug will stay in the stomach before it is emptied into the small intestine.

j. the decrease in hepatic enzyme activity that results in reduced metabolism of drugs.

k. a complex protein that catalyzes chemical reactions.

l. the transfer of drugs and their metabolites from the liver to the bile in the gall bladder, then into the intestine, and then back into circulation.

m. the process of metabolism and excretion.

n. the time the drug concentration is above the MEC.

o. a term sometimes used to refer to all the ADME processes together.

p. when different molecules associate or attach to each other.

q. the movement of drugs from an area of lower concentration to an area of higher concentration; requires cellular energy.

r. the movement of drug from the dosage formulation to the blood.

s. drugs that activate receptors to accelerate or slow normal cellular function.

t. drugs that bind with receptors but do not activate them.

u. fat-like substance.

REVIEW

                                           the answer key begins on page 511

1. metabolite ____

2. minimum effective concentration (MEC) ____

3. minimum toxic concentration (MTC) ____

4. nephron ____

5. onset of action ____

6. passive diffusion ____

7. pharmaceutical alternative ____

8. pharmaceutical equivalent ____

9. protein binding ____

10. receptor ____

11. selective (action) ____

12. site of action ____

13. therapeutic equivalent ____

14. therapeutic window ____

a. the attachment of a drug molecule to a protein, effectively making the drug inactive.

b. the cellular material which interacts with the drug.

c. the movement of drugs from an area of higher concentration to lower concentration.

d. the characteristic of a drug that makes its action specific to certain receptors.

e. the location where an administered drug produces an effect.

f. the blood concentration needed for a drug to produce a response.

g. the time MEC is reached and the response occurs.

h. a drug's blood concentration range between its MEC and MTC.

i. the upper limit of the therapeutic window.

j. the substance resulting from the body's transformation of an administered drug.

k. the functional unit of the kidney.

l. drug products that contain identical amounts of the same active ingredient in the same dosage form.

m. pharmaceutical equivalents that produce the same effects in patients.

n. drug products that contain the same active ingredient but not necessarily in the same salt form, amount, or dosage form.

CHOOSE THE BEST ANSWER   *the answer key begins on page 511*

1. The place where a drug causes an effect to occur is called the
   a. site of action.
   b. site of administration.
   c. therapeutic window.
   d. minimum toxic concentration (MTC).

2. When a drug produces an effect, it is acting at a/an _____ level.
   a. tissue
   b. atomic
   c. molecular
   d. organ

3. Drug action can be caused by a
   a. physical action, such as a protective ointment.
   b. chemical action, such as an antacid neutralizing acidity.
   c. osmotic action, such as moving water out of tissues into blood.
   d. all of the above.

4. An antagonist will
   a. not bind to a receptor.
   b. accelerate a normal body process.
   c. prevent other drugs from binding to a receptor.
   d. cause extended stimulation of receptors.

5. In a blood concentration–time curve, the range between the minimum toxic concentration (MTC) and the minimum effective concentration (MEC) is called the
   a. onset of action.
   b. concentration at site of action.
   c. duration of action.
   d. therapeutic window.

6. The time a drug's blood concentration is above the MTC is called the
   a. onset of action.
   b. duration of action.
   c. concentration at site of action.
   d. none of the above

7. When studying concentration and effect, the _____ is the time MEC is reached and the response occurs.
   a. therapeutic window
   b. MTC
   c. onset of action
   d. duration of action

8. Which drug would not typically be monitored with peak and trough blood concentrations?
   a. vancomycin
   b. valproic acid
   c. promethazine
   d. phenytoin

9. If the blood concentration–time profile reflects the amount of drug at the site of action, the maximum therapeutic response would occur
   a. at the onset of action.
   b. at the MEC.
   c. at the peak blood concentration.
   d. when elimination is the predominant process.

10. The transfer of a drug out of a dosage form and into the blood is called
    a. absorption.
    b. dissolution.
    c. metabolism.
    d. elimination.

11. Blood concentrations are the result of _____ simultaneously occurring processes, which together are referred to as _____.
    a. two, passive diffusion
    b. four, disposition
    c. three, elimination
    d. five, absorption

12. Unionized drugs are
    a. actively transported.
    b. hydrophobic drugs.
    c. passively diffused through membranes.
    d. hydrophilic drugs.

REVIEW

13. Which processes can influence the absorption of drugs given orally?
    a. first-pass metabolism
    b. intestinal transit time
    c. gastric emptying
    d. all of the above

14. Which formulation does not have an absorption step?
    a. intravenous solution
    b. intramuscular emulsion
    c. topical cream
    d. vaginal suppository

15. When drug molecules are bound to plasma or tissue proteins they are
    a. more potent.
    b. metabolized.
    c. inactive.
    d. excreted.

16. An enzyme is a complex _____ that catalyzes chemical reactions.
    a. lipid
    b. mineral
    c. protein
    d. atom

17. When some drugs are chronically administered, the liver will decrease its enzyme activity. This is called
    a. enzyme induction.
    b. enzyme inhibition.
    c. enzyme secretion.
    d. first pass metabolism.

18. Enterohepatic recycling occurs when a
    a. drug is metabolized to a metabolite.
    b. drug is secreted to the intestines along with the bile.
    c. drug is secreted into the intestines along with the bile and reabsorbed back into the blood circulation.
    d. all of the above

19. Elimination is
    a. absorption and metabolism.
    b. metabolism and excretion.
    c. distribution and excretion.
    d. distribution and metabolism.

20. Which set of circumstances will result in a drug undergoing urinary reabsorption?
    a. basic drug in high urine pH
    b. basic drug in low urine pH
    c. acidic drug in high urine pH
    d. none of the above

21. The amount of drug excreted in the urine is the amount
    a. filtered + secreted + reabsorbed.
    b. filtered + secreted - reabsorbed.
    c. filtered - secreted + reabsorbed.
    d. filtered - secreted - reabsorbed.

22. The percentage or fraction of the administered dose of a drug that actually reaches the systemic circulation and the rate at which this occurs is the drug's
    a. bioequivalence.
    b. bioavailability.
    c. biotransformation.
    d. biopharmaceutics.

23. To determine the bioavailability of a drug product, it must be compared to another product containing the same drug. If the second product is an intravenous solution, the bioavailability is termed
    a. relative.
    b. bioequivalent.
    c. redundant.
    d. absolute.

24. For elimination of a drug to be essentially complete, ____ times the half-life must elapse.
    a. two
    b. three
    c. five
    d. seven

11

FACTORS AFFECTING DRUG ACTIVITY

LEARNING OBJECTIVES

At the completion of study, the student will:

➡ enumerate physiological factors that influence drug disposition and lead to variation in drug response.

➡ describe how common disease states can lead to altered drug response.

➡ understand common adverse drug reactions and that reactions can occur in one patient but not another.

➡ describe the mechanisms of drug–drug interactions that affect the disposition of one or both drugs and result in either increases or decreases in therapeutic or side effects.

➡ explain the types of drug–drug interactions that do not alter the drugs' disposition but interact at the site of action.

➡ describe drug–diet interactions that alter drug disposition.

HUMAN VARIABILITY

Human variability in biopharmaceutics and disposition can significantly alter blood concentration-time profiles and drug efficacy. Differences in age, weight, genetics, and gender are among the variables that influence the differences in disposition and response to medications.

Age

Human life is a continuous process but it is usually characterized as having stages. The distinctions between the stages are open to individual interpretation, but they are often based on physiological characteristics. The stages are generally considered as:

➡ Neonate, up to one month after birth

➡ Infant, between the ages of one month and two years

➡ Child, between the ages of two and twelve years

➡ Adolescent, between the ages of 13 and 19 years

➡ Adult, between 20 and 70 years

➡ Elder, older than 70 years

Neonates and Infants

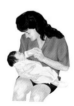

Drug distribution, metabolism, and excretion are quite different in the neonate and infant than in adults because their organ systems are not fully developed. They are not able to eliminate drugs as efficiently as adults. Older infants reach approximately adult levels of protein binding and kidney function, but liver function and the blood-brain barrier are still immature.

Children

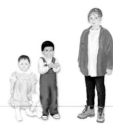

Children metabolize certain drugs more rapidly than adults. Their rate of metabolism increases between 1 year and 12 years of age depending on the child and the drug. Afterwards, metabolism rates decline with age to normal adult levels. Some of the drugs eliminated faster in children include clindamycin, valproic acid, ethosuximide, and theophylline.

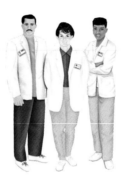

Adults

Adults experience a decrease in many physiological functions between 30 to 70 years of age, but these decreases and their affects on drug activity are gradual.

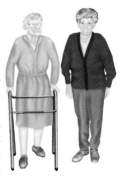

The Elderly

The elderly typically consume more drugs than any other age group. They have a greater incidence of chronic illnesses and multiple disease states. This requires the elderly to take multiple medications, which leads to a higher incidence of drug interactions.

They also experience more physiological changes that significantly affect drug action:

➡ Changes in gastric pH, gastric emptying time, intestinal motility, and gastrointestinal blood flow all tend to slow the rate of absorption.

➡ Changes in the cardiovascular system (including lower cardiac output) tend to slow distribution of drug molecules to their sites of action, metabolism, and excretion.

➡ Though there is probably a decrease in the liver's production of metabolizing enzymes, the metabolism of most drugs does not appear to decrease.

➡ A decline in kidney function (including glomerular filtration and secretion) occurs which in turn tends to slow urinary excretion of drugs.

pharmacogenetics a field of study which defines the hereditary basis of individual differences in absorption, distribution, metabolism, and excretion (the ADME processes).

Gender

For many years, women were excluded from clinical drug investigations. One reason had been to avoid exposing a fetus or potential fetus to unknown risks. What resulted was an inappropriate application of data collected from male subjects or patients to women. The FDA and NIH issued guidelines in 1993–94 stating that women will be included in clinical drug investigations unless a clear and compelling reason is known not to do so.

Since then, many studies have been completed in both genders that show differences in drug disposition depending on the drug. For example, males and females have similar elimination for cimetidine and lorazepam, but women eliminate propranolol, isosorbide dinitrate, diazepam, and temazepam more slowly than men. Acetaminophen and clofibric acid are eliminated more rapidly in women than men.

Some gender-based differences in drug response appear to be related to hormonal fluctuations in women during the menstrual cycle. For women with clinical depression, for example, higher dosages of antidepressant medication may be necessary when menstrual symptoms are worse.

Drug distribution may also be somewhat different between men and women simply as a result of differences in body composition (males have more muscle, women more fat).

Pregnancy

A number of physiological changes including delayed gastric emptying and decreased gastrointestinal tract motility occur in women in the later stages of pregnancy. These changes tend to *reduce the rate of absorption.*

Drug plasma protein binding may be reduced and metabolism increased in pregnant women for a number of drugs. The rate of urinary excretion for a number of drugs is much greater in pregnant women than in non-pregnant women.

Drugs can also readily transport from the maternal to the fetal circulation. Because the fetus has underdeveloped mechanisms to handle drug exposure, drug concentrations may be greater in the fetus than in the mother.

Genetics

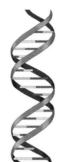 Genes determine the types and amounts of proteins produced in the body, with each person being somewhat different. Since drugs interact with proteins in plasma, tissues, receptor sites, and elsewhere, genetic differences can result in differences in drug action.

A field of study, **pharmacogenetics**, defines the hereditary basis of individual differences in absorption, distribution, metabolism and excretion (the ADME processes.) The largest contributing factor to inherited variability is metabolism. For example, people with certain genetic characteristics will not metabolize a drug that most people metabolize, or will metabolize it at an abnormal rate. In such cases, the individual may experience no therapeutic effect at all, or perhaps even an adverse or toxic effect instead.

Body Weight

Dosage adjustments based on weight are generally not made for adults who are slightly overweight. However, weight is often considered in infants, children, or unusually small, emaciated, or obese patients. Adults who are obese (i.e., body fat content greater than 30% of total body weight) will have significant changes in the distribution and renal excretion of a number of drugs.

Psychological Factors

Though the specific reasons are unknown, it is clear that psychological factors can influence individual responses to drug administration. For example, in clinical trials in which placebos are used, patients receiving them often report both therapeutic and adverse effects. This may account for some variability in patient responses to an administered non-placebo drug. At a fundamental level, it is a factor in patient willingness to follow prescribed dosage regimens.

DISEASE STATES

The disposition and effect of some drugs can be altered in one person but not in another due to the presence of diseases other than the one for which a drug is used.

Drug action can be altered when the normal functioning of organs involved in the ADME of the drug is changed. A pathological condition in any of these organs may have both a direct effect on the drug action or a secondary effect through other organs. Numerous studies have shown the effect of disease on drug action. However, it is not always possible to predict the outcome.

HEPATIC

There are a variety of liver diseases that affect hepatic function differently. Some, but not all, hepatic diseases require that the patient be monitored when receiving certain drugs.

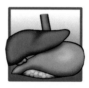

Cirrhosis and **obstructive jaundice** appear to decrease hepatic metabolism and thereby diminish drug elimination. With **acute viral hepatitis,** changes in drug disposition generally are of little significance, and return to normal as the condition clears.

The effect of hepatic disease on drug absorption is not well understood. However, to the extent that liver activity is decreased, it appears that first-pass metabolism is also reduced. This results in increased bioavailability for drugs that are usually severely degraded by first-pass metabolism. Another factor that increases bioavailability is that patients with cirrhosis can develop a condition in which a significant amount of the blood coming from the intestine bypasses liver cells and enters the circulatory system directly. When this happens, the bioavailability of drugs that would otherwise be degraded by first-pass metabolism rises substantially.

Selected Drugs with Decreased Elimination in Cirrhosis

➠ Encainide	➠ Caffeine
➠ Lidocaine	➠ Diazepam
➠ Meperidine	➠ Metronidazole
➠ Metropolol	➠ Theophylline
➠ Verapamil	➠ Erythromycin

CIRCULATORY

Circulatory disorders at the extreme can result in either a change in the magnitude of blood flow to and through an organ, or a regional redistribution of the cardiac output. Generally, these disorders tend to moderate between the extremes and typically cause a diminished blood flow to one or more organs of the body.

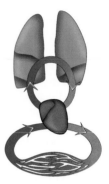

These changes in blood flow influence drug absorption, distribution, and elimination and therefore have the potential to alter the effect of a drug.

Decreased blood flow from cardiovascular disorders can have widespread effects on absorption. Possible factors that can be changed include edema in the large intestine, decreased splanchnic blood flow, delayed gastric emptying, decreased intestinal motility, changes in gastrointestinal pH, and changes in the bacterial flora of the intestine. These changes lead to delayed or erratic drug absorption. Those drugs that are normally well absorbed would be expected to be most affected by the blood flow changes.

Decreased blood flow can affect several factors responsible for metabolizing drugs in the liver. For drugs that are hepatically eliminated in proportion to the organ's blood flow, a diminished blood flow would suggest a decreased clearance. However, other physiological changes do occur in the liver as blood flow is decreased. For example, both external and internal hepatic anastomoses are formed which shunt the blood away from functioning hepatic cells. Also, there are changes in the ability of certain drugs to move from the blood into hepatic cells that contain metabolizing enzymes.

Changes in renal blood flow have less effect on the elimination of drugs than blood flow changes in the liver. It would be expected that decreased renal perfusion would reduce the renal excretion of most drugs. However, it appears that renal excretion can change significantly for those drugs that have a high renal clearance.

RENAL

Reduced renal function, especially end-stage renal disease, can affect the elimination of many drugs and affect the plasma protein binding of drugs.

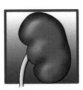

Effects on drug elimination: As renal function decreases, the dosage of a drug that is eliminated by the kidney should be reduced to avoid accumulation of the drug in the body.

Effects on plasma protein binding: The plasma protein binding of acidic drugs is markedly reduced in severe renal insufficiency. Albumin is the major plasma and tissue protein that is responsible for acidic drug binding. Normally, the kidneys do not allow the elimination of albumin. But in chronic renal disease, excessive protein filtration may occur, which leads to a loss of albumin from the body.

Orosomucoid is a plasma protein that is rapidly produced when the body is injured. It also is a protein that many basic drugs bind to in the body. In chronic renal disease, orosomucoid blood concentrations are higher than normal and this results in increased basic drug binding.

Decreases in renal function can be measured by monitoring the amount of creatinine excreted in the urine. Creatinine is produced by muscles in the body, and is excreted at a constant rate primarily by glomerular filtration. In diseased kidneys, the rate of creatinine excretion decreases.

THYROID

Changes in thyroid function can affect many of the aspects of absorption, excretion, and metabolism.

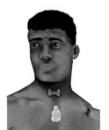

In **hypothyroidism** (a condition in which the thyroid is underactive), the bioavailability of a few drugs (e.g., riboflavin, digoxin) is increased. In **hyperthyroidism** (an overactive thyroid condition) their bioavailability is decreased because of changes in gastrointestinal motility.

Some other changes affected by thyroid conditions are:

➥ Renal blood flow is decreased in hypothyroidism and increased in hyperthyroidism.

➥ The activity of metabolizing enzymes in the liver is reduced in hypothyroidism and increased in hyperthyroidism.

➥ The metabolism of theophylline, propranolol, propylthiouracil, and methimazole is increased by hyperthyroidism.

Bioavailabilty of Selected Drugs in Patients with Renal Disease

➥ Decreased	Furosemide
➥ Increased	Propranolol
➥ Unchanged	Cimetidine, ciprofloxacin, digoxin, labetalol, sulfamethoxazole, trimethoprim

---

ABCD *cirrhosis* a chronic and potentially fatal liver disease causing loss of function and increased resistance to blood flow through the liver.

acute viral hepatitis an inflammatory condition of the liver caused by viruses; the effects are less than in cirrhosis but long term exposure can progress into chronic disease with the same characteristics.

obstructive jaundice an obstruction of the bile duct that causes hepatic waste products and bile to accumulate in the liver.

hypothyroidism a condition in which thyroid hormone secretions are below normal, often referred to as an underactive thyroid.

hyperthyroidism a condition in which thyroid hormone secretions are above normal, often referred to as an overactive thyroid.

ADVERSE DRUG REACTIONS

Because of human variability, adverse drug reactions can occur in one person but not another.

An **adverse drug reaction** can be any undesired symptom and can involve any organ. It may be common or rare, localized or widespread, mild or severe depending on the drug and the patient. Some adverse drug reactions occur with usual doses of drugs (often called side effects). Others are more likely to occur only at higher than normal dosages.

COMMON ADVERSE DRUG REACTIONS

Central Nervous System Effects

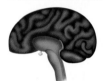

CNS effects may result from CNS stimulation (e.g., agitation, confusion, delirium, disorientation, hallucinations) or CNS depression (e.g., dizziness, drowsiness, sedation, coma, impaired respiration and circulation).

Hepatotoxicity

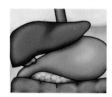

Hepatotoxicities (liver toxicities) include hepatitis, hepatic necrosis, and biliary tract inflammation or obstruction. These are relatively rare but potentially life-threatening. Commonly used hepatotoxic drugs include acetaminophen, halothane, isoniazid, chlorpromazine, methotrexate, nitrofurantoin, phenytoin, and aspirin.

Hypersensitivity or Allergy

Almost any drug, in almost any dose, can produce an allergic or hypersensitive reaction in a patient. This generally happens because a patient developed antibodies while previously taking the drug or a drug with a similar chemical structure. The drug will interact with the antibodies, releasing histamine and other substances that produce reactions that can range from mild rashes to potentially fatal **anaphylactic shock.**

Allergic reactions can occur within minutes or weeks of drug administration. Anaphylactic shock occurs within minutes. It is a hypersensitivity reaction that can lead to cardiovascular collapse and death if untreated. Its symptoms include severe respiratory distress and convulsions. Immediate emergency treatment with epinephrine, antihistamines, or bronchodilator drugs is required.

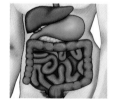

Gastrointestinal Effects

Anorexia, nausea, vomiting, constipation, and diarrhea are among the most common adverse reactions to drugs. More serious effects include ulcerations and colitis (e.g., irritable bowel disease).

adverse drug reaction an unintended side effect of a medication that is negative or in some way injurious to a patient's health.

hypersensitivity an abnormal sensitivity generally resulting in an allergic reaction.

anaphylactic shock a potentially fatal hypersensitivity reaction producing severe respiratory distress and cardiovascular collapse.

safety you should know

Pharmaceutical manufacturers are legally required to report any serious unlabeled (i.e., unexpected) adverse drug reactions through the FDA MedWatch Program. If the product presents a significant threat to consumer safety, that product can be recalled. A numerical classification (Class I, II, or III) indicates the potential hazard of the product. Note that adverse reactions to vaccines are not reported through MedWatch but instead through the Vaccine Adverse Event Reporting System (VAERS) maintained by the Centers for Disease Control (CDC).

Nephrotoxicity

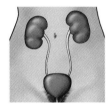

Kidney failure can occur with gentamicin and other aminoglycosides, and with ibuprofen and other nonsteroidal antiinflammatory drugs.

Drug Dependence

Chronic usage of narcotic analgesics, sedative-hypnotic agents, antianxiety agents, and amphetamines can result in physiological or psychological dependence. Physiological dependence is accompanied by unpleasant physical withdrawal symptoms when the dose is discontinued or reduced. Psychological dependence involves an emotional or mental fixation on drug usage.

Idiosyncrasy

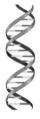

Idiosyncrasy is the unexpected reaction to a drug the first time it is given to a patient. Such reactions are thought to be caused by genetic characteristics that alter the patient's drug metabolizing enzymes.

Teratogenicity

This is the ability of a substance to cause abnormal fetal development when given to pregnant women. Drug groups considered teratogenic include analgesics, diuretics, antihistamines, antibiotics, and antiemetics.

Hematological Effects

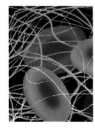

Blood coagulation, bleeding, and bone marrow disorders are potentially life threatening and can be caused by various drugs. Anticoagulants can cause excessive bleeding. Antineoplastic drugs may cause bone marrow depression.

Carcinogenicity

This is the ability of a substance to cause cancer. Several drugs are carcinogens, including some hormones and anticancer drugs.

idiosyncrasy an unexpected reaction the first time a drug is taken, generally due to genetic causes.

carcinogenicity the ability of a substance to cause cancer.

DRUG-DRUG INTERACTIONS

A drug's effect can be altered by a drug–drug interaction.

The probability of a drug–drug interaction increases with the number of drugs a patient takes and in certain disease states. Many drug–drug interactions can affect the disposition of one or both drugs and *result in either increases or decreases in therapeutic or side effects*. Following are some examples of drug–drug interactions that occur because their disposition is altered.

ABSORPTION

There are several means by which one drug may affect the extent or rate of gastrointestinal absorption of another drug:

Complexation

Some drugs can form nonabsorbable complexes by binding to other drugs, resulting in decreased absorption. For example, iron salts can affect the absorption of several tetracyclines, methlydopa, and levodopa in this way. Antacids and sucralfate appear to reduce the absorption of norfloxacin and ciprofloxacin by this mechanism.

Gastric Emptying

Certain drugs will affect gastric emptying and therefore the absorption of other drugs. For example, use of propantheline will delay acetaminophen absorption by slowing the rate of gastric emptying. On the other hand, use of metoclopramide will increase acetaminophen absorption, since metoclopramide increases the rate of gastric emptying. Another problem with reducing gastric emptying time is that drugs that are degraded by gastric acid have a longer time to degrade, resulting in a decreased amount of drug available for absorption from the intestine.

Gastric pH

Drugs that alter the gastrointestinal pH can have varied effects on other administered drugs. Some of the factors affected by pH are the amount of unionized drug available for absorption; the rate of dissolution; intestinal motility; and degradation.

Intestinal Metabolism

Alterations in metabolism are involved in the interaction between oral contraceptives and oral antibiotic therapy. The antibiotic kills the normal bacterial flora in the GI tract, which disrupts the enterohepatic recycling of the oral contraceptive's estrogens.

DISTRIBUTION

Displacement

One drug can displace another from a plasma protein binding site and so increase the amount of the free drug available for distribution. This will increase its pharmacological effect and its elimination, since more of the free drug is available for metabolism and excretion.

Such displacement interactions generally occur within the first week or two of administration. When they do occur, many turn out to be self-correcting after a few days, at which point the concentration of displaced drug often returns to pre-interaction levels, even if the patient continues to take both drugs.

The biggest consequence of displacement interactions is the *change in pharmacological effect*. If drugs are highly protein bound, displacement tends to have a greater effect than with drugs that are not highly bound. For example, warfarin is 98% plasma protein bound, with only 2% free or unbound. If a drug interaction displaces only 2% of the bound warfarin, then 96% will be bound, but 4% will now be free. That is a 100% increase in the free concentration of warfarin, and it might double its pharmacological effect. By comparison, for a drug that is only 60% bound, displacing 2% will cause only a 5% increase in the concentration.

ABCD *complexation* when two different molecules associate or attach to each other.

displacement a drug that is bound to a plasma protein is removed when another drug of greater binding potential binds to the same protein.

enzyme inhibition the decrease in hepatic enzyme activity that results in reduced metabolism of drugs.

enzyme induction the increase in hepatic enzyme activity that results in greater metabolism of drugs.

METABOLISM

Enzyme Induction

Some drugs are capable of increasing the concentration of metabolizing enzymes in the liver. This process is called enzyme induction. It increases the metabolism of drugs that use the same enzyme system and usually results in a *reduction in pharmacological effect.* Examples of enzyme inducers include phenobarbital, carbamazepine, phenytoin, and rifampin. Cigarette smoking and chronic alcohol use may also induce metabolism.

The time course of drug interactions from enzyme induction is slower than for many other types of interactions. Though enzyme induction may be dose related, it can also be influenced by age, genetics, or liver disease. As a result, it is a difficult type of interaction to predict.

Enzyme Inhibition

Another alteration in metabolism is called enzyme inhibition, which usually occurs when two drugs compete for binding sites on the same metabolizing enzyme. This generally *increases the plasma concentration (and consequently the pharmacological effect) of at least one of the drugs.* Enzyme inhibition is one of the most common drug interactions. In fact, if a drug is known to be metabolized by the liver, manufacturers often study its potential for enzyme inhibition early in the drug development process. Examples of enzyme inhibitors include allopurinol, cimetidine, erythromycin, disulfiram, isoniazid, ketoconazole, and verapamil.

Unlike enzyme induction, which has a much slower time course, enzyme inhibition has a rapid onset, generally within 24 hours, and tends to disappear quickly once the inhibitor is discontinued. Enzyme inhibition is also easier to predict since it appears to be dose related. It is also true that drugs that share a similar chemical structure often share the potential for enzyme inhibition.

EXCRETION

Glomerular Filtration

Drug interactions that actually change the filtration rate itself are rare. Changes in the filtration rate are more likely to occur in response to specific drugs, such as those that change the systemic blood pressure, for example. Whatever the cause, changes in the filtration rate will also change the rate of drug excretion.

Renal Secretion

There are different secretory systems in the kidneys for basic drugs and acidic drugs. Basic drugs do not seem to compete for the acidic drug transport system, or visa versa. However, two basic drugs or two acidic drugs may compete for the same transport system and this can cause one or both of the drugs to accumulate in the blood. For example, probenecid competes with penicillin and reduces penicillin's secretion. Probenecid also inhibits the secretion of cephalosporins. The interaction between NSAIDS and methotrexate is another example. Some of these interactions can increase methotrexate concentrations two- to three-fold. An example of such a competition involving basic drugs is quinidine and digoxin. Quinidine reduces digoxin excretion by 30% to 50%.

Urinary Reabsorption

Urinary reabsorption, a passive transport process, is influenced by the pH of the urine and the extent of ionization of the drug. In acidic urine, acidic drugs tend to be reabsorbed while basic drugs are not. As a result, basic drugs are excreted in the urine. In alkaline urine, acidic drugs will not be reabsorbed but will instead be excreted in the urine, while basic drugs will be reabsorbed. An example of these interactions is quinidine, which is a base. The excretion of quinidine is reduced nearly 90% when the urine pH is increased from less than 6.0 to over 7.5.

DRUG-DRUG INTERACTIONS (cont'd)

Some drug–drug interactions do not alter the drugs' disposition but interact at the site of action.

Sometimes, the drugs directly compete for the same receptor. But other times, the interaction is more indirect and involves interfering with normal physiological processes. These interactions are commonly called "additive," "summative," "synergistic," or "potentiation" and have precise pharmacological definitions. But most often these definitions are used as synonyms because it is difficult to quantify the extent of altered drug activity.

➡ **Additive effects** occur when two drugs with similar pharmacological actions result in an effect equal to the sum of the individual effects.

Example: trimethoprim + sulfamethoxazole for antibiotic effect.

Sulfamethoxazole and trimethoprim are commonly used in combination for treating *Pneumocystis carinii* pneumonia, an opportunistic infection in AIDS patients.

Example: amiodarone + dofetilide for prolongation of heart's QT interval.

Many drugs affect the electrical activity of the heart. Amiodarone and dofetilide are two drugs that prolong repolarization as part of their therapeutic effect. But phenothiazines (tranquilizers) and some antibiotics slow repolarization as an undesired effect. If these drugs are used together, repolarization may be delayed too long, and arrhythmias may occur.

➡ **Synergism** occurs when two drugs with similar pharmacological actions produce greater effects than the sum of individual effects.

Example: aspirin + warfarin = increased anticoagulation.

Aspirin increases the risk of bleeding in anticoagulated patients because it inhibits platelet function and causes gastric erosions. Large doses of aspirin (3 g/day or more) can increase the entire anticoagulation response. However, low doses of aspirin appear to primarily increase minor bleeding, and so the combination of aspirin and warfarin is used intentionally in many patients.

Example: vancomycin + gentamicin = increased anti-bacterial effects of gentamicin.

Enterococcus fecalis is a gram-negative microorganism that is not susceptible to gentamicin. But if another antibiotic (e.g., vancomycin) is given that inhibits the synthesis of the microorganism's cell walls, the effect of gentamicin is increased.

additive effects the summation in effect when two drugs with similar pharmacological actions are taken.

synergism when two drugs with similar pharmacological actions produce greater effects than the sum of individual effects.

potentiation when one drug with no inherent activity of its own increases the activity of another drug that produces an effect.

antidote a drug that antagonizes the toxic effect of another.

➥ **Potentiation** occurs when one drug with no inherent activity of its own increases the activity of another drug that produces an effect.

> **Example:** amoxicillin + clavulanic acid = increased duration of amoxicillin's antibiotic effect.

> Clavulanic acid inhibits the enzyme that degrades amoxicillin, and thereby allows amoxicillin to be more potent than if used alone.

➥ An **antidote** to a particular drug is given to block or reduce its toxic effects.

> **Example:** naloxone + morphine = relief of morphine induced respiratory depression. Naloxone displaces morphine from their receptor sites, preventing morphine from causing further depressive effects.

> **Example:** vitamin K + warfarin = opposition of the anticoagulant effect of warfarin and a return to normal blood clotting time.

> The anticoagulation effects of warfarin can be reduced or abolished by the concurrent use of vitamin K. Vitamin K can be given as a drug, but can also be consumed by the patient in some green vegetables such as spinach, brussel sprouts, or broccoli. Some liquid dietary supplements (e.g., Ensure-Plus, Nutrilite 330) contain vitamin K and can also cause the interaction.

> **Example:** Protamine sulfate is given as an antidote to heparin overdose. Protamine combines with heparin to form a stable complex, which leads to the decrease in the anticoagulant activity of both drugs.

> **Example:** Flumazenil is a benzodiazepine antagonist that reverses the sedative effects of diazepam, midazolam, and zolpidem. Flumazenil competes for the same receptors as the benzodiazepines, and displaces them.

Time Course of Drug Interactions

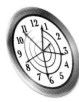
The time it takes for drug–drug interactions to occur can vary substantially. Some interactions occur almost immediately while others may take weeks. Knowing the time course of an interaction allows quick identification and treatment of potential interactions. It also allows clinicians to evaluate the relative importance of an interaction from two drugs compared to their therapeutic effects. For example, if an interaction requires one to two weeks to occur, short term administration over a few days will not cause a significant adverse effect.

DRUG–DIET INTERACTIONS

Dietary intakes and patterns vary widely and can contribute to variability in the disposition and effects of drugs.

Differences may be attributed to various factors including food preferences and availability, diets designed for weight gain or loss, and variations for seasonal, religious, and therapeutic reasons.

ABSORPTION

The physical presence of food in the gastrointestinal tract can alter absorption in several ways:

- interacting chemically (e.g., tetracycline and iron);
- improving the solubility of some drugs by increasing bile secretion;
- affecting the performance of the dosage form (e.g., altering the release characteristics of polymer coated tablets);
- altering gastric emptying;
- altering intestinal motility;
- altering liver blood flow.

As a result, some drugs have increased bioavailability and some have decreased bioavailability in the presence of food. For example, the bioavailability of propranolol, metoprolol, hydralazine, erythromycin, and phenytoin is enhanced by the presence of food.

The bioavailability of a drug is generally decreased when the presence of food slows absorption. For example, when tablets or capsules are taken with food, they dissolve more slowly, slowing absorption as a result.

Food may also combine with a drug to form an insoluble drug–food complex. This is how tetracycline interacts with dairy products, such as milk and cheese. It combines with the calcium in milk products to form an insoluble, nonabsorbable compound that is excreted in the feces. In general, dietary fiber decreases the absorption of drugs.

DISTRIBUTION

The presence of food can also influence drug distribution. For example, high fat meals can increase fatty acid levels in the blood. The fatty acids bind to the same plasma protein binding sites as many drugs. This displaces the previously bound drug and increases the free concentration of that drug, leading to an increased effect.

There are also differences in the plasma protein binding of certain drugs between well nourished and undernourished people.

ADMINISTRATION TIMES

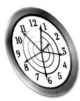

Interactions that alter drug absorption can be minimized by separating the administration of drugs and food intake by about 2 hours.

drug–diet interactions when elements of ingested nutrients interact with a drug and this affects the disposition of the drug.

METABOLISM

Most foods are complex mixtures of carbohydrate, fat, and protein. Research studies designed to determine the influence of diet on drug metabolism use diets in which one of these nutrients is increased, another decreased, and the third nutrient and total caloric intake are kept constant. In general, high protein (low carbohydrate) diets are associated with accelerated metabolism while high carbohydrate (low protein) diets appear to decrease metabolism. The substitution of fat calories for carbohydrate seems not to affect drug metabolism rates.

In general, mildly or moderately undernourished adults have normal or enhanced metabolism of drugs and severely malnourished adults have decreased drug metabolism. As with any diet, however, there are many variables in malnourishment that can produce an affect on metabolism.

EXCRETION

Increasing protein in the diet appears to increase glomerular filtration, decrease reabsorption, and decrease secretion in the kidney. The total effect of restricted protein intake will depend on the urinary excretion characteristics of the specific drug.

Effect of Dietary Factors on Metabolism

Change in Food Composition	Effect on Metabolism
increased protein	increased metabolism
increased carbohydrate	decreased metabolism
increased fat	no effect
decreased calories	decreased metabolism

SPECIFIC FOODS

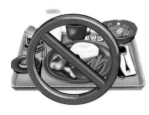 Some foods contain substances that react with certain drugs. For example, eating foods containing tyramine while using monoamine oxidase (MAO) inhibitors may produce severe hypertension or intracranial hemorrhage. MAO inhibitors include isocarboxazid, phenelzine, and procarbazine. Foods containing tyramine include beer, red wine, aged cheeses, yeast products, chicken livers, and pickled herring.

Certain cruciferous vegetables (i.e., brussels sprouts, cabbage) stimulate the metabolism of a few drugs. Other foods that might also have the similar effect are alfalfa, turnips, broccoli, cauliflower, or spinach. Some of the same foods are also involved with an interaction with oral anticoagulants such as warfarin. Spinach and other greens contain vitamin K, and vitamin K inhibits the action of oral anticoagulants. A patient ingesting foods containing vitamin K while taking an anticoagulant would not receive the full therapeutic effect from warfarin.

REVIEW

KEY CONCEPTS

HUMAN VARIABILITY

✔ Differences in age, weight, genetics, and gender are among the significant factors that influence the differences in medication responses among people.

✔ Drug distribution, metabolism, and excretion are quite different in the neonate and infant than in adults because their organ systems are not fully developed.

✔ Children metabolize certain drugs more rapidly than adults.

✔ The elderly typically consume more drugs and have a higher incidence of drug interactions than other age groups. They also experience more physiological changes that significantly affect drug action.

✔ Genetic differences can cause differences in the types and amounts of proteins produced in the body, which can result in differences in drug action.

DISEASE STATES

✔ The disposition and effect of some drugs may be altered in one patient but not another by the presence of diseases other than the one for which a drug is used.

ADVERSE DRUG REACTIONS

✔ Almost any drug, in almost any dose, can produce an allergic or hypersensitive reaction in a patient. Anaphylactic shock is a potentially fatal hypersensitivity reaction.

✔ Anorexia, nausea, vomiting, constipation, and diarrhea are among the most common adverse reactions to drugs in the GI tract.

DRUG–DRUG INTERACTIONS

✔ Many drug–drug interactions affect the disposition of one or both drugs and result in either increases or decreases in therapeutic or side effects.

✔ Decreased intestinal absorption of oral drugs occurs when drugs complex to produce nonabsorbable compounds.

✔ Displacement of one drug from protein binding sites by a second drug increases the effects of the displaced drug.

✔ Drugs that induce liver metabolism may also increase metabolism of other drugs that use the same metabolizing enzymes.

✔ Some drugs increase excretion by altering urinary pH and lessening renal reabsorption.

✔ Some drug–drug interactions do not alter a drug's disposition but interact at the site of action.

✔ Additive effects occur when two drugs with similar pharmacological actions result in an effect equal to the sum of the individual effects.

✔ Synergism occurs when two drugs with similar pharmacological actions produce greater effects than the sum of the individual effects.

DRUG–DIET INTERACTIONS

✔ Some foods contain substances that react with certain drugs, e.g., foods containing tyramine can react with monoamine oxidase (MAO) inhibitors.

SELF TEST

MATCH THE TERMS   the *answer key begins on page 511*

1. acute viral hepatitis ____

2. additive effects ____

3. adverse drug reaction ____

4. anaphylactic shock ____

5. antidote ____

6. carcinogenicity ____

7. cirrhosis ____

8. complexation ____

9. displacement ____

10. drug–diet interactions ____

11. enzyme induction ____

12. enzyme inhibition ____

13. hypersensitivity ____

14. hyperthyroidism ____

15. hypothyroidism ____

16. idiosyncrasy ____

17. obstructive jaundice ____

18. pharmacogenetics ____

19. potentiation ____

20. synergism ____

a. when two different molecules associate or attach to each other.

b. an abnormal sensitivity generally resulting in an allergic reaction.

c. a potentially fatal hypersensitivity reaction producing severe respiratory distress and cardiovascular collapse.

d. an unexpected reaction the first time a drug is taken, generally due to genetic causes.

e. the ability of a substance to cause cancer.

f. when two drugs with similar pharmacological actions result in an effect equal to the sum of the individual effects.

g. when two drugs with similar pharmacological actions produce greater effects than the sum of the individual effects.

h. a drug that antagonizes the toxic effect of another drug.

i. a chronic and potentially fatal liver disease causing loss of function and increased resistance to blood flow through the liver.

j. an inflammatory condition of the liver caused by viruses.

k. when elements of ingested nutrients interact with a drug and this affects the disposition of the drug.

l. an obstruction of the bile duct that causes hepatic waste products and bile to accumulate in the liver.

m. a condition in which thyroid hormone secretions are above normal, often referred to as an overactive thyroid.

n. a condition in which thyroid secretions are below normal, often referred to as an underactive thyroid.

o. a field of study which defines the hereditary basis of individual differences in the ADME processes.

p. an unintended side effect of a medication that is negative or in some way injurious to the patient's health.

q. an effect produced when one drug with no inherent activity of its own increases the activity of another drug.

r. a drug bound to a plasma protein is removed when another drug of greater binding potential binds to the same protein.

s. the decrease in hepatic enzyme activity that results in reduced metabolism of drugs.

t. the increase in hepatic enzyme activity that results in greater metabolism of drugs.

REVIEW

the answer key begins on page 511

CHOOSE THE BEST ANSWER

1. Drug distribution, metabolism, and excretion are quite different in _____ than in adults because their organ systems are not fully developed.
   a. infants and adolescents
   b. neonates and infants
   c. children and adolescents
   d. elders

2. Children between the ages of _____ metabolize certain drugs more rapidly than adults.
   a. 0 and 6 months
   b. 6 and 18 months
   c. 1 and 2 years
   d. 1 and 12 years

3. Which physiological change is typically seen with pregnant women that affects drug disposition?
   a. decreased rate of absorption
   b. decreased urinary excretion
   c. increased plasma protein binding
   d. decreased rate of metabolism

4. The distribution of drugs may be different between men and women due to
   a. normal fluctuations.
   b. age.
   c. body composition.
   d. activity.

5. The placebo effect is a
   a. psychological variable.
   b. gender variable.
   c. hypersensitive reaction.
   d. drug dependence variable.

6. Adults have a gradual decline in many physiological functions between the ages of
   a. 12–20 years.
   b. 20–40 years.
   c. 30–70 years.
   d. 40–75 years.

7. Adults that have greater than _____ body fat have significant changes in drug distribution and renal excretion.
   a. 10%
   b. 20%
   c. 30%
   d. 40%

8. In end-stage renal disease, _____ levels increase and _____ levels decrease.
   a. albumin, orosomucoid
   b. orosomucoid, albumin
   c. anastomoses, orosomucoid
   d. albumin, thyroid

9. Which endogenous compound is used to monitor renal function?
   a. ciprofloxacin
   b. creatinine
   c. cimetidine
   d. caffeine

10. When hepatic function is decreased by a hepatic disease, it is expected that
    a. first-pass metabolism will increase.
    b. urinary excretion will decrease.
    c. first-pass metabolism will decrease.
    d. hepatic blood flow will increase.

11. Acute viral hepatitis is an inflammatory condition caused by
    a. chronic alcohol abuse.
    b. glomerular filtration.
    c. decreased renal blood flow.
    d. viruses.

12. Examples of CNS stimulation include
    a. agitation, confusion, coma.
    b. disorientation, hallucinations, confusion.
    c. delirium, dizziness, hallucinations.
    d. dizziness, drowsiness, and impaired respiration.

13. _____ is accompanied by an emotional fixation on drug usage.
    a. Psychological dependence
    b. Teratogenicity
    c. Physiological dependence
    d. Hypersensitivity

14. An unexpected adverse effect to a drug the first time it is given to a patient is considered what type of reaction?
    a. hypersensitivity
    b. anaphylaxis
    c. idiosyncrasy
    d. autoimmune

15. Anaphylactic shock usually occurs within
    a. minutes.
    b. hours.
    c. days.
    d. weeks.

16. The rate of absorption is generally increased by
    a. decreased gastric emptying.
    b. increased GI tract motility.
    c. increased first-pass metabolism.
    d. changes in gastric pH.

17. Displacement drug interactions occur at
    a. hepatocytes.
    b. nephrons.
    c. protein binding sites.
    d. glomerulus.

18. If a drug is _____ plasma protein bound, a displacement interaction will probably be significant.
    a. 10%
    b. 30%
    c. 60%
    d. 90%

19. Enzyme inhibition reactions generally occur in
    a. 24 hours.
    b. 4 days.
    c. 1 week.
    d. 1 month.

20. In acidic urine, acidic drugs are reabsorbed and basic drugs are not. This occurs because
    a. acidic drugs are more unionized in acidic urine.
    b. acidic drugs are more ionized in acidic urine.
    c. basic drugs are more unionized in acidic urine.
    d. basic drugs are more ionized in basic urine.

21. When two drugs with similar pharmacological actions produce an effect equal to the sum of the individual effects, the interaction is called
    a. an additive effect.
    b. a complexation effect.
    c. an induction effect.
    d. a displacement effect.

22. A/an _____ is a drug that antagonizes the toxic effects of another drug.
    a. agonist
    b. synergist
    c. antidote
    d. inducer

REVIEW

23. Drug–diet interactions that alter drug absorption can be minimized by separating the administration of the drug and food intake by
    a. 15 minutes.
    b. 30 minutes.
    c. 2 hours.
    d. 4 hours.

24. A high carbohydrate (low protein) diet would be expected to _____ the metabolism of many drugs.
    a. decrease
    b. have no effect
    c. increase

25. Spinach and other green vegetables contain vitamin _____ that inhibits the action of oral anticoagulants.
    a. A
    b. C
    c. B-complex
    d. K

12

INFORMATION

LEARNING OBJECTIVES

At the completion of study, the student will:

➡ understand the three types of literature.

➡ become familiar with pharmacy references and understand how to use them.

➡ know what is meant by the World Wide Web, its place in pharmacy, and key pharmacy web sites.

➡ be familiar with references that provide information on the pharmacy technician profession.

CHAPTER OUTLINE

INFORMATION

The tremendous amount of drug research done each year results in the appearance of many new drugs on pharmacy shelves. As a pharmacy technician, you may find it difficult to absorb and keep up with pharmaceutical information. Becoming familiar with the various pharmaceutical information sources will allow you to keep current with the information necessary to perform your job on an on-going basis.

Pharmacy literature can be thought of as a pyramid divided into three sections.

Primary literature sits at the base. It provides the foundation for the development of secondary and tertiary sources of professional literature.

Of the three types of reference materials, pharmacists and technicians usually find the tertiary sources the easiest and most convenient to use.

However, no single tertiary reference source contains all the information that will be needed by the pharmacy department. Also, view tertiary references carefully, since authors may misinterpret or misquote the original literature. Finally, keep in mind that tertiary references are usually published one or more years after the original literature and therefore may no longer be current.

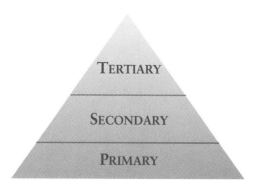

primary literature original reports of clinical and other types of research projects and studies.

secondary literature general reference works based upon primary literature sources.

tertiary literature condensed works based on primary literature, such as textbooks, monographs, etc.

PHARMACY LITERATURE

Primary Literature

Primary literature provides direct access to the largest amount of and most current information from contemporary research. It includes original reports of scientific, clinical, technological, and administrative research and is found in professional and scientific journals such as the *journal of Pharmacy Technology*. The need for large storage spaces and the varying quality of journal articles constitute the greatest disadvantages of this type of literature. Specific information in primary literature can be found with database searches on pubmed (pubmed.gov), a service of the US National Library of Medicine, using topics, authors, or journals.

Secondary Literature

Secondary literature references aid in identifying and locating primary literature and consist of **abstracting services**, indexing or bibliographic services, and microfiche systems.

Abstracting services (e.g., *Drugdex*) summarize information contained in some professional and scientific journals. Indexing or bibliographic services (e.g., *Index Medicus*) provide more comprehensive listings of current articles in worldwide professional and scientific journals. A lag time of 1–12 weeks exists for secondary literature, You can usually find these indexing services in hospital or university libraries as well as online.

Tertiary Literature

Tertiary literature sources contain condensed and compact information based on established knowledge in primary literature. This type of literature reference includes textbooks, monographs, standard reference books, and review articles.

abstracting services services that summarize information from various primary sources for quick reference.

LEGAL ASPECTS

Federal

At present, no federal law mandates that pharmacies maintain professional drug information literature. The Occupational, Safety, and Health Administration (OSHA) does however require pharmacies to have a Material Safety Data Sheets (MSDS) for each hazardous chemical they stock. A pharmacy can obtain MSDSs from the manufacturers or the local OSHA area office. A MSDS provides information you need to ensure the implementation of proper protective measures for exposure to hazardous chemicals. The National Institute for Occupational Safety and Health (NIOSH) develops recommendations for occupational safety and health standards such as the 2004 alert "Preventing Occupational Exposures to Anti-Neoplastic and Other Hazardous Drugs in Health Care Settings."

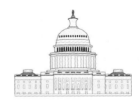

For drugs manufactured and marketed in the United States, the U.S. Food, Drug and Cosmetic Act recognizes the USP-NF general chapters <1> to <999> as enforceable by the Food and Drug Administration. The USP-NF is available in print, on CD, and on-line at www.usp.org.

The Health Insurance Portability and Accessibility Act (HIPAA) of 1996 affects many of the daily activities that take place in the pharmacy. The act's privacy regulation, *HIPAA Privacy Standards: A Compliance Manual for Pharmacies*, was created to protect the privacy of patient health records and requires pharmacies to set boundaries on the use and disclosure of patients' protected health information (PHI).

State

Most states have Pharmacy Statutes and State Board of Pharmacy Rules and Regulations that require pharmacies to maintain specific professional literature references. Pharmacy technicians should know which are mandated by their state regulatory agencies. Examples might include the current edition of *21 Code of Federal Regulations (CFR) Part 1300 to End* or a state's *Uniform Controlled Substances Act*.

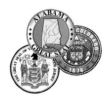

Legal References

An awareness of the legal aspects of pharmacy protects both the pharmacy technician and the patients. The pharmacy law references described below provide information on laws concerning controlled substances, drug control, and other laws critical to the practice of pharmacy.

➥ *Pharmacy Law Digest of Facts and Comparisons* (bound) provides an overview of the legal system as it affects pharmacy practice, including information on controlled substances, government inspections, regulation of pharmaceuticals, civil liability, and business laws. It also contains a review of legal cases involving the practice of pharmacy, and reprints of the National Association of Boards of Pharmacy (NABP) law tables.

➥ *Legal Handbook for Pharmacy Technicians* by Dione Davey, PharmD, JD, teaches technicians the essentials on how pharmacy is regulated.

COMMON REFERENCES

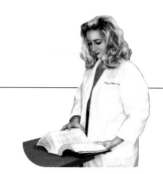

The tertiary literature sources described below are the most commonly available references in pharmacies and drug information centers in the United States.

Some of these references focus on specific areas, while others seek to be very comprehensive. As such, there is overlap in the kinds of information these references provide. You may be able to find what you are looking for in more than one source. At the same time, it is helpful to know if one reference will be particularly useful for certain kinds of information, which we have noted in *green italics* in the following descriptions.

Drug Facts and Comparisons (DFC) (www.factsandcomparisons.com)

The DFC, a preferred reference for comprehensive and timely drug information, contains information about prescription and OTC products presented in easy-to-use comparative tables of therapeutic groups. *It is used to compare medications in the same therapeutic class.* A loose-leaf edition provides the most up-to-date drug reference through monthly updates. The drug information is also available online and on monthly and annual CDs through *Facts and Comparison 4.0.*

Martindale, *The Complete Drug Reference*

Formerly known as Martindale, *The Extra Pharmacopoeia,* contains international drug monographs with drug names, manufacturers, country of origin, active constituents, and licensed indications. *Use Martindale to research foreign drugs.*

AHFS Drug Information (www.ashp.org/ahfs)

The American Hospital Formulary Service (AHFS) is accepted as the source of comparative, unbiased, and evidence-based drug information. It groups drugs by therapeutic use and is updated electronically and in an annual print update. *Use AHFS when investigating* **off-label medication indications.** *PDA* and *Desktop* formats are available.

Handbook on Injectable Drugs (www.ashp.org)

This is a collection of monographs on commercially available parenteral drugs. *It includes information on preparation, storage, administration, compatibility, and stability of injectable drugs.* It is available through ASHP in print and CD formats.

Red Book: Pharmacy's Fundamental Reference

The *Red Book* is the guide to accurate product information and prices on prescription drugs, OTC items, and reimbursable medical supplies. *It provides the latest pricing information, including nationally-recognized AWP's and suggested retail prices for OTC products.* It also contains NDC numbers for all FDA-approved drugs; buying groups and billing standards; directories for manufacturers, wholesalers and third party administrators; complete package information; guide to herbal medicines; common lab values; drug interaction information; and product listings for patients with special needs.

"Orange Book" the common name for the FDA's *Approved Drug Products with Therapeutic Equivalence.*

off-label indication a use of a medication for an indication not approved by the FDA.

King's Guide to Parenteral Admixtures (www.kingguide.com)

This reference provides information on injectable drug compatibility and stability, updated quarterly. It is available in print, online, and in PDA and wall chart formats.

American Drug Index

This bound index published by Facts and Comparisons provides quick access to a comprehensive list of drugs and drug products. Drug names are cross-referenced with monographs that provide generic pronunciations, manufacturer, strength, composition, package size, dosage forms, uses, and common abbreviations. *Use this reference to find trade and generic names.*

The Merck Index (www.merck.com)

Provides information on chemicals, drugs, and biologicals via monographs, supplemental tables, and organic name reactions. It includes chemical, common and generic names; chemical structures; molecular formula; physical and toxicity data; therapeutic and commercial uses; and caution and hazard information. *Use* The Merck Index *when information on chemical attributes of drugs is needed.* The printed edition includes a companion CD.

Physicians' Desk Reference (PDR) (www.pdr.net)

The PDR provides FDA regulation information on prescription drugs. *The information is similar to pharmaceutical manufacturer's drug package inserts since manufacturers prepare the essential drug information found in the PDR.* It contains drug usage information and warnings, drug interactions, and full size color photos of drugs. The PDR electronic library is available on CD. PDR.net membership includes FDA-approved product labeling, the *PDR e-book*, resource centers, study abstracts, *Medline* and *Stedman's Medical Dictionary* and PDA downloads and CME.

USP Pharmacist's Pharmacopeia Product Information (www.usp.org)

The *USP Pharmacist's Pharmacopeia* provides comprehensive information for pharmacy, veterinary, and other health care professionals on compounding, packaging, labeling, and storage of pharmaceutical preparations. It is published bi-annually with five interim supplements available on the USP website or in pdf downloads. *Use USP to prepare for regulatory surveys and to comply with standards of practice regarding compounding sterile and non-sterile preparations.*

"Orange Book" (www.accessdata.fda.gov/scripts/cder/ob/docs/querytn.cfm)

"Orange Book" is the common name for the FDA's *Approved Drug Products with Therapeutic Equivalence Evaluations. Use the Orange Book to determine the therapeutic equivalence of a brand and generic drug.* Drugs with Code A are considered equivalent while drugs with Code B are documented as nonequivalent.

Tech Manual Section VI: Chapter 2, Controlling Occupational Exposure to Hazardous Drugs or ASHP Tech Assistance Bulletin on Handling Cytotoxic and Hazardous Drugs

These references are needed if a pharmacy compounds cytotoxic products.

OTHER REFERENCES

Professional Practice Journals

These journals are official publications of pharmacy organizations and can reflect the political views or policies of these groups. They also reflect changes in standards of practice and indicate trends in the profession. They may publish some original research studies. Examples are *Today's Technician* (NPTA), *America's Pharmacist* (NCPA), *American Journal of Health-System Pharmacy* (ASHP) and the *Journal of the American Pharmacists Association* (APhA).

Trade Journals

Trade journals are published commercially for pharmacists but are not produced by any professional association. They tend to contain large amounts of advertising material. Examples are: *Pharmacy Times* (www.pharmacytimes.com) and *US Pharmacist* (www.uspharmacist.com).

Indexes of Primary Literature

Primary literature can be accessed by printed indexes and abstracts or by CD and online database searching. The continuing development of online and CD databases has increased the efficiency of the access, retrieval, and storage of information. *Thomson Reuter's Micromedex* Healthcare Series (www.micromedex.com) and PubMed (www.pubmed.gov) are two databases of importance to the pharmaceutical researcher. *Micromedex* is a subscription to full-text databases covering drug information, toxicology, and critical care. It includes *Drugdex*, *Poisondex*, *Diseasedex*, *Kinetidex*, *IVdex*, and *Identidex* as well as *Index Nominum*, *Martindale*, *The Physicians' Desk Reference* (PDR), *Red Book*, *MSDS*, and *Carenotes*. *PubMed/*MedlinePlus contributes the most comprehensive index of international medical literature and clinical trials.

Newsletters

Newsletters are published rapidly and frequently and provide a useful source of current information. *The Medical Letter* and *The Pink Sheet* are a few examples of the many newsletters available to pharmacy personnel.

➡ *The Medical Letter on Drugs and Therapeutics* (www.medicalletter.org) contains short abstracts from journal articles. It also provides information on clinical trials and profiles on products recently granted New Drug Application (NDA) status.

➡ *The Pink Sheet: Prescription Pharmaceuticals and Biotechnology* (www.thepinksheet.com) reports on important regulatory issues, business and finance, as well as research and development and new products.

 Many of these resources (including a considerable amount of primary literature) are available (at least in part) over the internet. For more information on using the internet, see page 304.

Textbooks

Textbooks can provide basic information on a particular topic or a range of topics. As with any publications, there is a wide range in the quality, level, and usefulness of textbooks. It is important to not accept the information in them as the last word on a subject. However, textbooks are very useful for explaining basic concepts and in refreshing your understanding of a topic. The texts below are noted for their authoritativeness and reliability in providing pharmaceutical information.

➡ ***Handbook of Nonprescription Drugs: An Interactive Approach to Self Care (www.otchandbook.com***

> The *Handbook* provides a quick access to OTC drug information, complementary therapies, non-drug measures, treatment algorithms, assessment and triage techniques, and patient counseling tips. It serves both as a textbook for the pharmacy student and an information source for the practicing pharmacist. A searchable e-book in pdf format can be downloaded.

➡ **Remington,** *The Science and Practice of Pharmacy*

> Published every 5 years since 1885, Remington is the most comprehensive work in the pharmaceutical sciences. It covers all aspects of pharmacy for students, practitioners and researchers, including ethical principles, technology and automation, professional communication, specializations in pharmacy practice, and medication errors. Drug monographs are categorized by drug class. The companion CD is essentially a scanned version of the entire book.

➡ ***Goodman and Gilman's The Pharmacological Basis of Therapeutics (www.goodmanandgilman.com)***

> This is a principal pharmacy text on pharmacology and therapeutics, emphasizing clinical pharmacy practice. The digital edition with PDA download capability, combines both the print and online presentations.

Personal Digital Assistants (PDA's)

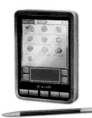

A PDA is a fully functioning computer the size of a paperback book. In 1996, the original Palm Pilot™ was introduced and since then PDA's have evolved into machines for downloading information from the Internet. Pharmacists use PDAs to provide drug information to patients and health care professionals. PDAs have a touch screen for entering data, a memory card/slot for data storage, and wired or wireless connectivity. Newer PDAs can also be used as mobile phones, media players, and web browsers. Pharmacy software is available on the Internet from a variety of sources including www.epocrates.com, www.micromedex.com, www.lexi.com, and www.ashp.org.

REVIEW

KEY CONCEPTS

INFORMATION

✔ Primary literature provides direct access to the most current contemporary research. Secondary literature primarily consists of general reference works based upon primary literature sources. Tertiary literature sources contain condensed information based on primary literature.

✔ OSHA requires pharmacies to have Material Safety Data Sheets (MSDS) for all their hazardous chemicals.

✔ The USP-NF Chapters <1> through <999> are enforced by the FDA.

✔ State laws and State Board of Pharmacy rules and regulations require pharmacies to maintain specific professional literature references.

COMMON REFERENCES

✔ *Drug Facts and Comparisons* (DFC) is a preferred reference for comprehensive and timely drug information, containing information about prescription and OTC products.

✔ Martindale, *The Complete Drug Reference* provides the best source of information on drugs in clinical use internationally.

✔ *AHFS* is accepted as the authority for drug information questions. It groups drug monographs by therapeutic use and provides off-label medication uses.

✔ The "Orange Book" is the common name for the FDA publication titled *Approved Drug Products with Therapeutic Equivalence Evaluations*.

✔ The *Handbook on Injectable Drugs* is a collection of monographs on commercially available parenteral drugs that include concentration, stability, dosage, and compatibility information.

✔ The *Red Book: Pharmacy's Fundamental Reference* is the pharmacist's guide to products and prices and provides annual price lists of drug products, as well as manufacturer, package size, strength, and wholesale and retail prices.

OTHER REFERENCES

✔ *Today's Technician*, a professional practice journal, is the official publication of the NPTA.

✔ A personal digital assistant (PDA) is a fully functioning computer the size of a paperback book. Pharmacists use it to provide drug information. Pharmacy software for PDA's can be downloaded from the internet.

THE INTERNET

✔ The Internet is a supernetwork, with many networks from around the world all connected to each other by telephone lines, cable, or satellite and all using a common "language."

✔ A search engine will search the Web for specific information you enter.

TECHNICIAN REFERENCES

✔ The Pharmacy Technician Certification Board (PTCB) administers the National Pharmacy Technician Certification Exam (PTCE). The PTCB website at www.ptcb.org provides information regarding exam application and preparation.

✔ Once certified as a Pharmacy Technician, the PTCB requires you to obtain 20 hours of continuing education credit every two years to maintain your certification. At least one of the 20 hours must be in pharmacy law.

SELF TEST

MATCH THE TERMS

the answer key begins on page 511

1. abstracting services ____

2. browser ____

3. Digital Subscriber Line (DSL) ____

4. HIPAA ____

5. Internet Service Provider (ISP) ____

6. modem ____

7. off-label indication ____

8. "Orange Book" ____

9. PDA ____

10. primary literature ____

11. search engine ____

12. secondary literature ____

13. tertiary literature ____

14. trade journals ____

15. Uniform Resource Locator (URL) ____

16. World Wide Web ____

a. original reports of clinical and other types of research projects and studies.

b. journals published commercially for pharmacy but not produced by any professional association.

c. condensed works based on primary literature, such as textbooks, monographs, etc.

d. services that summarize information from various primary sources for quick reference.

e. regulation created to protect the privacy of patient health records.

f. a fully functioning computer the size of a paperback book.

g. a collection of electronic documents at an internet address.

h. a company that provides access to the Internet.

i. software that searches the web for information related to criteria entered by the user.

j. provides Internet connections that are faster than telephone modem connections.

k. general reference works based upon primary literature sources.

l. the common name for the FDA's Approved Drug Products publication.

m. computer hardware that enables a computer to communicate through telephone lines.

n. a software program that allows users to view web sites on the World Wide Web.

o. a web address.

p. a use of a medication for an indication not approved by the FDA.

REVIEW

the answer key begins on page 511

CHOOSE THE BEST ANSWER

1. _____ contain(s) a comprehensive listing of current articles from international professional journals.
   a. Primary literature
   b. Indexing services
   c. Secondary literature
   d. AHFS Drug Information

2. _____ literature contains general reference works based upon primary literature sources.
   a. Primary
   b. Tertiary
   c. Secondary
   d. Abstract

3. The Occupational, Safety and Health Administration (OSHA) requires pharmacies to have this literature on hand:
   a. Material Safety Data Sheets
   b. *The Merck Index*
   c. policy and procedure manuals
   d. Remington, *The Science and Practice of Pharmacy*

4. _____ develops recommendations for occupational safety and health standards.
   a. The FDA
   b. HIPAA
   c. NIOSH
   d. OSHA

5. The general chapters <1> through <999> of the USP-NF are enforced by the
   a. DEA.
   b. FDA.
   c. OSHA.
   d. HIPAA.

6. Which common reference would a pharmacy technician search to compare medications in the same therapeutic class for a patient on a restricted formulary?
   a. *American Hospital Formulary Service*
   b. *Drug Facts and Comparisons*
   c. *Physicians' Desk Reference*
   d. *USP DI*

7. Which reference would you use to identify a drug that a patient purchased in England?
   a. *Drug Facts and Comparisons*
   b. Martindale, *The Complete Drug Reference*
   c. *The Merck Index*
   d. *USP-NF*

8. To what pharmacy reference would you direct a physician who is looking for prescription information on major pharmaceuticals similar to drug package inserts?
   a. *The Merck Index*
   b. *Drug Facts and Comparisons*
   c. *Physicians' Desk Reference*
   d. *USP-NF*

9. Which pharmacy drug reference would you search for an indication for an off-label medication?
   a. *Drug Facts and Comparisons*
   b. *Physicians' Desk Reference*
   c. *AHFS Drug Information*
   d. Martindale, *The Complete Drug Reference*

10. Where would a pharmacy technician look for nationally recognized AWPs and NDCs for FDA approved drugs?
   a. *AHFS*
   b. "Orange Book"
   c. *Red Book*
   d. *USP-NF*

11. *The Medical Letter on Drugs and Thera-peutics* is an example of a
    a. pink sheet.
    b. trade journal.
    c. professional practice journal.
    d. newsletter.

12. The common name for the FDA's *Approved Drug Products with Therapeutic Equivalent Evaluations* is the
    a. "Medical Book."
    b. "Orange Book."
    c. "Red Book."
    d. "USP-NF."

13. A patient would like to order their medications online. To which web site would a pharmacy technician direct them?
    a. ashp.org
    b. nabp.org
    c. osha.gov
    d. ptcb.org

14. The most comprehensive text covering pharmaceutical sciences is
    a. Remington, *The Science and Practice of Pharmacy.*
    b. *Goodman and Gilman's The Pharmacological Basis of Therapeutics.*
    c. the "Orange Book."
    d. the *American Drug Index.*

15. Safari and Microsoft Explorer are examples of a
    a. browser.
    b. DSL.
    c. ISP.
    d. URL.

16. A company that provides access to the Internet is a/an
    a. browser.
    b. ISP.
    c. search engine.
    d. URL.

17. Google is an example of a
    a. modem.
    b. browser.
    c. search engine.
    d. uniform resource locator.

18. _____ is a family of technologies that provide digital data transmission over the telephone network.
    a. WWW
    b. ISP
    c. DSL
    d. URL

19. The Bureau of Labor Statistics provides information about pharmacy careers on the internet in the
    a. *Occupational Outlook Handbook.*
    b. "Orange Book."
    c. *Red Book.*
    d. *Pink Sheet.*

20. The directory of accredited technician training programs can be found at the website for
    a. JCAHO.
    b. ASHP.
    c. APhA.
    d. NABP.

REVIEW

21. A pharmacy technician searching for PTCE information, a practice exam, and a guidebook to help prepare for the PTCE should contact which organization?
    a. ASHP
    b. AAPT
    c. NPTA
    d. PTCB

22. As a member of NPTA, a pharmacy technician will receive which bimonthly journal that provides information and continuing education specifically for pharmacy technicians?
    a. *journal of Pharmacy Technology*
    b. *Today's Technician*
    c. *Pharmacy Times*
    d. *The Pink Sheet*

23. How many contact hours of continuing education in pharmacy law is required every two years to maintain your certification?
    a. one
    b. three
    c. five
    d. ten

24. Which reference would a pharmacy technician choose to research the compatibility of IV cefazolin and heparin running through the same IV line?
    a. *Drug Facts and Comparisons*
    b. *King's Guide to Parenteral Admixtures*
    c. Martindale, *The Complete Drug Reference*
    d. PDR

25. Which pharmacy reference would a pharmacy technician compounding a product consult to find the solubility properties of a chemical in water?
    a. *American Drug Index*
    b. Martindale, *The Complete Drug Reference*
    c. *The Merck Index*
    d. *Red Book*

13

INVENTORY MANAGEMENT

INVENTORY MANAGEMENT

An *inventory* is a listing of the goods or items that a business will use in its normal operation.

Pharmacies generally develop an inventory of medications based upon what they expect to need. Rarely used medications might not be kept in inventory but instead ordered as needed.

The goal of inventory management is two-fold: to ensure drugs are available when needed and that contract or special pricing is followed.

Because medication needs are often urgent, pharmacies must maintain good control of their stock or inventory. This means that all drugs which are likely to be needed are both on hand and usable—that is, they have not expired or been damaged, contaminated, or otherwise made unfit for use. The technician plays a critical role in inventory management, but there are many participants in the process—the pharmacy, the institution, the wholesaler, the manufacturer, the government, insurers, and other third parties.

Inventory management is an integral part of the technician's job responsibility.

Each technician is required to master the specific inventory system in use at their workplace. In some cases, inventory management may be the technician's primary responsibility, and the technician has the opportunity to become a "pharmaceutical buyer." At hospitals and other institutions, for example, a purchasing/inventory technician is often responsible for obtaining and maintaining the institution's medication and device supply.

Why Use Wholesalers?

The thousands of medications that a pharmacy stocks represent many manufacturers. Obtaining them from individual manufacturers would be a difficult and costly process. Besides the paperwork involved (individual purchase orders, invoices, payments, etc.), there would be many different procedures to learn: how orders could be placed, how they would be shipped, returns policies, and so on.

Wholesalers stock inventories of the most used medications, obtain less-used medications as they are needed, and make frequent deliveries, often on a daily basis. They also provide added-value services such as emergency delivery, automated inventory systems, automated purchasing systems, generic substitution options, private label products, and many others. Obtaining most medications from a single wholesaler greatly simplifies the purchasing process and reduces the staff needed for it.

THE INVENTORY ENVIRONMENT

There are many participants in the inventory process—the pharmacy, the institution, the wholesaler, the manufacturer, the government, insurers and other third parties.

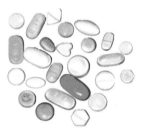

The Formulary

Many hospitals, HMOs, insurers, and other health-care systems maintain a list of medications called a **formulary.** These are the medications that are approved for use in the system.

➡ An **open formulary** is one that allows purchase of any medication that is prescribed.

➡ A **closed formulary** is a limited list of approved medications. A physician must receive permission to use a medication that is not on the list. Closed formularies are generally used as a cost savings tool, in which less expensive substitutes are stocked. Though these substitutes are mainly generic equivalents, in some hospitals a drug on the formulary that is **therapeutically equivalent** (chemically different but with similar actions and effects) may be substituted for a drug not on the formulary.

➡ Formulary medications are routinely reviewed when new information is available about side effects or contraindications. In addition, Look-Alike and Sound-Alike medications may be stored, labeled, or marked separately to prevent mix-ups. Medications may be removed from the formulary or from public access if significant side effects are found.

inventory a list of goods or items a business uses in its normal operations.

formulary a list of medications approved for use.

open formulary a system that allows a pharmacy to use any prescribed medication.

closed formulary a limited list of approved medications.

therapeutic equivalent pharmaceutical equivalents that produce the same effects in patients.

The Government

In the United States, the Drug Enforcement Administration (DEA) regulates the distribution of controlled substances and has various distribution, inventory, record keeping, and ordering requirements. Schedule II—V substances can either be stocked separately in a locked cabinet or dispersed with non-controlled drugs. Schedule II drugs require a special reorder form. Controlled substances stock must be continually monitored and documented. All records must be kept on hand for two years, unless state law requires a longer time frame.

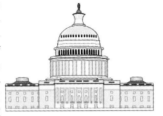

The Pharmacy

Individual pharmacies (whether in community or institutional environments) may use their own inventory system or one provided by another party such as a wholesaler or a corporate parent if they are part of a chain. When drugs need to be purchased, pharmacies buy them directly from wholesalers and sometimes manufacturers, or participate in large purchasing groups known as GPOs (group purchasing organizations) that buy drugs in bulk for its members. Because of the savings that bulk purchasing provides, independent pharmacies and hospitals often join buying groups that negotiate bulk contracts.

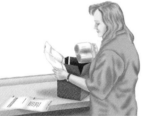

Drug manufacturers

When drugs are not available from wholesalers due to expense, storage requirements, or other reasons, they can be obtained directly from the manufacturer. In this case, a purchasing account for the pharmacy must be set up with the manufacturer.

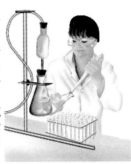

Wholesalers

More than three-quarters of pharmaceutical manufacturers' sales are directly to drug wholesalers,* who in turn resell their inventory to hospitals, pharmacies, and other pharmaceutical dispensers. Wholesalers stock tens of thousands of items from hundreds of manufacturers, everything from disposable razors to Activase®, a life saving emergency use drug. They are government-licensed and regulated and offer their customers dependable one-stop-shopping for most of their medication needs. Using wholesalers simplifies the drug purchasing process and saves time, effort, and expense.

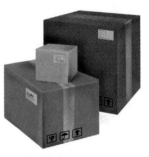

Source: National Wholesale Drug Association

 safety you should know

It is important to deal only with well-known or established wholesalers and suppliers who can document the pedigree or path of a drug from manufacturer to consumer. Unscrupulous manufacturers have made counterfeit medications, which may look like an established drug but which have little or no active ingredients, and then sell them to lesser known wholesalers or suppliers.

INVENTORY SYSTEMS

Apharmaceutical inventory system tracks inventory, forecasts needs, and generates reorders to maintain adequate inventory. The goal of a good inventory system is to have the right amount of stock at the right price available at all times. Too many drugs on hand involves unnecessary cost and maintenance and may result in spoilage. Too few drugs means that medications won't be available when needed.

In order to maintain an adequate supply of medications, pharmacies use a *perpetual inventory system*.

A perpetual inventory system maintains a continuous record of every item in inventory so that it always shows the stock on hand. This is a requirement for Schedule II substances, but it is also important for many medications since their availability has health consequences.

Spoilage

Time or storage conditions may cause the chemical compounds in medications to break down, resulting in either lost potency or changed function. This is called inventory spoilage. Use of such medications may be dangerous.
Medications carry expiration dates and storage requirements that must be honored. It is an important task of the pharmacy technician to constantly check all stock for drugs going out of date.

✔ **Note:** As an expiration date approaches, it may already be too late to dispense the medication, since it must be used before the date passes. If an expiration date for a medication has passed, or the medication cannot be completely used before that date, the medication must be appropriately disposed of or returned to the supplier for credit. In some cases, wholesalers will not accept expired drugs, but the drug manufacturer will. When returned, packages must generally be unopened.

Disposal of Non-Returnable Medications

Federal legislation such as in the Safe Water Drinking Act requires safe disposal of medications. Companies such as Stericylce (www.stericycle.com) can assist with complying with OSHA, EPA, and DOT regulations for disposing of non-returnable medications.

INVENTORY CONCEPTS

Turnover

The turnover rate is the number of days it takes to use the complete stock of an item. Besides quality and spoilage issues, there is also a financial consideration. If a supplier's payment terms are "thirty days net" and stock turnover averages less than thirty days, the stock will be sold before the supplier must be paid, which lowers the cost of the stock.

Fast Movers and Slow Movers

A general rule is that 20% of your stock will account for 80% of your orders or prescriptions. To keep inventory dollars low, focus on keeping a 1–2 week supply of fast moving drugs and a month's supply of slower moving drugs.

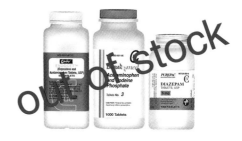

Availability

Besides monitoring stock on hand, it is important to monitor the market availability of medications. A particular drug may be unavailable due to manufacturing difficulties, raw material unavailability, recalls, etc. This can increase market demand for substitutes for the unavailable drug, sometimes causing shortages in the substitutes as well. For instance, in the fall of 2009 the slower than anticipated delivery of the H1N1 Swine Flu vaccine substantially increased demand for Tamiflu®.

perpetual inventory a system that maintains a continuous record of every item in inventory so that it always shows the current amount of stock on hand.

turnover the rate at which inventory is used, generally expressed in number of days.

point of sale system (POS) an inventory system in which the item is deducted from inventory as it is sold or dispensed.

reorder points minimum and maximum stock levels which determine when a reorder is placed and for how much.

TOOLS FOR PERPETUAL INVENTORY

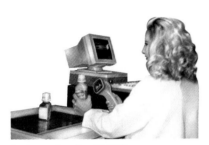

Point of sale (POS)

Pharmacy operations generally use a point of sale system in which the item is deducted from inventory as it is sold or dispensed. The transaction is often triggered by the scanning of a bar code on the medication packaging, though it can also be keyed into the system.

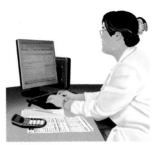

Automated Reports

Computerized inventory systems provide a continuous picture of the inventory situation through automated reports that allow users to analyze and monitor their inventory in a variety of ways. They automatically update stock amounts, track turnover, produce purchase orders based on reorder points, and forecast future needs.

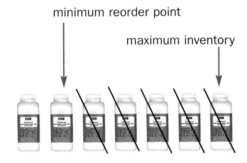

minimum reorder point

maximum inventory

Reorder Points

In order to maintain adequate inventory for their needs, community and institutional pharmacies maintain computer databases of their inventory using drug reorder points. These are maximum and minimum inventory levels for each drug. As the minimum reorder point of a medication is reached, most computer systems will generate an automatic purchase order for more of it. What medications should be ordered (and how much) is automatically identified on a daily basis. The order amount will be calculated to reach the maximum reorder point. Reorder points for any item can generally be set according to the needs of the facility.

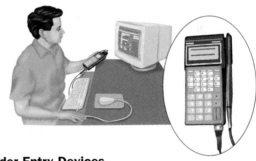

Order Entry Devices

Portable hand-held devices are widely used to enter ordering data. When inspection of stock shows that a drug is approaching the minimum inventory level, the reorder can be made using one of these devices. The drug's ID number is entered by hand or scanned into the device using a bar coded shelf tag and the wand attached to the device. A desired quantity, generally enough to reach the maximum inventory level, is then entered to complete the order. The data is sent to the institution's ordering computer. Confirmation is received to verify stock will be sent.

COMPUTERS & INVENTORY

There are many different kinds of computer systems in retail and hospital pharmacy.

Among the many available options, these systems can automate the printing of the label, coordinate billing and pricing with insurance, use bar codes to check medication identification when filling prescriptions, check for allergies and possible drug interactions, print medication information for the patient and in some hospital systems also calculate weight-based dosing and provide disease-specific alerts based on lab values, provide drug information for the pharmacists and nurses, and of course automate filling prescriptions and medication orders and managing inventory.

Computerized inventory systems automatically adjust inventory and generate orders based on maintaining set inventory levels.

The inventory system is often a component of a comprehensive pharmacy management system that includes elements like patient profiling, management reporting, and so on. In many cases, the drug wholesaler provides the system to its customers as part of the wholesaler service. The customer's system interacts with the wholesaler's so that various types of information (pricing, order information, etc.) can be exchanged automatically between the two systems.

Entering correct information is essential to any computer system.

Computerized systems may automatically create and maintain records based on each inventory transaction. However, many of these transactions are manually entered into the system. So there is always a possibility of error. For this reason, each system produces reports that cover virtually every aspect of the inventory process from stock to turnover to reorders. These reports can be read on screen or in printed form so that errors can be detected.

To protect against possible abuses, users are given passwords to access different features of the system.

This not only protects the employer, but the employee as well. It prevents unauthorized activities and also documents who did what and when.

KEY COMPUTER CONSIDERATIONS

System Care and Maintenance

Computer systems have become very durable, but they need care and maintenance. It is important to know and follow the operating instructions for any system. Some factors that can cause damage to computers are temperature, dust, moisture, movement, vibrations, and power surges.

System Backup

Each system's **database** of information is a critical component of the pharmacy or institution in which it functions. These files must be regularly backed-up or copied to an appropriate storage media. There are many types of such media but whatever the media, it is important to know its reliability. Depending on the operation, back up may need to be performed daily.

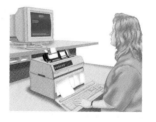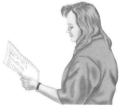

Manual Checking

Checking reports manually is an important step in ensuring that records are correct. Simple data entry errors can result in serious mistakes affecting orders, stock availability, prices, and other issues. For example: If a box containing 150 u/d tablets of Tylenol® is set up in the system as one unit, but is incorrectly keyed into the system as 150 units, the system's information will be grossly incorrect.

automated dispensing system a system in which medications are dispensed, upon confirmation of an order communicated from a centralized computer system, at their point-of-use.

database a collection of information structured so that specific information within it can easily be retrieved and used.

AUTOMATED DISPENSING SYSTEMS

Baker Cells® is an example of an automated counting/filling device that is sometimes used by pharmacies to process a high volume of prescriptions. These devices have cells, each of which is filled with a particular drug. When a drug is ordered, the device quickly counts the appropriate amount of capsules or tablets into the a prescription vial. Some robotic dispensing machines such as Parata RDS® also produce the prescription label. Technicians keep the cells stocked and must record all drug lot numbers.

The Pyxis Med/Supply Station® is like an ATM for medications. There are several manufacturers of such devices and they are generally known as automated dispensing machines (ADM). ADMs make floor stock available to nurses within a hospital. A network of storage stations are located throughout a facility and are connected to a Pyxis® server which in turn links to the hospital's ADT, billing, and materials management information systems. The system not only tracks inventory per se but keeps a record of which drugs/supplies were taken by which nurse for which patient.

Homerus® is an example of a centralized robotic unit-dose dispensing device. It can individually package and store large amounts of medications from bulk supplies, deliver bar-coded medications to 24-hour patient-specific medication bins, and return medications to storage after a patient is discharged.

Some hospitals have mobile robots that travel throughout a facility delivering drugs to various nursing units and departments.

Carousels are used to efficiently store bulk or unit dose medications. They use bar codes to track medications placed in the machine. This system allows quick removal and returning of medications through computerized access panels.

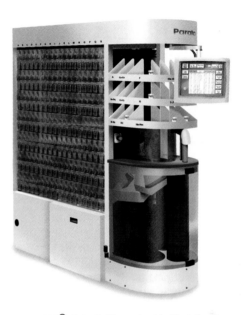

Parata RDS® (Robotic Dispensing Machine) Courtesy of Parata Systems, LLC

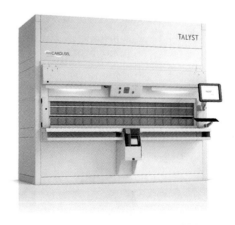

Talyst AutoCarousel. Photo courtesy of Talyst.

ORDERING

Ordering systems involve automated and manual activities.

Much of the work is done by computer systems. However, manual checking, editing, and confirmation are essential to making such systems work as required.

AUTOMATED ORDERING

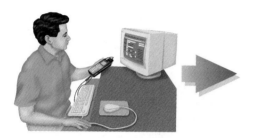 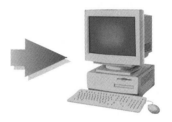

Orders can be generated using an order entry device or automatically generated by the system based on stock levels and reorder points. These reports must be checked and confirmed. If changes are needed, they can be made manually. The system then produces a revised order, which should again be checked and edited until it is ready for sending to the supplier.

When an order is ready, the ordering system and the supplier's system are connected over phone lines or Internet connection so the order can be "downloaded" from one system to the other.

The supplier's computer system analyzes the order line by line to determine if it can be filled as requested. It checks to see if there is enough of each item in the supplier's inventory to fill the order. If there is more than one warehouse in the system, it may check multiple locations to see if the items are available.

➥ If the order can be filled as ordered, a message will automatically confirm the order to the ordering system. This confirmation can be read onscreen by the orderer but should also be printed for their records.

➥ If the order cannot be filled exactly as ordered, a message containing the exceptions will be sent. This report should be printed and appropriate action taken to fill the order. It may be necessary to create a second purchase order, talk with the supplier personally, or find an alternative supplier. Some common reasons for omissions are: temporary out-of-stocks, back-ordered drugs, or the item may no longer be carried.

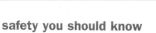 **safety you should know**

Good ordering practices set up checks and balances so that the same person does not perform both ordering and receiving. This is especially important with controlled substances.

Material Safety Data Sheets (MSDS) OSHA required notices on hazardous substances which provide hazard, handling, clean-up, and first aid information.

ORDER DETAILS

Shipping

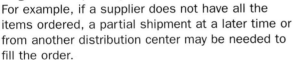

The type of shipping indicated by the purchaser determines the time and cost of shipping.

Orders may be delivered in single or multiple shipments. For example, if a supplier does not have all the items ordered, a partial shipment at a later time or from another distribution center may be needed to fill the order.

Material Safety Data Sheets (MSDS) indicate when special shipping is required for hazardous substances such as chemotherapeutic agents. The Postal Service, Federal Express, United Parcel Service, and others all have specific policies for shipping hazardous substances that must be followed. Some substances are not allowed to be shipped by plane, because the Federal Aviation Administration (FAA) will not allow them on board. Often these drugs are shipped via a courier.

Credits/Returns

Each supplier has policies and procedures that must be followed in order to receive the credit on returns. Documentation must be carefully checked item by item. A printed copy must be kept on file in addition to any electronic version.

Companies known as "reverse distributors" specialize in returns of expired and discontinued drugs to the manufacturer. They complete each manufacturer's return form and package, mail and track the drugs. They also return and fill out the paper work for C-II drugs and other controlled substances. Their fee is generally a percentage of the return credit, and is deducted automatically from the refund so there is not a separate bill.

 safety you should know
Stock that has expired, been damaged, recalled, or has otherwise been targeted for return or disposal must be segregated and clearly marked to avoid contamination and/or mix-up with the good stock.

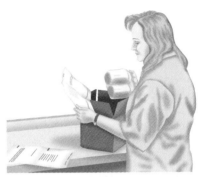

Receiving

Accuracy is essential in checking in the medications received from suppliers. It is important to be alert for drugs that have been incorrectly picked, received damaged, are outdated or missing entirely from the supplier. In many settings, items are stickered with bar codes that can be scanned to do an automatic count.

✔ Shipments, invoices and purchase orders must be reconciled item by item.

✔ The strength and amount of each item must be checked to make sure they are correct. A common mistake is an item sent in bulk instead of unit dose (or the reverse).

✔ Shipment prices on the supplier invoice should match the purchase order exactly. Individual price changes must be identified and may have to be entered into the system manually to make sure the system has the correct information.

✔ Broken or damaged stock must be brought to the attention of the supplier. Broken items should be removed, bagged, or otherwise separated to help prevent contamination or damage to other stock.

✔ If there are any discrepancies, the supplier should generally be notified immediately.

✔ Controlled substances are shipped separately and should be checked in by a pharmacist.

Receiving Chemotherapy Drugs

The National Institute for Occupational Safety and Health (NIOSH) publishes very detailed guidelines on how to safely and legally handle chemotherapy and other hazardous drugs.

NIOSH Publication No. 2004-165: *Preventing Occupational Exposure to Antineoplastic and Other Hazardous Drugs* can be downloaded from http://www.cdc.gov/niosh/docs/2004-165/.

FORMS

The Online Ordering Screen

Online ordering systems generally contain abbreviated descriptions of drug products in the formulary. The technician uses a "Select" (or similar) function to choose products and may then "Add" it to an order. Quantities may be manually entered or edited—if they have been automatically recorded by the system.

The system automatically assigns to each order a **purchase order number** for identification. Once the order is finished, checked, and ready, it is sent to the supplier's system.

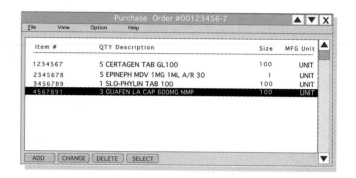

The Confirmation Printout

When an online purchase order is received by the supplier, the supplier's system checks the order to see what items it will be able to ship to the orderer. Once it completes this process, a confirmation of the order is sent back to the orderer's system. This confirmation indicates which items will be shipped, which will not (due to unavailability), and what the cost of the items and any related costs may be. The confirmation comes in the form of a file that is saved on the system, but is also printed out so a hard copy of the confirmation is available for checking.

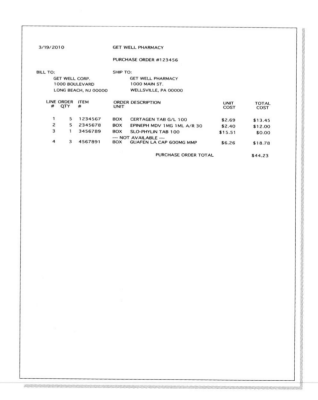

purchase order number the number assigned to each order for identification.

The Shipping Invoice

When the items are shipped, the supplier includes an invoice listing the items in the shipment, items that may be shipped separately, items that are unavailable, and the cost of the shipment. The invoice must be checked item by item against the items in the shipment to make certain nothing is missing.

WHOLESALE DRUG 100 MIDDLETOWN RD. MIDDLETOWN, NY 00000	PHONE: (800) 123 - 4567 DEA: XYG102436		**INVOICE** BATCH: 000		BILLING DATE: 3/19/2010 42 AJ 42 AJ DEM: E		
SOLD TO GET WELL PHARMACY 1000 MAIN ST. WELLSVILLE, PA 00000	DEA: AB1234563		P.O.BILL ONLY-LG PHCY: NONE	123456		ROUTE STOP	
	INVOICE DATE 3/19/2010	INVOICE NO.		CUSTOMER		PAGE	

DIRECTS & SPECIAL PURCHASES

All product discounts earned or granted under Wholesale Drug programs, including off-invoice allowances, may be subject to certain state and federal laws and regulations regarding reporting and/or disclosure requirements and may be required to be reflected in the costs claimed or charges made by your pharmacy under Medicaid, Medicare or any other health care reimbursement program or provider plan.

DEPT	ITEM NUMBER	QTY ORD	UN	ITEM DESCRIPTION	UNIT PRICE	TOTAL
AB	1234567	5	BOX	CERTAGEN TAB G/L 100	$2.69	$13.45
CD	2345678	5	BOX	EPINEPH MDV 1MG 1ML A/R 30	$2.40	$12.00
EF	3456789	1	BOX	SLO-PHYLIN TAB 100	$15.51	$0.00
				— NOT AVAILABLE —		
GH	4567891	3	BOX	GUAFEN LA CAP 600MG MMP	$6.26	$18.78

SUBTOTAL 44.23
NET PAYABLE BY STMT DUE DATE 44.23

LINES 4	CASES 0	PIECES 13	THIS INVOICE IS PAYABLE TO WHOLESALE DRUG CO. AT THE ABOVE ADDRESS. CLAIMS MUST BE MADE WITHIN FIVE DAYS AND SHOW DATE OF INVOICE.

THIS IS TO CERTIFY THAT ABOVE NAMED ARTICLES ARE PROPERLY CLASSIFIED, DESCRIBED, PACKAGED, MARKED AND LABELED TO THE APPLICABLE REGULATIONS OF THE DEPARTMENT OF TRANSPORTATION.

The Returns Form

Preprinted multi-part forms are often used for returns, though some computer inventory systems generate their own form. When returning items, the following information is usually required:

➥ original p.o. number
➥ item number
➥ quantity
➥ reason for return

Reasons for returning products can include overshipments, damaged or expired products, or changed needs.

WHOLESALE DRUG 100 MIDDLETOWN RD. MIDDLETOWN, NJ 00000	OFFICE USE ONLY CREDIT NO. CREDIT DATE:	**RETURN GOODS FORM**				052805
ACCOUNT NAME: ADDRESS: CITY/STATE: ACCT. No.:	VENDOR NAME: ADDRESS: CITY/STATE: ACCT. No.:		DATE PREPARED: DATE RECIEVED: WAREHOUSE DATE WORKED: RETURN GOODS NARCOTIC FORM No.:			

PKR	(1) INVOICE DATE MO DAY YR	(2) INVOICE NO.	(3)	(4) ITEM NUMBER	(5) QTY	(6) DESCRIPTION	(7) QTY REC'D	CHECKED BY	COST	SELL	DISC.
P.O.No.						REASON FOR RETURNING: ☐ Short ☐ Long (rec. but not billed) ☐ Damaged ☐ Outdated ☐ Too many on hand ☐ Do not need					
P.O.No.						REASON FOR RETURNING: ☐ Short ☐ Long (rec. but not billed) ☐ Damaged ☐ Outdated ☐ Too many on hand ☐ Do not need					
P.O.No.						REASON FOR RETURNING: ☐ Short ☐ Long (rec. but not billed) ☐ Damaged ☐ Outdated ☐ Too many on hand ☐ Do not need					
P.O.No.						REASON FOR RETURNING: ☐ Short ☐ Long (rec. but not billed) ☐ Damaged ☐ Outdated ☐ Too many on hand ☐ Do not need					
P.O.No.						REASON FOR RETURNING: ☐ Short ☐ Long (rec. but not billed) ☐ Damaged ☐ Outdated ☐ Too many on hand ☐ Do not need					
P.O.No.						REASON FOR RETURNING: ☐ Short ☐ Long (rec. but not billed) ☐ Damaged ☐ Outdated ☐ Too many on hand ☐ Do not need					

I CERTIFY THAT THE ABOVE ITEMS HAVE BEEN STORED IN ACCORDANCE WITH PRODUCT LABEL SPECIFICATION, AND MAINTAINED UNDER PROPER CONDITIONS FOR STORAGE, HANDLING AND SHIPPING TO PREVENT MISBRANDING, ADULTERATION, OR REDUCTION IN PRODUCT EFFICACY.

STORE SIGNATURE: _____ DATE PICK UP: _____ BY: _____

TO ENSURE PROPER CREDIT, INVOICE DATE AND ITEM NUMBER MUST BE INCLUDED, SEE INSTRUCTIONS ON REVERSE SIDE.

STOCKING & STORING

Most medications are received from the supplier in bulk "stock bottles" that carry FDA required information on the label.

This information includes the brand name, generic name, prescription legend, storage requirements, dosage form, quantity, controlled substance mark, manufacturer's name, lot number, expiration date, and NDC (National Drug Code) number.

Some medications, particularly in hospitals, are packaged in individual doses called *unit-dose packaging.*

Unit dose packaging allows the dispensing of individual doses. Because the dose information is on each dose, it is easily checked before leaving the pharmacy. In many settings, technicians prepare unit-dose packaging under the supervision of a pharmacist as part of their job.

The USP and state laws provide regulations for repackaging medications.

Many states follow the USP guidelines and require using the manufacturer's original expiration date or a date of no more than 12 months from the date the medication is repackaged, whichever is shorter. A repackaging log must be maintained, depending on state law, to track all repackaged medications back to their original manufacture and lot number.

Drugs must be stored according to manufacturer's specifications.

Most drugs are kept in a fairly constant room temperature of 59°–86°F (and not below, unless stated by the manufacturer to do so). The storage room must have adequate ventilation or proper air distribution. Drug shelves should allow for proper air flow around the medications and room.

Bar codes are used to quickly identify a product.

On most medications, the bar code includes the product's NDC number which in turn identifies the product and package size. Many computer systems use bar codes to provide a double check for pharmacists and technicians when filling prescriptions. Bar codes are also used in hospitals for Bedside Medication Verification (BMV): When administering a medication, a nurse scans their own bar-coded name badge, the patient's bar-coded arm band, and the medication; the computer then verifies that that is the correct medication to give to that patient at that time.

PACKAGING

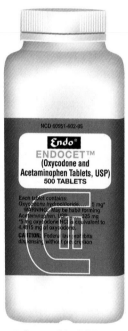

bulk container with 500 tablets of Endocet

Unit-Dose Packaging

Unit-dose packaging can take many forms: plastic packs, vials, tubes, ampules, etc. Some are packaged in individual bubbles on cards containing ten or more doses. Each unit-dose package contains the name of the drug, its strength, and the expiration date. All unit-dose containers must comply with USP requirements.

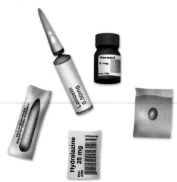

unit-dose packaging a package containing a single dose of a medication.

STORAGE

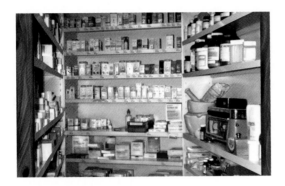

Physical Organization

Drugs may be organized by various methods. Storing by manufacturer would locate the drug using its brand name and is often done in a retail pharmacy. Storing alpha-generically organizes drugs alphabetically by their generic names. For example, if the generic name "cimetidine" is on the shelf, Tagamet® may be placed there along with the generic.

Whatever the overall organization, the following basic guidelines should be met:

✔ Each medication should be organized such that the oldest items are dispensed first.

✔ The location of each drug should be quickly identifiable through a locator system in which each drug is assigned a location number that is stored in the computer system.

✔ Enough space should be provided to minimize breakage and to help prevent accidentally selecting the wrong medication.

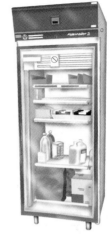

Refrigeration

Some drugs must be stored at a constant temperature in a controlled commercial refrigerator designed for medications. If refrigerated or frozen medications are left out for a period of time longer than stated in the literature, they may begin to break down chemically and/or lose potency. Commercial refrigerators and freezers have gauges on the outside that indicate the internal temperature and allow it to be monitored. The temperature of refrigeration should generally be 40–42°F.

The refrigerator or freezer should be plugged into a wall receptacle that is marked for emergency use and will switch to emergency power generators if there is a power failure. If any medication is left out of refrigeration beyond the recommendations of the manufacturer, it should be discarded.

Point-of-Use Stations

In hospitals and other settings, medications are stocked in dispensing units throughout the facility that may be called supply stations or med-stations. Since they are at the point-of-use, they greatly simplify the dispensing of medications to patients.

Items stocked in these stations differ based upon the needs of the patients. For example, a station in an operating room would contain many anesthetics.

All withdrawals and restocks of stations are recorded just as they would be from a central dispensary. As discussed earlier in this chapter, some stations may be linked into the facility computing system so the information can be automatically communicated to it.

Durable and Non-Durable Equipment Supplies

Durable medical equipment, also known as DME, is often stocked in retail pharmacies. This includes items such as walkers, wheel chairs, crutches, and bedpans. These products are often large and take up space and so sometimes are ordered on a next-day basis from wholesalers. In hospitals, these items are found in central supply or distribution departments.

Non-durable medical supplies and equipment include items such as syringes, needles, ostomy supplies, povidine iodine, antiseptics, and other disposable medical devices.

REVIEW

KEY CONCEPTS

INVENTORY MANAGEMENT

- ✔ Good inventory management ensures that drugs which are likely to be needed are both on hand and usable—that is, not expired, damaged, contaminated, or otherwise unfit for use.

- ✔ An open formulary is one that allows purchase of any medication that is prescribed. A closed formulary is a limited list of approved medications.

- ✔ Schedule II substances must be stocked separately in a secure place and require a special order form for reordering. Their stock must be continually monitored and documented.

- ✔ Formularies must be routinely reviewed to evaluate newer products and safety profiles of current medications.

- ✔ More than three-quarters of pharmaceutical manufacturers' sales are directly to drug wholesalers, who in turn resell their inventory to hospitals, pharmacies, and other pharmaceutical dispensers.

INVENTORY SYSTEMS

- ✔ A perpetual inventory system maintains a continuous record of every item in inventory so that it always shows the stock on hand.

- ✔ Turnover is the rate at which inventory is used.

- ✔ Pharmacy operations generally use a point of sale system in which the item is deducted from inventory as it is sold or dispensed.

- ✔ Drug reorder points are maximum and minimum inventory levels for each drug.

- ✔ Important reports (especially purchase orders) should be regularly printed out and filed as hard copy both for convenience and as a backup record-keeping system.

COMPUTERS AND INVENTORY

- ✔ Pharmacy computer files must be regularly backed-up or copied to an appropriate storage media.

- ✔ In a computerized inventory system, orders can be generated using an order entry device or automatically generated by the system based on stock levels and reorder points.

ORDERING

- ✔ In an online ordering system, if an order can be filled as ordered, a message from the supplier will automatically confirm the order to the ordering system. The system automatically assigns to each order a purchase order number for identification.

- ✔ Material Safety Data Sheets (MSDS) for hazardous substances such as chemotherapeutic agents indicate when special handling and shipping is required.

- ✔ Controlled substances are shipped separately and should be checked in by a pharmacist.

- ✔ Good ordering practices assign separate personnel for ordering and receiving steps or processes.

STOCKING AND STORING

- ✔ Most medications are received from the supplier in bulk "stock bottles."

- ✔ Drugs must be stored according to manufacturer's specifications.

- ✔ Most drugs are kept in a fairly constant room temperature of 59°–86°F. The temperature of refrigeration should generally be 40–42°.

- ✔ Medications should be organized in a way that will dispense the oldest items first.

- ✔ In hospitals and other settings, medications are stocked in dispensing units throughout the facility that may be called supply stations or automated dispensing machines.

SELF TEST

MATCH THE TERMS   *the answer key begins on page 511*

1. automated dispensing system _____

2. closed formulary _____

3. database _____

4. formulary _____

5. inventory _____

6. Material Safety Data Sheets (MSDS) _____

7. open formulary _____

8. perpetual inventory _____

9. point-of-sale system (POS) _____

10. purchase order number _____

11. reorder points _____

12. therapeutic equivalent _____

13. turnover _____

14. unit-dose packaging _____

a. a system that allows purchase of any medication that is prescribed.

b. a limited list of approved medications.

c. the rate at which inventory is used, generally expressed in number of days.

d. an inventory system in which the item is deducted from inventory as it is sold or dispensed.

e. minimum and maximum stock levels which determine when a reorder is placed and for how much.

f. a collection of information structured so that specific information within it can easily be retrieved and used.

g. OSHA required notices that provide hazard, handling, clean-up, and first aid information.

h. the number system assigned to each order for identification.

i. a package containing a single dose of a medication.

j. a system that maintains a continuous record of every item in inventory so that it always shows the stock on hand.

k. a list of goods or items a business uses in its normal operations.

l. pharmaceutical equivalents that produce the same effects in patients.

m. a system in which medications are dispensed at their point of use upon confirmation of an order communicated from a centralized computer system.

n. a list of medications approved for use.

CHOOSE THE BEST ANSWER   *the answer key begins on page 511*

1. A list of the goods or items a business will use in its normal operation is called a(an)
   a. purchasing.
   b. inventory.
   c. open formulary.
   d. closed formulary.

2. A goal of inventory management is
   a. to ensure that drugs are available when they are needed.
   b. to maintain MSDS sheets.
   c. to develop closed formularies.
   d. to increase use of wholesalers.

REVIEW

3. In an open formulary, when a medication is ordered that is not on the formulary
   a. the medication may be ordered without obtaining additional permission.
   b. the patient must obtain the medication at another pharmacy.
   c. the physician must first receive permission to use the medication.
   d. the pharmacist is required to choose a therapeutic equivalent.

4. Formulary medications are routinely reviewed to
   a. add more quantity of the same product.
   b. review safety of older products and evaluate newer products.
   c. make room on the shelves.
   d. add a product upon request of the manufacturer.

5. A therapeutically-equivalent drug is
   a. chemically the same.
   b. chemically different but with similar actions and effects.
   c. the generic version of a trade drug.
   d. a drug that a physician must get approval to use.

6. "Fast Movers" account for approximately what percent of a pharmacy's orders and prescriptions?
   a. 5%
   b. 30%
   c. 40%
   d. 80%

7. Wholesalers who provide medications to hospitals, pharmacies, and other medication dispensers account for about _____ of pharmaceutical manufacturers' sales.
   a. half
   b. one-quarter
   c. three-quarters
   d. one-third

8. As an expiration date approaches, the pharmacy technician should be aware that it must be _____ before the expiration date passes.
   a. returned to the manufacturer for credit
   b. dispensed
   c. used
   d. returned to the wholesaler for credit

9. If a supplier's terms are thirty days net,
   a. it would be best to have a turnover less than thirty days.
   b. it would be best to have a turnover equal to thirty days.
   c. it would be best to have a turnover greater than thirty days.
   d. none of the above.

10. _____ is an inventory system in which the item is deducted from inventory as it is sold or dispensed.
    a. Point of sale system
    b. Turnover
    c. Automated reports
    d. Reorder point system

11. Minimum and maximum stock levels used to determine when a reorder is placed and for how much are
    a. reorder points.
    b. automatic ordering.
    c. POS.
    d. turnovers.

12. Checking of order reports to ensure the order contains no gross errors is done
    a. by computer.
    b. manually.
    c. by the corporate office.
    d. by the wholesaler.

13. Hard copies of order reports
   a. are only needed if there is a computer failure.
   b. are not needed since everything is on the computer.
   c. are kept for an established amount of time for business and legal reasons.
   d. are only needed if there is a power failure.

14. All of the following are used to store medications except
   a. automated dispensing machines.
   b. carousels.
   c. glove boxes.
   d. Pyxis® machines.

15. A bar code on a product from a manufacturer
   a. indicates the medication's price.
   b. ensures the patient receives the correct medication.
   c. keeps count of the medications stocked.
   d. includes the product's NDC number.

16. Material Safety Data Sheets (MSDS) provide
   a. protocols for fire hazards in the pharmacy setting.
   b. safety codes by OSHA in the storage of inventory.
   c. information concerning hazardous substances.
   d. none of the above.

17. In receiving an order, it is important to be alert for drugs that have been incorrectly picked, received damaged, are outdated, or missing, so orders are reconciled
   a. once per month.
   b. item by item.
   c. every two years.
   d. once per year.

18. When reconciling an order, if a technician detects a discrepancies, the supplier should be notified
   a. immediately.
   b. before the end of the current reporting period.
   c. before the end of the month.
   d. before the end of the week.

19. A purchase order number is
   a. a number that is used to identify the pharmacy.
   b. is the same on all orders from a given pharmacy.
   c. is assigned by the FDA.
   d. a number used to identify an order.

20. Most drugs are kept at room temperature between
   a. 59–86°C.
   b. 33–45°C.
   c. 59–86°F.
   d. 33–45°F.

21. A package that contains a single dose of a medication is called a(an)
   a. MSDS package.
   b. single use package.
   c. POS package.
   d. unit-dose package.

22. In an alpha-generic organization, drugs are stored alphabetically by
   a. generic name with corresponding trade versions placed next to the generic drug.
   b. trade name with the corresponding generic version placed next to it.
   c. manufacturer.
   d. drug classification.

REVIEW

23. The temperature of a refrigerator in a pharmacy should generally be
    a. 40–42°F.
    b. 28–32°C.
    c. 40–42°C.
    d. 28–32°F.

24. A generic term used for computerized medication dispensing machines used in hospitals is a/an
    a. ADM.
    b. CART.
    c. Pyxis®.
    d. PAR.

25. Proper disposal or destruction of non-returnable medications includes
    a. placement in regular trash.
    b. flushing down sink or water system.
    c. using a company that meets EPA regulations.
    d. selling the medications at a discount.

26. Best practices for ordering medications include
    a. having the same person place the order and check it in.
    b. having different people place the order and check it in.
    c. having the pharmacy manager check in all products.
    d. having anyone available place and receive orders.

27. Safe handling of chemotherapy medications can be found in a publication by
    a. the DEA.
    b. JCAHO.
    c. SAFRX.
    d. NIOSH.

28. An example of Durable Medical Equipment (DME) could be
    a. ostomy supplies.
    b. crutches.
    c. syringes.
    d. antiseptics.

14

FINANCIAL ISSUES

FINANCIAL ISSUES

Financial issues have a substantial influence on health care and pharmacy practice.

In 1985, the average prescription price was approximately $10. By 2008 the average prescription price exceeded $70. The increase is due to a number of reasons, including inflation and the aging of the population. It is also due to the use of new medications that enhance the quality of health care, but which are often costly.

The use of third party programs to pay for prescriptions has also increased dramatically.

Third party programs are simply another party besides the patient or the pharmacy that pays for some or all of the cost of medication: essentially, an insurer. Although many individuals are uninsured, most people have some form of private or public health insurance. These include both public programs such as Medicaid and Medicare and private programs such as HMOs and basic health insurance. Many but not all such programs include prescription drug coverage. While the growth of these programs is largely a response to the rising costs of health care, in many cases third party programs allow patients to benefit from new and often more expensive drug therapies than they would otherwise be able to afford.

Because of the pharmacy technician's role in the prescription filling process, he or she must understand the different types of health insurance and how drug benefits differ among the programs.

A patient's prescription drug program determines important considerations for filling their prescription. Generic substitution may be required. There may be limits on the quantity dispensed (tablets, capsules, etc.) per fill, or on the frequency and number of refills, and so on.

PHARMACY BENEFIT MANAGERS

Regardless of how the claims are submitted and processed, participating pharmacies must sign contracts with insurers or pharmacy benefit managers before patients can get their prescriptions filled at that pharmacy and billed to their insurer or pharmacy benefit manager. A **pharmacy benefit manager (PBM)** is a company that administers drug benefit programs. Many insurance companies, HMOs, and self-insured employers use the services of more than 50 PBMs to manage drug benefit coverage for employees and health plan members. The following are the names of some pharmacy benefit managers (PBMs).

- ➡ Argus
- ➡ Caremark
- ➡ Cigna Healthcare
- ➡ Express Scripts
- ➡ Medco Health Solutions
- ➡ MedImpact
- ➡ ScripNet
- ➡ Walgreens Health Solutions

pharmacy benefit managers companies that administer drug benefit programs.

online adjudication the resolution of prescription coverage through the communication of the pharmacy computer with the third party computer.

co-insurance an agreement for cost-sharing between the insurer and the insured.

co-pay the portion of the price of medication that the patient is required to pay.

maximum allowable cost (MAC) the maximum price per tablet (or other dispensing unit) an insurer or PBM will pay for a given product.

U&C or UCR the maximum amount of payment for a given prescription, determined by the insurer to be a usual and customary (and reasonable) price.

dual co-pay co-pays that have two prices: one for generic and one for brand medications.

COMPUTERS AND THIRD PARTY BILLING

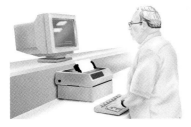

Procedures used by pharmacies to submit third party claims vary. Most insurers or pharmacy benefit managers mail checks to pharmacies (or their accounts receivable departments) at regular intervals along with listings of the prescriptions covered and those not covered (i.e., rejected).

Before the computer age, prescriptions were billed to third parties using paper claims. Although paper claims are still used, most claims are now filed electronically by online claim submission and **online adjudication** of claims. This electronic submission and adjudication process benefits both third party programs as well as pharmacies. The online communication between the prescription-filling computer in the pharmacy and the claim-processing computer of the insurer or pharmacy benefit manager results in improved accuracy and control. It is also much faster and more direct than processing paper claims. The benefits of computerizing the claims process have also been a factor in the rise of third party programs.

CO-PAYS

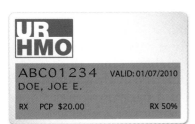

One of the common aspects of many third party programs is **co-insurance**, which is essentially an agreement between the insurer and the insured to share costs. One aspect of this is the requirement for the patient to **co-pay** for the filled prescription. That is, the patient must pay a portion of the price of the medication and the insurance company is billed for the remainder.

The amount paid by the insurer is not equal to the retail price normally charged, but is determined by a formula described in a contract between the insurer and the pharmacy. There is a **maximum allowable cost (MAC)** per tablet or other dispensing unit that an insurer or PBM will pay for a given product. This is often determined by survey of the **usual and customary (U&C)** prices for a prescription within a given geographic area. This is also referred to as the **UCR (usual, customary, and reasonable)** price for the prescription.

Many third party plans have **dual co-pays**, which means that a lower co-pay applies to prescriptions filled with generic drugs and a higher co-pay applies to prescriptions filled with brand name drugs that have no generic equivalent. Some plans have three different co-pays: the lowest co-pay applies to prescriptions filled with generic drugs, a higher co-pay applies to prescriptions filled with brand name drugs which have no generic equivalent, and a third higher co-pay applies to prescriptions filled with brand name drugs which have a generic equivalent.

THIRD PARTY PROGRAMS

PRIVATE HEALTH INSURANCE

Basic private health insurance policies may pay for prescribed expenses (such as prescriptions) when the patient is covered by a supplementary comprehensive major medical policy or when the patient's coverage includes an additional prescription drug benefit. Patients covered by comprehensive major medical policies pay out-of-pocket for their prescriptions. Once a **deductible** is met, the insurer may pay a portion of the cost of prescriptions filled the rest of the year. In other words, once a patient has paid a certain dollar amount for prescribed medical expenses (usually including prescriptions), the insurance company will reimburse a portion of the cost of filled prescriptions for the rest of the year. Whether or not a patient is required to get generic drugs when they are available is determined by individual plans and may not be obvious before filling the prescription. Major medical claims frequently involve paper claims. However, the use of electronic claim processing for major medical claims is growing.

Prescription Drug Coverage

Some traditional health insurance policies have the added benefit of prescription drug coverage. Patients with prescription drug coverage through a private insurance company are issued **prescription drug benefit cards** to carry in their wallets. These cards contain necessary billing information for pharmacies, including the patient's identification number, group number, and co-pay amount.

As with other prescription plans, there may be various types of co-pays and patients may be required to get generic drugs (when available). Many third party programs for prescription drugs have drug formularies. A **drug formulary** is a list of medications that are covered by a third party program; patients are given their formulary information when they register for benefits. Additionally, some third party programs have different **tiers** or categories of drugs with corresponding differences in co-pays, depending on which tier a specific drug is in.

Most prescription claims are processed through online adjudication: the pharmacy computer communicates with the insurer's or PBM's computer to determine the prescription drug benefit. When the claim is adjudicated or processed by the insurer or pharmacy benefit manager it becomes obvious if generic substitution is mandatory.

deductible a set amount that must be paid by the patient for each benefit period before the insurer will cover additional expenses.

prescription drug benefit cards cards that contain third party billing information for prescription drug purchases.

formulary a list of medications covered by third party plans.

tier categories of medications that are covered by third party plans.

MANAGED CARE PROGRAMS

Managed care programs include health maintenance organizations (HMOs), point-of-service programs (POS), and preferred provider organizations (PPOs). Managed care programs provide all necessary medical services (usually including prescription coverage) in return for a monthly premium and co-pays. Most managed care prescription drug plans require generic substitution when a generic is available. Some managed care plans have single co-pays, some have dual co-pays, and some have three types of co-pays.

HMOs

HMOs are made of a network of providers who are either employed by the HMO or have signed contracts to abide by the policies of the HMO. HMOs usually will not cover expenses incurred outside their participating network. *HMOs often require generic substitution.*

POSs

POS programs are made of a network of providers contracted by the insurer. Patients enrolled in a POS choose a primary care physician (PCP) who is a provider in the insurer's network. Patients may receive care outside of the POS network, but the primary care physician is required to make referrals for such care. POSs often partially reimburse expenses incurred outside of their network. *POSs usually require generic substitution.*

PPOs

PPOs are also a network of providers contracted by the insurer. Of the managed care options, PPOs offer the most flexibility for their members. PPOs often partially reimburse expenses incurred outside of their participating network and do not require a primary care physician within their network to make referrals. *PPOs usually require generic substitution.*

Patients with prescription drug coverage through managed care organizations are issued prescription drug benefit cards with billing and co-pay information. Most claims for these programs are processed through online adjudication. Many HMOs, POSs, and PPOs use pharmacy benefit managers (PBMs) to manage drug benefit coverage.

 HMOs a network of providers for which costs are covered inside but not outside of the network.

POSs a network of providers where the patient's primary care physician must be a member and costs outside the network may be partially reimbursed.

PPOs a network of providers where costs outside the network may be partially reimbursed and the patient's primary care physician need not be a member.

THIRD PARTY PROGRAMS
(cont'd)

PUBLIC HEALTH INSURANCE

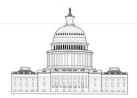

The largest public health insurance plans in the United States are Medicare and Medicaid.

Medicare

Medicare is a federal program that covers people over the age of 65, as well as disabled people under the age of 65, and people with kidney failure. Medicare Part A basically covers inpatient hospital expenses for patients who meet certain conditions, and it may also cover some hospice expenses. Medicare Part B basically covers doctors' services as well as some other medical services that are not covered by Part A. Medicare beneficiaries who pay a monthly premium for this medical coverage are covered by Medicare Part B.

Medicare beneficiaries may choose to enroll in the Medicare Prescription Drug Plan, also known as Medicare Part D. The Medicare Prescription Drug Plan requires participants to pay a monthly premium and also meet certain deductibles and co-payments. Medicare beneficiaries that do not participate in the Medicare Prescription Drug Plan may have prescription drug coverage through a current or former employer. Some Medicare beneficiaries may not have any prescription drug coverage if they do not participate in either the Medicare Drug Plan or a prescription drug plan from a current or previous employer. Furthermore, some Medicare beneficiaries may qualify for Medication Therapy Management Services (MTMS) provided by pharmacists.

Medicaid

Medicaid is a federal-state program for eligible individuals and families with low incomes. State welfare departments usually operate Medicaid. Each state decides who is eligible for Medicaid benefits and what services will be covered. A prescription drug formulary is a listing of the drugs that are covered by Medicaid. Prescription drug formularies for Medicaid recipients are determined by each state. *Medicaid programs do not automatically cover drugs that are not on the state formulary.* Completion of a prior authorization form is sometimes required to justify the need for a medication that is not on the state Medicaid formulary. Completion of the form does not imply the drug will be covered. Medicaid recipients can also qualify for HMO programs.

OTHER PROGRAMS

Workers' Compensation

In the United States, the federal government and every state have enacted workers' compensation laws. Under workers' compensation legislation, procedures for *compensation for employees accidentally injured on-the-job* are established. Administrative guidelines require that accidents be reported to a public board that grants compensation awards to injured workers.

In recent years, state workers' compensation programs have been broadened to provide for coverage of occupational diseases. Prescriptions related to the occupational injury or disease can be billed to the state's bureau of workers' compensation or to the employer (if the employer is self-insured). Many workers' compensation claims can be processed through online adjudication. However, some claims require paper claims. It is important to realize the billing procedure can be slightly different for self-insured claims. Pharmacy benefit managers (PBMs) may administer workers' compensation prescription drug benefits.

Patient Assistance Programs

Patient assistance programs are programs offered by some pharmaceutical manufacturers to help needy patients who require medication they cannot afford and do not have insurance coverage. Patient assistance programs require patients and their physicians to complete applications and submit them to the pharmaceutical manufacturer offering the program. Patients who qualify for patient assistance programs are often given cards issued by pharmacy benefit managers.

Medicare a federal program providing health care to people with certain disabilities or who are over age 65; it includes basic hospital insurance, voluntary medical insurance, and voluntary prescription drug insurance.

Medicaid a federal-state program, administered by the states, providing health care for the needy.

workers' compensation an employer compensation program for employees accidentally injured on the job.

patient assistance programs manufacturer sponsored prescription drug programs for the needy.

ONLINE ADJUDICATION

In online adjudication, the technician uses the computer to determine the exact coverage for each prescription with the appropriate third party. The pharmacy computer communicates with the insurer's or pharmacy benefit manager's computer to determine this. Most community pharmacy computer programs are designed so the prescription label does not print until confirmation of payment is received from the insurer or PBM.

THE ONLINE PROCESS

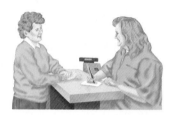

While non-patient information (NABP number, prices, co-pay, etc.) is provided by the computer system, it is generally the pharmacy technician's responsibility to obtain the patient, prescription, and billing information. In a typical community pharmacy, a patient presents a prescription (and often a prescription drug card) to a technician who must then obtain all of the patient and billing information required to enter the prescription and claim. If the patient has had prescriptions filled previously at the pharmacy, much of this information will be in the system already (though it is important for the technician to verify that this information is still correct).

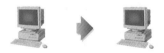

Once the necessary information is obtained, the pharmacy technician enters it into the pharmacy computer. Billing information for the prescription is then transmitted to a processing computer for the insurer or PBM. If all information has been entered correctly and is in agreement with data on-file with the insurer, the prescription claim is processed using online adjudication and an online response is received in less than one minute in the pharmacy. The claim-processing computer instantly determines the dollar amount of the drug benefit and the appropriate co-pay.

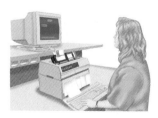

The pharmacy technician usually has an opportunity to review the data provided by the claim-processing computer before giving the OK for the prescription label and receipt to print in the pharmacy. The receipt indicates how much of the price of the prescription the patient must pay as determined by the insurer. The prescription can then be filled. The pharmacy technician should carefully review this adjudication information before proceeding to make sure the claim was processed properly. The pharmacy may be underpaid if the drug dispensed has a generic equivalent. The pharmacy technician should also look for claim processing messages such as drug or disease interaction alerts.

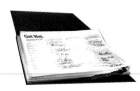

When prescriptions are billed online, pharmacies must keep records to verify that prescriptions were actually dispensed. Insurers or PBMs require pharmacies to maintain hard copies of each prescription that must be readily retrievable upon request. Insurers or PBMs also require pharmacies to maintain signature logs for all claims submitted electronically that must be readily retrievable upon request.

ONLINE CLAIM INFORMATION

Although there are many different types of health care insurance, the information required for online processing of claims is remarkably similar. The following information is usually required for online claim processing:

➡ cardholder identification number (usually the social security number of the employee or a variation of this number)

➡ group number (a number assigned by the insurer to the employer of the cardholder)

➡ name of patient

➡ birth date

➡ sex (M or F)

➡ relationship to cardholder (cardholder (C), spouse (S), dependent (D), other (O))

➡ date RX written

➡ date RX dispensed

➡ is this a new or refill prescription

➡ national drug code (NDC) of drug

➡ DAW indicator

➡ amount or quantity dispensed

➡ days supply

➡ identification number of prescribing physician

➡ identification of the pharmacy; effective May, 2007, pharmacies are identified by the National Provider Identifier (NPI)

➡ ingredient cost

➡ dispensing fee

➡ total price

➡ deductible or co-pay amount

➡ balance due

Dispense As Written (DAW)

When entering patient and prescription information, it is important to verify whether the patient's plan covers the brand name of a particular drug or if the patient is required to get generic drugs. When brand name drugs are dispensed, numbers corresponding to the reason for submitting the claim with brand name drugs are entered in a DAW (Dispense as Written) indicator field. Most health plan members have a choice between brand and generic drugs.

In some programs, if a patient receives a brand name drug when a generic is available, the patient must pay the difference between the cost of the brand and the cost of the generic. The following lists DAW indicators.

0 No DAW (No Dispense As Written)

1 DAW handwritten on the prescription by the prescriber

2 Patient requested brand

3 Pharmacist selected brand

4 Generic not in stock

5 Brand name dispensed but priced as generic

6 N/A

7 Substitution not allowed; brand mandated by law

8 Generic not available

 Billing special medications such as compounded prescriptions requires somewhat different procedures. These procedures are different for each insurer or PBM. When billing compounded medications or special medications the pharmacy technician should refer to informational booklets provided to the pharmacy by the insurer or PBM or call the pharmacy help desk as listed on the prescription drug card.

REJECTED CLAIMS

In the online adjudication process, the insurer sometimes rejects the claim as submitted.

This occurs before the prescription is dispensed and provides an opportunity to resolve the problem before it becomes larger. There are various reasons for rejections, and most problems can be resolved by telephoning a representative of the insurer or discussing the rejection with the patient. Rejections are best resolved during normal business hours.

REJECTIONS

At right are common reasons for rejection of pharmacy third party claims and suggestions on how to correct such rejections.

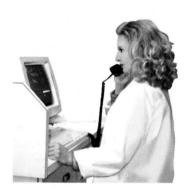

Resolving Rejections

When there is a question on coverage, the pharmacy technician can telephone the insurance plan's pharmacy help desk to determine if the patient is eligible for coverage. Pharmacy help desk personnel are often very helpful in resolving problems. If an employer has changed insurers, sometimes pharmacy help desk personnel can advise the pharmacy technician who the new insurer is. Many pharmacies maintain a list of phone numbers for insurers and their processors. If the prescription drug card is not available, the pharmacy technician can obtain the phone number of the insurer from this list.

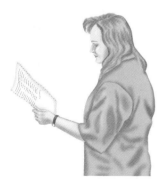

Handling Paper Claim Rejects

When paper claims are rejected by third parties, rejections often do not appear for several weeks after the claim was submitted. Rejections of paper claims are almost always accompanied by an explanation of the rejection and give details on what the technician can do to obtain successful payment of the claim. In many cases, the paper claim form was not completed correctly, information is missing, and the technician needs to only complete the missing information and resubmit the claim. Sometimes a telephone call must be made to the patient and/or the insurer to resolve the problem.

Dependent exceeds age limit as specified by plan

Many prescription drug plans have age limitations for children or dependents of the cardholder. Often, full-time college students are eligible for coverage as long as appropriate paperwork is on file with the insurer.

Invalid birth date

The birth date submitted by the pharmacy sometimes does not match the birth date in the insurer's computer. To solve this problem, first double-check that you have the correct birth date for the patient.

Invalid person code

The person code (e.g. 00,01,02,03) does not match the person code for the patient with the same sex and birth date information in the insurer's computer.

Invalid sex

The sex (M or F) submitted by the pharmacy does not match the sex in the insurer's computer for the patient. To solve this problem, change the sex code (if M change to F) and resubmit the claim.

Prescriber is not a network provider

This type of reject is common to Medicaid programs and is sometimes seen with HMO programs. Simply stated, only prescriptions issued by network prescribers are covered by the insurer.

Unable to connect with insurer's computer

Sometimes, due to computer problems, an insurer's computer may be unavailable for claim processing. Under these circumstances, the technician must follow the guidelines of their employer.

Patient not covered (coverage terminated)

This can occur when a patient has a new insurance card, whether the new card is issued by the same insurer or a new one. If the insurer has not changed, perhaps billing numbers have changed (new cardholder identification number, group number, etc.).

Refill too soon

Most third party plans require that most of the medication has been taken before the plan will cover another dispensing of the same medication. Early refills should always be brought to the attention of the pharmacist. If the pharmacist thinks it is appropriate to dispense a refill early (for example, if a patient is going on vacation), the next step is to contact the insurer to determine if it will pay for an early refill.

Refills not covered

Many managed care health programs require mail order pharmacies to fill prescriptions for maintenance medications. Patients often are not aware of mail order requirements of their prescription drug coverage. Ideally the employer is responsible to explain mail order requirements if their employees are required to use mail order for maintenance medications. Sometimes, patients do not realize this restriction until prescription claims are rejected at their community pharmacy. In such cases, the pharmacy technician will have to contact the insurer to determine if emergency refills are covered at the community pharmacy.

NDC not covered

This type of rejection is common with state Medicaid programs and managed care programs with closed formularies. Ideally, the patient is aware that the insurer has a limited formulary for prescription drug coverage. However, often patients are not aware of how this works. The pharmacy technician can call the pharmacy help desk for specific information about drug coverage. Sometimes, the insurer will consider prior authorization to cover medications that are not on the formulary. Sometimes, the insurer will not cover the prescribed medication and a pharmacist may determine what should be done next.

OTHER BILLING PROCEDURES

PAPER CLAIMS FOR BILLING PRESCRIPTIONS

Processing paper claims usually involves the pharmacy and the patient completing a form that has been issued by the insurer. Most insurers require completion of a form that they provide. A **universal claim form** (UCF) is a standardized form accepted by many insurers. Before online claim submission, most pharmacy third party claims were submitted on universal claim forms. Instructions for completing paper claims (insurer provided forms as well as universal claim forms) are printed on the claim forms so that anyone can complete the forms as long as they have access to the required information. Usually there is a requirement for signature by the patient and the pharmacist or health care provider. Incomplete forms or forms that have not been completed following directions printed on the forms are returned to the pharmacy for correction before the insurer will consider paying the claim. Generally, the same type of information required for online claims is also required for paper claim processing.

IN-HOUSE BILLING PROCEDURES

Pharmacy billing is not limited to billing insurers. Some pharmacies have in-house billing procedures. For example, the finances of an elderly or disabled patient may be handled by a family member or legal representative who does not live with the patient. In these cases, a monthly bill is mailed to the family member or legal representative, who then pays the pharmacy. Most pharmacies do not have in-house billing. When a pharmacy does do in-house billing, the pharmacy technician must carefully follow the policies and procedures of the employer.

DISEASE STATE MANAGEMENT SERVICES

Disease state management services are evolving as a component of pharmaceutical care. PBMs are selling disease management services to employers and health plans. Conditions most often targeted for disease state management include diabetes, hypertension, asthma, smoking cessation, and cholesterol management.

Both electronic and paper billing systems can be used for billing disease state management services; however, currently, paper billing systems are more common. Pharmacy technicians must properly document services as well as submit and follow up on paper claims. Note that the paper claims for these services are submitted to a department within an insurance company or PBM that is different from the department that processes claims for prescription drugs. The claims should include a cover letter, a copy of the order for the service from the physician (also known as the statement of medical necessity), an appropriate billing form (usually the standard **CMS-1500 form**, formerly named the HCFA 1500 form, shown at right), and accurate documentation of the services provided by the pharmacy.

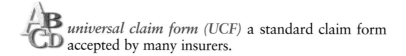

universal claim form (UCF) a standard claim form accepted by many insurers.

CMS-1500 (formerly HCFA 1500) form the standard form used by health care providers, such as physicians, to bill for services. It can be used to bill for disease state management services and is available at http://www.cms.hhs.gov/cmsforms/downloads/cms1500805.pdf.

1500

HEALTH INSURANCE CLAIM FORM

APPROVED BY NATIONAL UNIFORM CLAIM COMMITTEE 08/05

PICA

1. MEDICARE	MEDICAID	TRICARE CHAMPUS	CHAMPVA	GROUP HEALTH PLAN	FECA BLK LUNG	OTHER	1a. INSURED'S I.D. NUMBER	(For Program in Item 1)
(Medicare #)	(Medicaid #)	(Sponsor's SSN)	(Member ID#)	(SSN or ID)	(SSN)	(ID)		

2. PATIENT'S NAME (Last Name, First Name, Middle Initial)

3. PATIENT'S BIRTH DATE MM DD YY SEX M F

4. INSURED'S NAME (Last Name, First Name, Middle Initial)

5. PATIENT'S ADDRESS (No., Street)

6. PATIENT RELATIONSHIP TO INSURED Self Spouse Child Other

7. INSURED'S ADDRESS (No., Street)

CITY STATE

8. PATIENT STATUS Single Married Other

CITY STATE

ZIP CODE TELEPHONE (Include Area Code) ( )

Employed Full-Time Student Part-Time Student

ZIP CODE TELEPHONE (Include Area Code) ( )

9. OTHER INSURED'S NAME (Last Name, First Name, Middle Initial)

10. IS PATIENT'S CONDITION RELATED TO:

11. INSURED'S POLICY GROUP OR FECA NUMBER

a. OTHER INSURED'S POLICY OR GROUP NUMBER

a. EMPLOYMENT? (Current or Previous) YES NO

a. INSURED'S DATE OF BIRTH MM DD YY SEX M F

b. OTHER INSURED'S DATE OF BIRTH MM DD YY SEX M F

b. AUTO ACCIDENT? YES NO PLACE (State)

b. EMPLOYER'S NAME OR SCHOOL NAME

c. EMPLOYER'S NAME OR SCHOOL NAME

c. OTHER ACCIDENT? YES NO

c. INSURANCE PLAN NAME OR PROGRAM NAME

d. INSURANCE PLAN NAME OR PROGRAM NAME

10d. RESERVED FOR LOCAL USE

d. IS THERE ANOTHER HEALTH BENEFIT PLAN? YES NO If yes, return to and complete item 9 a-d.

READ BACK OF FORM BEFORE COMPLETING & SIGNING THIS FORM.

12. PATIENT'S OR AUTHORIZED PERSON'S SIGNATURE I authorize the release of any medical or other information necessary to process this claim. I also request payment of government benefits either to myself or to the party who accepts assignment below.

SIGNED DATE

13. INSURED'S OR AUTHORIZED PERSON'S SIGNATURE I authorize payment of medical benefits to the undersigned physician or supplier for services described below.

SIGNED

14. DATE OF CURRENT: MM DD YY ILLNESS (First symptom) OR INJURY (Accident) OR PREGNANCY(LMP)

15. IF PATIENT HAS HAD SAME OR SIMILAR ILLNESS. GIVE FIRST DATE MM DD YY

16. DATES PATIENT UNABLE TO WORK IN CURRENT OCCUPATION FROM MM DD YY TO MM DD YY

17. NAME OF REFERRING PROVIDER OR OTHER SOURCE

17a.
17b. NPI

18. HOSPITALIZATION DATES RELATED TO CURRENT SERVICES FROM MM DD YY TO MM DD YY

19. RESERVED FOR LOCAL USE

20. OUTSIDE LAB? YES NO $ CHARGES

21. DIAGNOSIS OR NATURE OF ILLNESS OR INJURY (Relate Items 1, 2, 3 or 4 to Item 24E by Line)
1. ___ . ___
2. ___ . ___
3. ___ . ___
4. ___ . ___

22. MEDICAID RESUBMISSION CODE ORIGINAL REF. NO.

23. PRIOR AUTHORIZATION NUMBER

24. A. DATE(S) OF SERVICE From MM DD YY To MM DD YY	B. PLACE OF SERVICE	C. EMG	D. PROCEDURES, SERVICES, OR SUPPLIES (Explain Unusual Circumstances) CPT/HCPCS MODIFIER	E. DIAGNOSIS POINTER	F. $ CHARGES	G. DAYS OR UNITS	H. EPSDT Family Plan	I. ID. QUAL.	J. RENDERING PROVIDER ID. #
1								NPI	
2								NPI	
3								NPI	
4								NPI	
5								NPI	
6								NPI	

25. FEDERAL TAX I.D. NUMBER SSN EIN

26. PATIENT'S ACCOUNT NO.

27. ACCEPT ASSIGNMENT? (For govt. claims, see back) YES NO

28. TOTAL CHARGE $

29. AMOUNT PAID $

30. BALANCE DUE $

31. SIGNATURE OF PHYSICIAN OR SUPPLIER INCLUDING DEGREES OR CREDENTIALS (I certify that the statements on the reverse apply to this bill and are made a part thereof.)

SIGNED DATE

32. SERVICE FACILITY LOCATION INFORMATION

a. NPI b.

33. BILLING PROVIDER INFO & PH # ( )

a. NPI b.

NUCC Instruction Manual available at: www.nucc.org

PLEASE PRINT OR TYPE

APPROVED OMB-0938-0999 FORM CMS-1500 (08-05)

OTHER BILLING PROCEDURES (cont'd)

MEDICATION THERAPY MANAGEMENT SERVICES

Medicare Part D provides opportunities for pharmacists to provide **Medication Therapy Management Services (MTMS)** to some Medicare beneficiaries that are taking multiple medications or have certain diseases. Pharmacy technicians have an important responsibility for billing these services, maintaining necessary documentation, and ensuring that payment is received. The CMS-1500 form is especially important for billing MTMS through **Prescription Drug Plans (PDPs)**.

In order to bill Prescription Drug Plans for MTMS using the CMS-1500 form, the pharmacist or pharmacy offering the services must be enrolled as a provider for the patient's PDP and also have a **National Provider Identifier (NPI)**. Applying for a NPI can be done online using the web-based NPI process (https://nppes.cms.hhs.gov) or by mailing the completed **CMS-10114** form to NPI Enumerator.

When completing the CMS-1500 form, the diagnosis code is needed and can be obtained from the physician. When billing MTMS, **Current Procedural Terminology Codes (CPT Codes)** provide a systematic way to bill for the services provided. Three different CPT Codes can be used to bill Prescription Drug Plans for MTMS provided by pharmacists: 99605, 99606, and 99607. Also, it is essential that documentation for services provided is carefully maintained.

CPT Codes for Pharmacist-Provided Services

➡ 99605 — Used for a first-encounter with a patient and may be billed in 1–15 minute increments.

➡ 99606 — Used for follow-up encounters and may be billed in 1–15 minute increments.

➡ 99607 — An add-on CPT Code to be used with 99605 or 99606 when additional 15 minute increments of time are spent face-to-face with a patient.

Medication Therapy Management Services (MTMS) services provided to some Medicare beneficiaries who are enrolled in Medicare Part D and who are taking multiple medications or have certain diseases.

Prescription Drug Plans (PDPs) third party programs for Medicare Part D.

National Provider Identifier (NPI) the code assigned to recognized health care providers; needed to bill MTMS.

Current Procedural Terminology Codes (CPT Codes) identifiers used for billing pharmacist-provided MTM Services.

CMS-10114 form the standard form used by health care providers to apply for a National Provider Identifier (NPI). This six-page form, page one of which is shown below, is available by calling EPI Enumerator at 1-800-465-3203.

DEPARTMENT OF HEALTH AND HUMAN SERVICES
CENTERS FOR MEDICARE & MEDICAID SERVICES

Form Approved
OMB No. 0938-0931

NATIONAL PROVIDER IDENTIFIER (NPI) APPLICATION/UPDATE FORM

Please PRINT or TYPE all information so it is legible. Do not use pencil. Failure to provide complete and accurate information may cause your application to be returned and delay processing of your application. In addition, you may experience problems being recognized by insurers if the records in their systems do not match the information you have furnished on this form.

SECTION 1 – BASIC INFORMATION

A. Reason For Submittal Of This Form (Check the appropriate box)

1. ❏ Initial Application
2. ❏ Change of Information (See instructions)
   NPI No._____

3. Deactivation NPI No._____
   REASON (Check one of the following)
   ❏ Death   ❏ Business Dissolved
   ❏ Other _____

B. Entity Type (Check the appropriate box)

1. ❏ An individual who renders health care. (Complete Sections 2A, 3, 4A and 5)
2. ❏ An organization that renders health care. (Complete Sections 2B, 3, 4B and 5)

SECTION 2 – IDENTIFYING INFORMATION

A. Individuals

1. Prefix (e.g.,Major, Mrs.)	2. First	3. Middle	4. Last
5. Suffix (e.g., Jr., Sr.)		6. Credential (e.g., M.D., D.O.)	

Other Name Information (If applicable. Use additional sheets of paper if necessary)

7. Prefix (e.g.,Major, Mrs.)	8. First	9. Middle	10. Last
11. Suffix (e.g., Jr., Sr.)		12. Credential (e.g., M.D., D.O.)	

13. Type of other Name
   ❏ Former Name   ❏ Professional Name   ❏ Other (Describe) _____

14. Date of Birth (mm/dd/yyyy)	15. State of Birth (U.S. only)	16. Country of Birth (If other than U.S.)

17. Gender
   ❏ Male   ❏ Female

18. Social Security Number (SSN)	19. IRS Individual Taxpayer Identification Number

B. Organizations and Groups

1. Name (Legal Business Name)	2. Employer Identification Number (EIN) or SSN

3. Other Name (Use additional sheets of paper if necessary)

4. Type of Other Name
   ❏ Former Legal Business Name   ❏ D/B/A Name   ❏ Other (Describe) _____

REVIEW

KEY CONCEPTS

FINANCIAL ISSUES

✔ Third party programs are simply another party besides the patient or the pharmacy that pays for some or all of the cost of medication: essentially, an insurer.

✔ A pharmacy benefit manager (PBM) is a company that administers drug benefit programs for insurance companies, HMOs, and self-insured employers.

✔ Co-insurance is essentially an agreement between the insurer and the insured to share costs. One aspect of it is the requirement for patients to co-pay a portion of the cost of prescriptions.

✔ The amount paid by insurers for prescriptions is not equal to the retail price normally charged, but is determined by a formula described in a contract between the insurer and the pharmacy.

THIRD PARTY PROGRAMS

✔ Prescription drug benefit cards contain necessary billing information for pharmacies, including the patient's identification number, group number, and co-pay amount.

✔ HMOs usually will not cover expenses incurred outside their participating network and often require generic substitution.

✔ POSs often partially reimburse expenses incurred outside of their network and usually require generic substitution.

✔ PPOs usually require generic substitution.

✔ Workers' compensation is compensation for employees accidentally injured on-the-job.

✔ Medicare covers people over the age of 65, disabled people under the age of 65 and people with kidney failure.

✔ Medicaid is a federal-state program for the needy.

ONLINE ADJUDICATION

✔ In online adjudication, the technician uses the computer to determine the exact coverage for each prescription with the appropriate third party.

✔ When brand name drugs are dispensed, numbers corresponding to the reason for submitting the claim with brand name drugs are entered in a DAW (Dispense as Written) indicator field in the prescription system.

REJECTED CLAIMS

✔ Many prescription drug plans have age limitations for children or dependents of the cardholder.

✔ Most third party plans require that most of the medication has been taken before the plan will cover a refill of the same medication.

✔ Many managed care health programs require mail order pharmacies to fill prescriptions for maintenance medications.

OTHER BILLING PROCEDURES

✔ When a claim is rejected, the pharmacy technician can telephone the insurance plan's pharmacy help desk to determine if the patient is eligible for coverage.

✔ Claims for disease state management services can be submitted using a paper system and often require follow-up.

SELF TEST

MATCH THE TERMS: I *the answer key begins on page 511*

1. CMS-1500 form _____

2. CMS-10114 form _____

3. co-insurance _____

4. co-pay _____

5. Current Procedural Terminology Codes (CPT Codes) _____

6. deductible _____

7. dual co-pay _____

8. formulary _____

9. HMOs _____

10. maximum allowable cost (MAC) _____

11. Medicaid _____

12. Medicare _____

13. Medication Therapy Management Services (MTMS) _____

14. National Provider Identifier (NPI) _____

15. online adjudication _____

a. the resolution of prescription coverage through the communication of the pharmacy computer with the third party computer.

b. the portion of the price of medication that the patient is required to pay.

c. the maximum price per tablet (or other dispensing unit) an insurer or PBM will pay for a given product.

d. a federal-state program, administered by the states, providing health care for the needy.

e. a cost-sharing agreement between the insurer and the insured.

f. co-pays that have two prices: one for generic and one for brand medications.

g. a set amount that must be paid by the patient for each benefit period before the insurer will cover additional expenses.

h. a network of providers for which costs are covered inside but not outside of the network.

i. the standard form used by health care providers, such as physicians, to bill for services. It can be used to bill for disease state management services.

j. a federal program providing health care to people with certain disabilities over age 65.

k. services provided to some Medicare beneficiaries who are enrolled in Medicare Part D and who are taking multiple medications or have certain diseases.

l. the code assigned to recognized health care providers; needed to bill MTMS.

m. identifiers used for billing pharmacist-provided MTM Services.

n. the standard form used by health care providers to apply for a National Provider Identifier (NPI).

o. a list of medications that are covered by a third party plan.

REVIEW

MATCH THE TERMS: II *the answer key begins on page 511*

1. patient assistance programs ____

2. pharmacy benefit managers ____

3. POSs ____

4. PPOs ____

5. prescription drug benefit cards ____

6. Prescription Drug Plans (PDPs) ____

7. tier ____

8. U&C or UCR ____

9. universal claim form ____

10. worker's compensation ____

a. companies that administer drug benefit programs.

b. a standard paper claim form accepted by many insurers.

c. the maximum amount of payment for a given prescription, determined by the insurer to be a usual and customary (and reasonable) price.

d. manufacturer sponsored prescription drug programs for the needy.

e. cards that contain third party billing information for prescription drug purchases.

f. a network of providers where the patient's primary care physician must be a member and costs outside the network may be partially reimbursed.

g. a network of providers where costs outside the network may be partially reimbursed and the patient's primary care physician need not be a member.

h. an employer compensation program for employees accidentally injured on the job.

i. third party programs for Medicare Part D.

j. categories of medications that are covered by a third party plan.

CHOOSE THE BEST ANSWER *the answer key begins on page 511*

1. Companies that administer drug benefit programs are called
   a. pharmacy benefit managers.
   b. MACs.
   c. HMOs.
   d. employers.

2. Another party, besides the patient or the pharmacy, that pays some or all of the cost of the medication is a(an)
   a. third party.
   b. co-insurance.
   c. MAC.
   d. UCR.

3. An agreement for cost-sharing between the insurer and the insured is called
   a. MAC.
   b. dual co-pay.
   c. co-insurance.
   d. co-pay.

4. The portion of the price of the medication that the patient is required to pay is called the
   a. co-insurance.
   b. co-pay.
   c. maximum allowable cost.
   d. Usual and customary price.

5. Pharmacies receive payment from third parties equal to
   a. the retail price of the drug.
   b. the manufacturer's cost.
   c. a wholesaler's price.
   d. none of the above.

6. Plans in which the patient pays a different amount depending on whether a generic or brand name medication is dispensed have
   a. dual co-pays.
   b. MAC.
   c. duplicate pricing.
   d. UCR.

7. If a third party plan has a dual co-pay, the patient usually pays _____ for generic drugs compared to brand name drugs.
   a. the same amount
   b. less
   c. more

8. HMOs, POS, and PPOs are examples of
   a. co-insurance.
   b. managed care programs.
   c. MAC.
   d. co-pays.

9. A(an) _____ is a network of providers for which costs are covered inside, but not outside of the network.
   a. POS
   b. HMO
   c. MAC
   d. PPO

10. A(an) _____ is a network of providers where costs outside the network may be partially reimbursed and the patient's primary care physician need not be a member.
    a. PPO
    b. HMO
    c. POS
    d. MAC

11. Which type of managed care program is least likely to require generic substitution?
    a. Medicare
    b. PPO
    c. Medicaid
    d. HMO

12. A drug formulary is
    a. a list of medications that are covered by a third party program.
    b. an official compendium of the FDA.
    c. a listing of the ingredients in a prescription.
    d. the price of a prescription under a third party program.

13. _____ is a federal-state program, administered by states, providing health care for the needy.
    a. Medicaid
    b. HMO
    c. Medicare
    d. PPO

14. Closed formulary programs, such as Medicaid, may cover drugs that are not on the formulary through a process called
    a. dual co-pay.
    b. co-insurance.
    c. POS.
    d. prior authorization.

REVIEW

15. Patient assistance programs are offered by
    a. HMOs.
    b. pharmacies.
    c. physicians.
    d. pharmaceutical manufacturers.

16. Which of the following information is generally not required in online claim processing?
    a. birth date
    b. weight
    c. sex
    d. group number

17. The DAW indicator that is appropriate for online adjudication if a physician has handwritten DAW on the prescription is
    a. 4.
    b. 2.
    c. 1.
    d. 3.

18. When there is a question on insurance coverage for an online claim, the pharmacy technician can
    a. telephone the insurance plan's pharmacy help desk.
    b. immediately refer the problem to the pharmacist.

19. When a technician receives a rejected claim "NDC Not Covered", this probably means
    a. the insurance plan has a closed formulary.
    b. the insurance plan has an open formulary.
    c. the birth date submitted does not match the birth date in the insurer's computer.
    d. the patient has mail order.

20. When a technician receives a rejected claim "Invalid Person Code," this probably means
    a. the patient is on Medicare.
    b. the patient has a mail order program.
    c. the person code entered does not match the birth date and/or sex in the insurer's computer.
    d. the patient is on Medicaid.

21. When a technician receives a rejected claim "Unable to Connect," this probably means
    a. the insurer has an incorrect birth date for the patient.
    b. the patient's coverage has expired.
    c. the connection with the insurer's computer is temporarily unavailable due to computer problems.
    d. the insurer has a closed formulary.

22. A standard form used by healthcare providers to bill for services is
    a. a universal claim form (UCF).
    b. a pdf.
    c. an NDC.
    d. CMS-1500.

23. The CPT Codes for billing Medication Therapy Management Services provided by pharmacists are
    a. ICD-9.
    b. MAC.
    c. PPO.
    d. 99605, 99606, and 99607.

15

COMMUNITY PHARMACY

COMMUNITY PHARMACY

Community or retail pharmacy practice is the practice of providing prescription services to the public.

In addition to prescription drugs, community pharmacies sell over-the-counter medications as well as other health and beauty products. A pharmacy may be owned independently or by a chain. Chains may specialize in pharmacy or be part of a broader mass merchandise or food store business.

One of the key characteristics of community pharmacy is the close interaction with patients.

The patient is a customer with alternatives as to where they can bring their business. So good customer service is a requirement, and for this, good **interpersonal skills** are needed.

Almost two thirds of all prescription drugs in the U.S. are dispensed by community pharmacies.

As a result, more pharmacists and technicians are employed in community pharmacy than any other area. An additional factor in employment is that the role of the community pharmacist in counseling and educating patients has been steadily increasing. This in turn has increased the role of the pharmacy technician in assisting pharmacists to dispense prescriptions. As a result, community pharmacy practice provides great opportunity for pharmacy technicians to find employment and serve the community.

Types of Community Pharmacies

There are about 60,000 community pharmacies in the United States which provide convenient access to medications and medication information. They are found in a variety of settings:

➡ **Independent Pharmacies**
   Individually owned local pharmacies.

➡ **Chain Pharmacies**
   Regional or national pharmacy chains such as CVS, Rite-Aid, Walgreens, and others.

➡ **Mass Merchandiser Pharmacies**
   Regional or national mass merchandise chains such as Walmart, KMart, Costco, Target, and others that sell various mass merchandise and have in-store pharmacies.

➡ **Food Store Pharmacies**
   Regional or national food store chains such as A&P, Giant Eagle, Kroger's, Pathmark, and others that have in-store pharmacies.

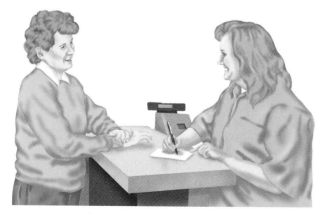

Customer Service

In contrast to institutional and other environments, technicians in the community pharmacy constantly interact with patients as customers. As a result, customer service is a major area of importance in the community pharmacy and technicians employed there must have strong interpersonal skills.

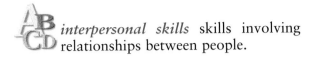
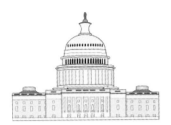

interpersonal skills skills involving relationships between people.

United States Government Regulations

The 1990 *Omnibus Budget and Reconciliation Act (OBRA)* requires community pharmacists to offer Medicaid patients counseling and instruction regarding prescription drug dosage, route of administration, and duration of administration; special directions; common severe side affects or interactions and therapeutic contraindications; proper storage; what to do if a dose is missed; and refill information.

The 1996 *Health Insurance Portability and Accountability Act (HIPAA)* requires all healthcare professionals to protect patients' privacy. Any information related to a patient or their medical condition is considered "protected health information" and must be kept confidential. This information includes but is not limited to the patient's name and address, date of birth, diagnosis, medical history, and medications.

Some practical ways of protecting patients' privacy include:

➡ Never discussing patients outside of the pharmacy setting.
➡ Shredding documents, papers, or labels with patient information (instead of discarding in regular trash).
➡ Speaking to patients and other healthcare professionals in the most private area possible.
➡ Never discussing patients with any individual unless the patient has provided written authorization to do so.

When working in any pharmacy, be sure to read and understand the pharmacy's HIPAA policy.

The 2003 *Medicare Prescription Drug Improvement and Modernization Act* provides a drug benefit program to senior citizens. Known as Medicare Part D, it relies on private prescription drug plan (PDP) companies to provide coverage to Medicare eligible individuals. The PDP's must operate within very detailed government guidelines but can design their own programs and compete with each other. PDP's use their own formularies or lists of covered drugs, non-covered drugs, and sometimes preferred drugs that may carry a lower copayment to the patient. The pharmacy staff needs to know how to assist patients when a drug is not covered and be involved with prescribers in making drug changes in accordance with formulary guidelines. Pharmacists and pharmacy technicians must also be familiar with online billing of these plans.

State Regulations

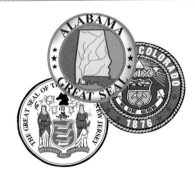

Community pharmacies are most closely regulated at the state level. For example, many states have mandated OBRA '90 counseling requirements for all patients, not just those on Medicaid. Also, states are increasingly requiring that technicians attain national pharmacy technician certification or they may have their own certifying process which may include registration with the state's board of pharmacy. States also regulate such things as the ratio of pharmacists to technicians; scope of technician practice; record keeping; equipment; and work areas.

ORGANIZATION

Prescription processing areas among community pharmacies may be organized differently, but they generally contain the same elements. A number of space and equipment requirements are dictated by State regulations.

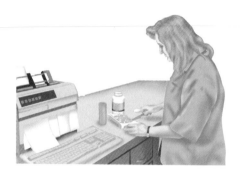

Prescription Counter

The prescription area of a pharmacy must have a counter area on which to prepare prescriptions. This counter should be kept orderly at all times.

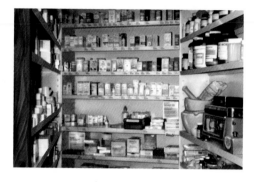

Storage

There must be adequate shelving, cabinets, or drawers for storage of medications. It is common to see several bays with shelving to hold bottles of medications. The medications may be arranged on the shelves alphabetically according to generic name or they may be arranged according to brand, or trade name.

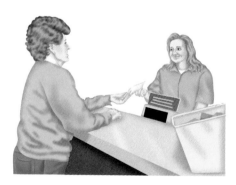

Transaction Windows

Pharmacies often have counter areas designated for intake of prescriptions being dropped off and may use the same or different counter area for dispensing the finished prescription. In accordance with HIPAA, **transaction windows** should be positioned so as to provide privacy for the patient. Some pharmacies are even establishing separate counseling rooms or booth areas.

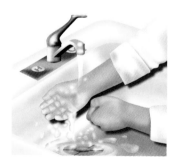

Sink

There must be an easily accessible sink that also must be kept clean at all times.

transaction windows counter areas designated for taking prescriptions and for dispensing them to patients.

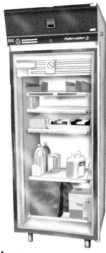

Refrigeration

There must also be a refrigerator in which to store medication that requires storage in temperatures between 2 and 8 degrees Celsius. The refrigerator must be designated for drugs only. No food products are allowed to be stored in the same refrigerator.

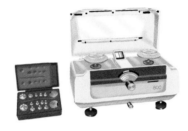

Equipment

Equipment that must be available for use in the pharmacy includes a prescription balance, a set of metric weights, a glass mortar and pestle, glass funnels, stirring rods, graduates for measuring liquids, spatulas, counting trays and or counting devices, ointment board or parchment paper for compounding creams, ointments, etc., prescription labels, and auxiliary or precautionary labels.

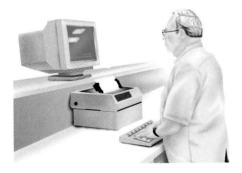

Computer System

There is an area for the computer monitor, keyboard, and printer.

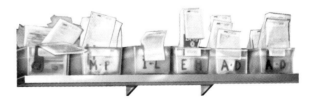

Prescription Bins or Shelves

Completed prescriptions that are not being immediately picked up are generally placed in bins or shelves alphabetized by customer.

CUSTOMER SERVICE

Customer satisfaction is the goal of customer service.

Good customer service requires presenting yourself to customers in a calm, courteous, and professional manner. It requires listening to and understanding customer requests for service and fulfilling those requests accurately or explaining to the customer's satisfaction why the request cannot be serviced.

The health of customers is a significant factor in their experience of community pharmacy service.

Customers may often feel sick or irritable and need their medication quickly. Having to wait in a line may be physically difficult or emotionally upsetting. The cost of the medication may be an additional worry. Consequently, though customer service is important in any type of retail store, it is particularly important in the community pharmacy setting.

It is important to respond to customers in a positive way at all times.

In any situation where a customer is angry, frustrated, or otherwise dissatisfied, it is especially important to give a positive response. This can be done in part by listening intently and making eye contact with the customer. Restating what the customer has said is also important, since it demonstrates that you have listened to their complaint. Use positive, not negative, terms to tell the customer what you can do, not what you can't do to solve their problem.

Involve the pharmacist in all difficult situations.

If after spending some time with the customer, you have been unable to resolve the problem, you should inform the pharmacist. This should be done immediately for serious complaints regarding problems with prescriptions. Remember that employees who possess well-developed interpersonal skills are good for business and will be appreciated by employers.

AT THE COUNTER

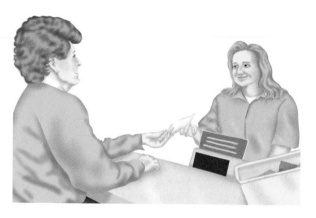

Since pharmacy technicians are generally responsible for handling the pharmacy counter, they have direct contact with customers and play a key role in assisting customers with their needs.

This involves taking in new and refill prescriptions, but also includes directing customers to requested over-the-counter products or answering other questions that do not require the pharmacist's judgment. The technician should be familiar with the layout of the store and know where various types of over-the-counter products are located so they can help customers find products quickly.

A pharmacy technician must know when to refer a customer to the pharmacist. It is a good idea to discuss such situations with the pharmacist regularly.

ON THE TELEPHONE

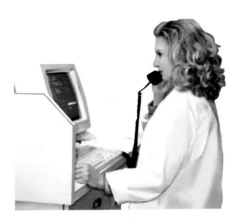

A significant part of the pharmacy technician's responsibilities includes answering the telephone. Calls must be answered in a pleasant and courteous manner, following a standard format that should be indicated by the store manager or pharmacist. Generally, this begins with stating the name of the pharmacy and your name. An example:

"Main Street Pharmacy, Joan speaking, may I help you?"

Many calls will concern the price or stock availability of prescription and over-the-counter products. Some will be to place refill requests. In that case, the same process is followed as when taking refill requests at the counter, except that the technician should also ask the patient when they plan to pick up the prescription.

Some calls will require the pharmacist's judgment. These should be directed immediately to the pharmacist. This applies to questions regarding medication or general health-related questions. When patients raise such questions, politely ask them to hold on the line while you get the pharmacist.

INTERPERSONAL TECHNIQUES

At the Counter

Techniques for interacting with customers at the counter include:

➡ listening carefully;
➡ making eye contact;
➡ repeating what the customer said;
➡ using positive rather than negative language to describe what you can do;
➡ calling the patient by name.

On the Phone

Techniques for interacting with customers on the telephone include:

➡ using a pleasant and courteous manner;
➡ stating the name of the pharmacy and your name;
➡ following the standard procedure indicated for your pharmacy;
➡ referring all calls that require a pharmacist's judgment to the pharmacist.

 safety you should know

Any time you are uncertain of whether a question requires the pharmacist's judgment, refer the question to the pharmacist.

PROCESSING PRESCRIPTIONS

A major responsibility of the pharmacy technician is to process new and refill prescriptions.

This is done using the pharmacy's computerized prescription system. Different pharmacies will use different systems. The pharmacist or another pharmacy technician will usually provide training on the system that is used. Learning to process prescriptions efficiently and accurately on the system is essential and will take some time and commitment.

PATIENT INFORMATION

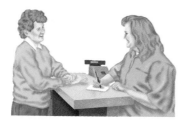

Among other features, the pharmacy's computerized prescription system contains patient profiles that provide complete information about patients, including their prescribers, insurer, medication history, and medical history, including allergies. The system also identifies drug interactions for patients taking multiple medications.

When taking in a new prescription, always ask whether the patient has ever had prescriptions filled at the pharmacy in the past. If the patient has not, be sure to get the following information for their profile:

- ➡ full name of the patient;
- ➡ address;
- ➡ telephone number;
- ➡ date of birth;
- ➡ any allergies to medication.

If a patient requests a prescription refill, *be sure to get the patient's name and the prescription number* which appears on the prescription bottle. If the prescription number is unavailable, ask for the name of the medication. Ask if the patient would like to wait while the prescription is filled or if they prefer to pick it up later; prioritize prescriptions for patients who wish to wait. Some pharmacies offer delivery service, which you can offer or let the patient request.

PRESCRIPTION INFORMATION

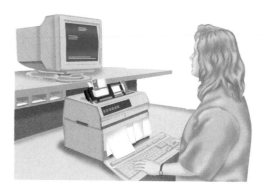

Different patients may have similar or even the same name, so always check the patient's address and date of birth to make sure you are working in the correct patient profile. When entering a new prescription into the system, enter the following information into the appropriate fields on the computer's dispensing screen:

- ➡ correct drug and strength;
- ➡ correct physician's name (and physician's DEA number for prescriptions for controlled substances or for prescriptions being billed to a third party that requires it);
- ➡ directions for use (the signa);
- ➡ quantity (i.e., the number of tablets or the metric quantity if dispensing a liquid, cream, inhaler, etc.);
- ➡ number of authorized refills;
- ➡ DAW code (indicates that a brand name or a generic product is being dispensed);
- ➡ initials of the dispensing pharmacist.

Scanning New Prescriptions

Many pharmacies are adding a scanning device to scan original prescriptions. Having a scanned copy of the original prescription allows for fast and efficient verification and accuracy checking. Note, however, that most states still require hard copy original prescriptions be physically stored in the pharmacy for a specified number of years.

ONLINE BILLING

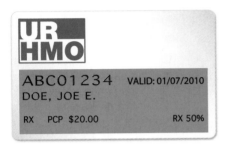

A major feature of computerized prescription systems is online billing of a prescription to a patient's insurance company or other third party. Since the majority of patients today have an insurance plan or third party coverage that will pay for the cost of their prescriptions, the technician must be familiar with all of the private, federal and state administered prescription plans, including Medicare Part D and Medicaid, that are accepted by the pharmacy. So entering a prescription also involves entering a code identifying the plan that will be billed. This generally includes:

➡ a plan number;
➡ a group number, which identifies the patient's employer;
➡ a patient or policy identification number, which is usually, but not always, the patient's social security number;
➡ a patient code, which indicates the specific patient covered under the plan (the primary card holder is usually 01, spouse is 02, and so on).

Once all third party billing information is entered, the technician can proceed with online billing. The third party will respond within a few moments by either stating that the claim has been paid or otherwise has been rejected. If a co-payment by the patient is required, the amount is indicated. If a rejection occurs, there will be a general message regarding why the claim has been rejected. If it is due to incorrect number entry, it can be easily corrected. Sometimes however, a call to the third party will be necessary to get the claim paid.

REFILLS

In the case of entering refill prescriptions, most pharmacy computer programs allow looking up a refill either by prescription number or through screening the patient profile for the medication. When processing a refill prescription, be sure to check that there are refills available. Most systems will indicate when no refills are available. If there are no refills, alert the pharmacist so that he or she can call the patient's physician for a new prescription. Prescriptions can be called in by a physician over the phone or faxed, and in some states they may be transmitted electronically from the prescriber to the pharmacy. Prescriptions ordered by telephone, fax, or electronic transmission have authenticity and security requirements that may call for handling by the pharmacist.

Note that when refilling prescriptions, be sure it is not too early to refill the medication. If it is more than a week early, many third parties will reject the claim. Also, refills for controlled substance medications should not be refilled early since they have the potential for abuse. In the case of a patient requesting an early refill of a controlled substance, involve the pharmacist right away.

SAFETY

Another important aspect of entering new and refill prescriptions has to do with screening for safety of prescription medication. Many computer software systems will flag drug interactions and allergy conflicts. When these flags occur, always alert the pharmacist so that he or she can evaluate the significance of the flag. The pharmacist may tell the pharmacy technician this is okay to proceed or will otherwise stop the process and may need to make a call to the patient's physician.

PREPARING THE PRESCRIPTION

The prescription system will print a prescription label based on the patient and prescription information that has been entered into it.

Once the label is generated, it is time to prepare the prescription. This begins with locating the medication and its container.

RETRIEVING & MEASURING

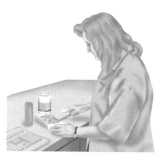

First, be sure to choose the correct drug and strength (i.e., ibuprofen 800 mg). One way to do this is to match the drug's unique 11-digit NDC (National Drug Code) number on the stock bottle to the NDC number on the prescription label. NDC numbers are also included in each product's bar code which can be scanned to further prevent errors.

If the product needed is a tablet or capsule, find the stock bottle on the shelf and count the correct number of pills using a **counting tray**. A counting tray has a side container-like area into which you count the correct number of pills or tablets. The pills to be dispensed can then slide easily into a prescription vial, and the remaining pills can slide back into the stock bottle.

The most common types of products are tablets and capsules, but there are many others such as creams and ointments, liquids, eye and ear drops, suppositories, injectables, and pediatric powders for reconstitution. Solutions are measured using volumetric glassware such as a graduate, pipet, flask, syringe or buret and ointments are weighed using a balance, weights, or weighing containers. *(See Chapter Nine for more information.)*

counting tray a tray designed for counting pills from a stock bottle into a prescription vial.

safety cap a child-resistant cap.

auxiliary labels labels regarding specific warnings, foods or medications to avoid, potential side effects, and other cautionary interactions.

CONTAINERS

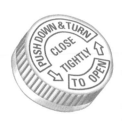

All prescription vials and bottles must have a **safety cap** or child resistant cap, unless the patient requests an easy-open cap. Most computer software programs have a field for recording the patient's preference. It is important to pay attention to which cap is indicated as some elderly or arthritic patients have extreme difficulty opening child-resistant caps.

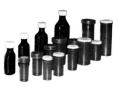

If preparing a liquid medication, select an appropriate size bottle and pour the correct volume of liquid into the bottle. For creams and ointments that are not pre-packaged, it will be necessary to transfer the product with a spatula to an ointment jar of the correct size.

AUTOMATED FILLING MACHINES

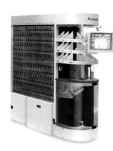

Some pharmacies use automated filling and dispensing machines such as the Parata Robotic Dispensing System® (shown at left) for their fastest-moving drugs. These machines automatically fill prescription bottles with correct quantities and label them. The pharmacy technician needs to maintain these machines on a daily basis by adding inventory to each cell, making sure the machine has a supply of labels, and keeping the machine clean. Note that a pharmacist must still check the final product even when dispensed by an automated filling machine. (*Photo Courtesy Parata Systems, LLC.*)

LABELS

Once the desired pills or other product is put in an appropriate container, the finished prescription label is placed on the product along with any **auxiliary labels** that may be necessary. These labels identify important usage information, including specific warnings or alerts on:

➡ administration
➡ proper storage
➡ possible side effects
➡ potential food and drug interactions

Examples include "take with food," "may cause drowsiness," and others shown at right. Some computer systems automatically identify which auxiliary labels are needed. If this is not the case, ask the pharmacist which labels should be applied.

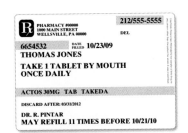

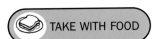 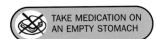

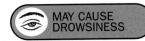 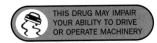

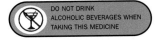 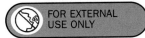

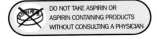 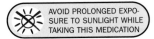

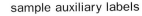

sample auxiliary labels

FINAL CHECK BY THE PHARMACIST

As the final step of the preparation process, organize the completed product and all paperwork, including the original prescription, for the pharmacist's final check. Leave stock bottles or other packaging next to the final product so the pharmacist can see that the correct product was chosen from stock. After the pharmacist has checked the prescription, the pharmacy technician returns any products used to their proper place on the shelf, cabinet, or drawer.

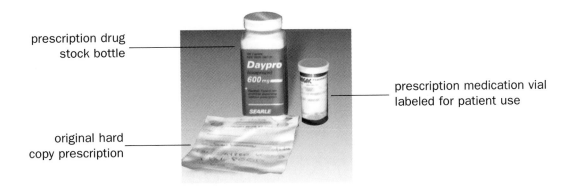

prescription drug stock bottle

prescription medication vial labeled for patient use

original hard copy prescription

CUSTOMER PICK-UP

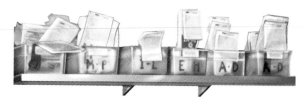

alphabetized prescription bins

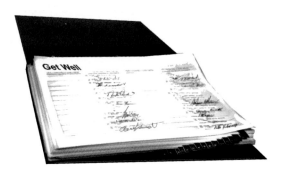

a signature log

 signature log a book in which patients sign for the prescriptions they receive, for legal and insurance purposes.

Picking Up the Prescription

Completed prescriptions are usually filed alphabetically by the patient's last name either in bins or another storage area. Always be sensitive to the confidential nature of prescription information and be sure to follow HIPAA privacy regulations. For instance, always speak in a quiet voice in the area specifically designated for prescription pick ups. Also, be careful not to inadvertently give out protected information. For instance, do not ask, "Would you also like to pick up your daughter's prescription while you're here?" Though this may seem helpful, it is a breach of HIPAA privacy regulations. Find only the prescription that was requested.

Signature Logs

Most community pharmacies have customers sign a log to record that the prescription was picked-up. The signature log will serve as proof to a third party payer such as Medicaid or a private insurer that the prescription was dispensed to the patient. It is common for third party payers to review the signature log when conducting audits at pharmacies.

The log may also record that patient medication counselling was offered. The usual process is to ask the patient if they would like the pharmacist to speak with them regarding their prescription. The patient is then asked to sign that they have either accepted or declined.

In addition, pharmacies may require a person picking up a Schedule II, and sometimes also a Schedule III, IV or V prescription, to show a driver's license. The driver's license number will be recorded either in the log or on the back of the prescription. This information will help in the event that the drug is used unlawfully.

Filing Hard Copy Original Prescriptions

Pharmacy technicians will often be responsible for filing hard copy original prescriptions by their prescription number. States laws vary, but most require that prescriptions for Class II controlled substances be filed separately. Again depending on state law, Class III, IV, and V prescriptions may be filed with or separately from prescriptions for non-controlled substances; if they are filed with non-controlled substance prescriptions, they may need to be stamped or marked with a red "C".

USING A CASH REGISTER

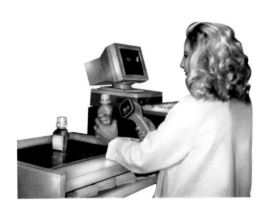

scanning a price

It is often a responsibility of the pharmacy technician to ring up prescriptions and over-the-counter products into the register and accept payment for them. Cash registers are integrated into the pharmacy's computerized system so prices for products can be automatically entered by using bar code scanners. Scanners can be hand-held or built into the counter. The scanner beam is targeted at the bar code and identifies the product for the register. The product's price (or discounted price if there is a prescription plan discount) is automatically entered into the register. If a mistake is made between the pricing on the product or shelf and the amount in the system, changes can be made manually, though each system is different, and technicians need to know and follow the procedures used at their pharmacy.

Operating a cash register also requires handling payments properly. When cash payment is made, it is it is important to count the payment within the customer's line of sight and to confirm the amount orally to the customer. This will avoid misunderstandings over what the customer thought they gave you. If change is necessary, the amount should be counted out loud and placed into the customer's hand. An example of such a transaction would be:

> A twenty dollar bill is given as payment for a bill of $14.50.

> ➡ The bill should be held or placed within the customer's line of sight and the amount confirmed as "That's Twenty dollars."

> ➡ The amount is then entered into the register and a receipt is produced.

> ➡ The change is counted out as it is placed into the customer's hand, i.e., "fifty cents makes fifteen dollars, and five dollars makes twenty dollars."

> ➡ After the customer has received their change and is given the receipt, the twenty dollar bill is placed into the register drawer.

Following this general procedure will avoid disputes, either out of confusion or intent to deceive, over whether a larger bill was tendered or the correct change given.

The pharmacy technician must also be able to handle checks and credit cards appropriately. It is very important to follow the store policy and procedure regarding handling of these transactions. Be sure to check the identification of the customer as instructed by the store manager or pharmacist.

OTHER DUTIES

The pharmacy technician should know the names and locations of the various over-the-counter products carried in the pharmacy.

The technician should be able to direct customers to any OTC product. Examples include cough and cold preparations, laxatives and antidiarrheals, medications for the treatment of indigestion, analgesics, vitamins, first aid supplies, dental and denture care products, and infant care products. Additionally, many pharmacies sell durable medical equipment such as canes, walkers, and wheelchairs.

The technician should not recommend OTC products to pharmacy customers, however.

With the exception of Behind-the-Counter OTC medications (see Chapter 3), OTC products may be bought freely by customers. However, they are not without risks. Incorrect dosages and drug-drug interactions with OTC products can produce significant adverse effects. For example, many cough and cold preparations contain ingredients that may increase blood pressure and worsen a diabetic condition. Therefore, the technician should *refer patients asking about OTC products to the pharmacist.* As always, the technician must involve the pharmacist whenever judgement is needed.

Pharmacy technicians are also responsible for reordering stock as needed.

The technician must know which products are used more frequently than others and reorder in appropriate quantities. For instance, a popular anti-hypertensive medication should be kept well stocked, while medications that are not as popular do not need to be available in large quantities.

The pharmacy technician is also generally responsible for keeping the pharmacy clean, neat, and in proper working order.

Periodically, the counting trays and the pharmacy counter should be wiped with alcohol. Pharmacy supplies, such as prescription bags, prescription vials and bottles, prescription labels and computer paper, must be stocked regularly. The stock bottles should periodically be rearranged so that all labels face front. At least monthly, the pharmacy technician should check all bottles for outdated expiration dates as it is unlawful to dispense outdated medications. Expired drugs must be sent back to the wholesaler or be destroyed.

RETAIL CONCEPTS

Community pharmacies do not just dispense prescriptions. They are retail businesses that sell over-the-counter medications and various other products. Retail businesses resell consumer ready products that they have purchased from wholesalers or manufacturers. To make a profit, the retailer sells the products at a **mark-up** from their purchase price. The mark-up is the amount of the retailer's sale price minus their purchase price. For example, if an over-the-counter medication is purchased at $5.00 a package, and the mark-up is 50%, the retailer's price to the consumer will be: $5.00 plus a $2.50 markup ($5.00 times 50%), or $7.50.

The mark-up represents the portion of sales that the retailer will clear after paying suppliers. This is what pays for the costs of doing business (building, equipment, salaries, etc.) and generates profits. So calculating the mark-up is very important to retailers. It is generally calculated by the pharmacy computer system and based on business costs and profit goals. They will differ by pharmacy and can differ by product. That is, some product lines may have lower or higher mark-ups than the standard products in the pharmacy. Each price that is stickered on a product includes the cost of the product and its mark-up.

Shelf Stickers

OTC products have **shelf-stickers** that can be scanned for inventory identification. They also indicate **unit price** information for consumers. A unit price is the price of a unit of medication (such as an ounce of a liquid cold remedy), rather than the price of the entire package. Unit prices protect the consumer from packaging and pricing that suggests that more is contained in the item than actually is.

mark-up the difference between the retailer's purchase price and their sale price.

shelf stickers stickers with bar codes that can be scanned for inventory identification.

unit price the price of a unit of medication, such as one ounce of a liquid cold remedy.

STOCK DUTIES

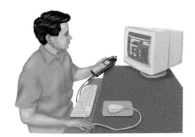

Ordering

Stock orders in most pharmacies are transmitted electronically to a drug wholesaler by either scanning or manually entering the product's stock number into a computer.

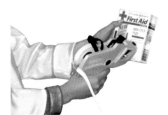

Stickering, Shelving, and Filing Invoices

Products are often stickered with pricing information and reorder numbers. These stickers may be applied with a stickering gun or by hand. Then the items need to be put on the shelves in their proper places. The invoices will also need to be filed for reference.

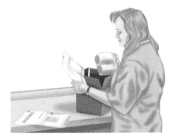

Receiving

The pharmacy technician is usually responsible for unpacking the order and check that all items on the invoice have been received. Each item must be checked to make sure the following are as ordered:

- ✔ drug product
- ✔ strength
- ✔ packaging
- ✔ quantity

In addition items must be inspected for:

- ✔ damage
- ✔ expiration dates

DISEASE STATE MANAGEMENT AND CLINIC SERVICES

Disease state management programs provide one-on-one pharmacist-patient consultation sessions to help manage chronic diseases or conditions such as diabetes. For example, the pharmacist may teach diabetes patients how to properly use blood glucose monitoring devices or the pharmacist may analyze a patient's blood-glucose readings on an on-going basis and recommend medication changes to the patient's physician. These programs are also offered for asthma/chronic obstructive pulmonary disease (COPD), anticoagulation, weight loss, smoking cessation and cholesterol reduction.

Some pharmacies also have walk-in clinics such as "Minute Clinics" at some CVS locations and "Take

Care" clinics at some Walgreens locations. These clinics are staffed by a nurse practitioner who can provide treatment for a limited number of common conditions such as common colds and minor injuries; administer flu shots or other vaccines; and possibly also write prescriptions for some medications, in accordance with applicable laws.

Fees for these services are either billed directly to the patient or to the patient's insurance. Pharmacy technicians may coordinate the billing, as well as schedule appointments and take patient information. As with all patient-related medical information, HIPAA regulations mandate complete confidentiality.

REVIEW

KEY CONCEPTS

COMMUNITY PHARMACY

✔ In addition to prescription drugs, community pharmacies sell over-the-counter medications as well as other health and beauty products.

✔ The role of the community pharmacist in counseling and educating patients has been steadily increasing.

ORGANIZATION

✔ Pharmacies have basic space and equipment requirements that may vary slightly from state to state but generally include a prescription counter to work on, proper storage areas for drugs, designated refrigerators for drugs, equipment for compounding, a sink, computer system and areas for dispensing prescriptions.

CUSTOMER SERVICE

✔ Technicians should always respond to customers in a positive and courteous way.

PROCESSING PRESCRIPTIONS

✔ In the case of a patient requesting an early refill of a controlled substance, involve the pharmacist right away.

✔ Processing new prescriptions involves entering patient information and prescription drug information, as well as billing information.

PREPARING THE PRESCRIPTION

✔ Whenever the prescription system flags drug interactions and allergy conflicts, alert the pharmacist so that he or she can evaluate the significance of the flag.

✔ Every drug product has a unique, eleven-digit National Drug Code (NDC) number that can be used when filling a prescription to verify the correct product has been retrieved from stock.

✔ All dispensed prescription vials and bottles must have a safety cap or child resistant cap, unless the patient requests an easy-open or non-child resistant cap.

✔ Auxiliary labels identify important usage information, including specific warnings or alerts on: administration, proper storage, possible side effects, and potential food and drug interactions.

✔ As a final step of the preparation process, the final product and all paperwork, including the original prescription, is organized for the pharmacist's final check.

CUSTOMER PICK-UP

✔ Customer signatures in a log are required for Medicaid and most third party insurers or HMO prescriptions, along with Schedule V controlled substances, poisons, and certain other prescriptions (depending upon the state).

OTHER DUTIES

✔ With the exception of Behind-the-Counter OTC Medications (see Chapter 3), OTC products may be bought freely by customers, but they are not without risks. The technician may direct customers to a product but should involve the pharmacist when making recommendations.

✔ Ordering stock is often a responsibility of the pharmacy technician.

✔ The pharmacy technician is generally responsible for keeping the pharmacy clean, neat, and in proper working order.

SELF TEST

MATCH THE TERMS   *the answer key begins on page 511*

1. automated filling machines ____

2. auxiliary labels ____

3. counting tray ____

4. interpersonal skills ____

5. mark-up ____

6. safety caps ____

7. shelf-stickers ____

8. signature log ____

9. transaction windows ____

10. unit price ____

a. skills involving relationships between people.

b. counter areas designated for taking prescriptions and for dispensing them to patients.

c. a child-resistant cap.

d. the price of a unit of medication (such as an ounce of a liquid cold remedy).

e. a tray designed for counting pills.

f. specific warnings that are placed on filled prescriptions.

g. a book in which patients sign for the prescriptions they receive, for legal and insurance purposes.

h. the amount of the retailer's sale price minus their purchase price.

i. stickers with bar codes that can be scanned for inventory identification.

j. automated machines that fill and label pill bottles with correct quantities of ordered drugs.

CHOOSE THE BEST ANSWER   *the answer key begins on page 511*

1. _____ are skills involving relationships between people.
   a. Computer skills
   b. Data management skills
   c. Transaction skills
   d. Interpersonal skills

2. About 2/3 of all prescription drugs in the U.S. are dispensed by
   a. community pharmacies.
   b. institutional pharmacies.
   c. hospital pharmacies.
   d. nursing home pharmacies.

3. More technicians and pharmacists are employed in _____ than any other type of pharmacy.
   a. community pharmacy
   b. hospital pharmacy
   c. mail order pharmacy
   d. long-term care

4. Community pharmacies that are individually owned local pharmacies are
   a. food store pharmacies.
   b. mass merchandiser pharmacies.
   c. chain pharmacies.
   d. independent pharmacies.

REVIEW

5. Community pharmacies, such as CVS and Walgreens, that are part of regional or national pharmacy chains are
   a. independent pharmacies.
   b. food store pharmacies.
   c. chain pharmacies.
   d. mass merchandiser pharmacies.

6. Community pharmacies that are part of regional or national food store chains such are Giant Eagle and Kroger are
   a. mass merchandiser pharmacies.
   b. food store pharmacies.
   c. chain pharmacies.
   d. independent pharmacies.

7. _____ require(s) community pharmacists to offer counseling to Medicaid patients regarding medications.
   a. Medicare Part D
   b. The 1990 Omnibus Budget and Reconciliation Act (OBRA)
   c. HIPAA
   d. The DEA

8. The HIPAA laws
   a. require pharmacists to provide counselling on all new medications.
   b. requires that health information be kept confidential.
   c. allows pharmacy staff to discuss a patient's health information outside the pharmacy.
   d. none of the above

9. Individual states
   a. do not regulate the practice of pharmacy.
   b. may require national pharmacy technician certification or may have their own registration and certification process.
   c. regulate the scope of pharmacy technician practice including the ratio of pharmacists to technicians.
   d. b & c

10. The refrigerator in a community pharmacy may be used to store
    a. drugs only.
    b. drugs and lunch of pharmacy personnel.
    c. drugs and sealed containers of soda pop.
    d. drugs and the pharmacist's lunch.

11. Good interpersonal skills include
    a. making eye contact.
    b. calling the customer by name.
    c. listening carefully.
    d. all of the above

12. A patient's question regarding medications or their general health
    a. can be handled by a technician.
    b. should be referred to the pharmacist.
    c. can be answered by the pharmacy technician or the pharmacist depending on state regulations.
    d. can sometimes be answered by the pharmacy technician and sometimes by the pharmacist depending on the technician's judgement.

13. Patient information that must be entered into the computer includes
    a. only the name of the patient.
    b. full name of patient, address, telephone number, date of birth, and any medication allergies.
    c. diagnosis made by the technician.
    d. diagnosis made by the pharmacist.

14. When entering a new prescription into the computer, the technician must enter the following information:
    a. the prescription number
    b. the metric quantity of the drug being dispensed
    c. the directions for use of the medication
    d. both b and c

15. When intaking a new prescription from a customer be sure to get which of the following information:
   a. full name of patient
   b. address
   c. date of birth
   d. all of the above

16. The group number in third party billing information usually identifies the
   a. employer.
   b. gender.
   c. family member.
   d. Social Security number of the insured.

17. An NDC number
   a. is nine digits long and is the same for some drugs.
   b. is the same as the prescription number.
   c. is an eleven digit number and is unique to each drug product.
   d. none of the above

18. All dispensed prescriptions must have a _____ cap unless that patient specifies a _____ cap.
   a. child resistant, non-child resistant
   b. child-resistant, child-resistant
   c. non-child resistant, non-child resistant
   d. non-child resistant, child-resistant

19. Labels that are placed on the prescription container in addition to the prescription label and provide specific warnings are
   a. warning stickers.
   b. flags.
   c. warning labels.
   d. auxiliary labels.

20. The pharmacist always checks the prescription
   a. after it is filled by the technician.
   b. when the patient signs the log.
   c. after it is rung on the cash register.
   d. as it is given to the patient.

21. The pharmacist _____ check the final product dispensed by an automated filling machine.
   a. must
   b. may
   c. does not need to

22. A(An) _____ is a book that patients sign for the prescriptions they receive.
   a. exempt narcotic book
   b. patient register book
   c. patient compliance book
   d. signature log

23. Ordering stock is a responsibility of the
   a. computer system.
   b. prescription counter.
   c. pharmacy technician.
   d. third party.

24. The _____ is generally responsible for keeping the pharmacy clean, neat, and in proper working order.
   a. staff pharmacist
   b. pharmacy manager
   c. pharmacy technician
   d. weekend pharmacist

25. The difference between the price the customer pays and the price the pharmacy pays for a product is called
   a. profit.
   b. overhead.
   c. margin.
   d. mark-up.

REVIEW

26. Unit price information is found on shelf stickers for
    a. Schedule III, IV, and V medications.
    b. Schedule II medications.
    c. OTC products.
    d. legend drugs.

27. Disease state management services are offered in
    a. private offices or areas.
    b. public access areas.
    c. the dispensing area of the pharmacy.
    d. waiting areas.

28. Coordinating of billing for disease state management services is a duty of the
    a. physician.
    b. third party.
    c. pharmacy technician.
    d. staff pharmacist.

29. Scheduling appointments for disease state management services is a duty of the
    a. registered nurse.
    b. pharmacy technician.
    c. physician.
    d. third party.

16

HOSPITAL PHARMACY

LEARNING OBJECTIVES

At the completion of study, the student will:

➡ list various members of the health care team.

➡ identify the variety of roles of a pharmacy technician.

➡ define hospital formulary and therapeutic exchange.

➡ summarize why unit dose medications are used in the hospital setting.

➡ discuss the components of a patient chart and/or electronic medical record.

➡ compare and contrast a hospital medication order and an outpatient prescription.

➡ differentiate manual verses automated order processing.

➡ outline the process of ordering and receiving drug inventory in the hospital.

➡ compare the difference between single dose and multidose vials of medication.

➡ explain the importance of Materials Safety Data Sheets (MSDS).

➡ demonstrate an understanding of hospital pharmacy calculations.

HOSPITAL PHARMACY

Hospital pharmacy technicians work as part of a team to help provide appropriate medication therapy for hospital patients.

Pharmacy technicians in the hospital work under the direct supervision of a pharmacist or supervising technician and play a vital role in the preparation, storage, and delivery of medications to patients. Most hospitals require a current state pharmacy technician license; however, some hospitals will train a person while in the process of applying for licensure. Training requirements may vary by state and hospital, but hospitals are increasingly seeking technicians who already received certification (CPhT).

To better understand the hospital pharmacy technician's roles and responsibilities, it is important to become familiar with the details of a hospital.

Though they may be organized differently, hospitals generally contain the same elements. Patient rooms are divided into groups called nursing units or patient care units. Patients with similar problems are usually located on the same unit. Often, names of specific units are referred to by their abbreviations. For example, a patient being treated for a heart attack would be treated in the Cardiac Care Unit (CCU) and a woman about to give birth would be admitted to the obstetrics (OB) ward.

The work station for medical personnel on a nursing unit is called the nurses' station.

The nurses' station is a communication center for patient care in the hospital. This area stores various items required for care of the patients on the unit, including medications.

There are several other areas of the hospital, called ancillary areas, that also provide patient care.

Each hospital has different ancillary areas, but some common ones are radiology, the cardiac catheterization lab, and the emergency room. These areas use medications and are serviced by the pharmacy department.

SOME HOSPITAL UNIT ABBREVIATIONS

- ➡ BMTU: Bone Marrow Transplant Unit
- ➡ CCU: Cardiac Care Unit or Coronary Care Unit
- ➡ ED: Emergency Department
- ➡ ER: Emergency Room
- ➡ ICU: Intensive Care Unit
- ➡ CT-ICU: Cardiothoracic ICU
- ➡ NICU: Neonatal ICU or Neurological ICU
- ➡ PICU: Pediatric ICU
- ➡ SICU: Surgical ICU
- ➡ OB: Obstetrics
- ➡ OR: Operating Room
- ➡ PAR: Post-Anesthesia Recovery
- ➡ PACU: Post-Anesthesia Care Unit
- ➡ PEDS: Pediatrics

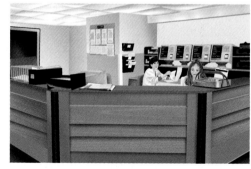

The nurses' station is a central storage and communication center for patient care in the hospital.

THE HEALTH CARE TEAM

It takes a team of many different types of health care professionals to meet the medication needs of patients, and individual patients generally receive care from a variety of these professionals. Most health care personnel are identified by abbreviations that indicate their discipline. Each individual profession plays a part on the multidisciplinary healthcare team. Their common objective is to care for patients and assist in their recovery. Pharmacy technicians interact with many of the following professions:

Physician

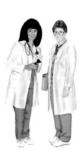

M.D., Medical Doctor
An MD examines patients, orders and interprets lab tests, diagnoses illnesses, and prescribes and administers treatments for people suffering from injury or disease. MD's write the majority of all medication orders.

D.O., Doctor of Osteopathy
A osteopathic physician has the same responsibilities as an MD but practices a "whole person" approach to medicine.

Other Staff

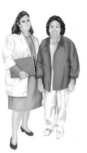

P.A., Physician's Assistant
A physician's assistant coordinates care for patients under the close supervision of a MD or DO. They are allowed to prescribe certain medications.

R.T., Respiratory Therapist
A respiratory therapist assists in the evaluation, treatment, and care of patients with breathing problems or illnesses. They may also administer respiratory drug treatments to patients.

P.C.T., Patient Care Technician
Person who works as a unit clerk or assists nursing in patient care activities. PCTs are often sent to the pharmacy to pick up medications that are needed for a patient in between pharmacy deliveries to the unit.

M.S.W., Master's of Social Work
A social worker is concerned with patient social factors such as child protection, coping capacities of patients and their families, and ability to pay for medications.

Nursing

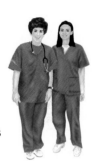

N.P., Nurse Practitioner
A nurse practitioner provides basic primary health care or can do further training to specialize in a specific area. The N.P. works closely with doctors and can prescribe various medications in most states.

R.N., Registered Nurse
A nurse who provides bedside care, assists physicians in various procedures, and administers medication regimens to patients.

L.P.N., Licensed Practical Nurse
A nurse who provides basic bedside care under the supervision of an RN. An LPN may administer medication to patients.

Pharmacy

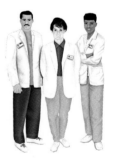

R.Ph., Registered Pharmacist
A pharmacist who is licensed to work by the state. Duties include reviewing patient drug regimens for appropriateness, dispensing medications, and advising the medical staff on the selection of drugs. An R.Ph. may have a bachelor of science in pharmacy (B.S. Pharm.) or a Doctor of Pharmacy (Pharm.D.) degree.

Pharm.D., Doctor of Pharmacy
The only degree now available to pharmacy school graduates. Pharm.D. requirements include more clinical sciences and experiential training than a B.S. Pharm.

TECHNICIAN ROLES

The hospital pharmacy technician has many responsibilities. Most pharmacy technicians are "cross-trained." This allows the technician to work in different areas of the pharmacy as needed. Some responsibilities may overlap between the different roles. Listed below are examples of various duties a pharmacy technician may have in the hospital setting.

Front Counter

Hospital pharmacy technicians are often assigned to work the front counter in the main pharmacy. This includes answering phone calls, helping other healthcare professionals at the pharmacy window, filling first doses of oral medications, and other duties as needed.

Cart Fill

In hospitals that have manual cart fill, technicians are assigned to fill the medication carts. The medication carts contain a 24 hour supply of patient medications in a patient cassette or drawer. In hospitals that utilize an automated dispensing cabinet or pharmacy "robot" to supply medications, this position may not exist or may be limited to filling a few medications that are not located in the automated dispensing cabinet or robot.

Order Processing

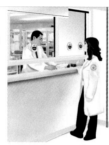

Order processing is another role often assigned to pharmacy technicians. In some hospitals, the technician is responsible for entering medication orders in the computer system. While entering orders, the technician may assist the pharmacist by screening the patient profile for allergies, duplicate therapies, and pertinent labs. By bringing this information to the pharmacist's attention, the technician can help prevent medication errors.

Monitoring Drug Therapy

A pharmacy technician is sometimes assigned to assist a pharmacist in monitoring patients' medication therapy. This role entails retrieving drug levels, labs values, or other patient specific information (e.g. blood pressure, fever, etc) from patient charts or the hospital computer system.

Narcotics

Many hospitals have a pharmacy technician who helps coordinate narcotic drug distribution. This involves ensuring the security of narcotics when receiving, preparing, and delivering them to nursing units or automated dispensing cabinets. The technician also reviews inventory reports, completes audits, reviews discrepancy reports, and confirms the hospital's compliance with state and federal controlled substances laws.

Delivery (hospital and clinics)

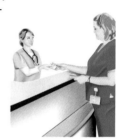

A delivery technician is responsible for transporting medications and other pharmacy supplies from the pharmacy to nursing units, other ancillary areas of the hospital and/or outpatient clinics. This role may include picking up new orders and bringing discontinued medications back to the pharmacy.

Automation

An automation technician is responsible for providing technical support for pharmacy systems. This role may entail operating a pharmacy "robot," assisting healthcare providers with use of automated dispensing cabinets, and assigning new users and passwords.

Quality Assurance (QA)

The quality assurance technician conducts inspections of nursing units and other areas of the hospital that store medications. During inspections, the technician makes sure that medications are stored and handled in compliance with hospital policy. This position may also include serving on various hospital committees.

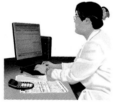

Investigational Drug Service

In hospitals that conduct drug studies, a pharmacy technician often assists the investigational drug pharmacist by preparing and delivering study medications for patients who are enrolled in specific drug studies.

Compounding/Unit Dosing

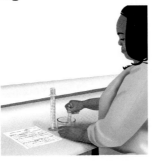

A pharmacy technician assigned to compounding is responsible for making medication formulations that are not available from a manufacturer. This is done by using specific recipes provided by the pharmacy. Duties also include reconstituting bottles of commercially available medications and drawing up unit-doses from bulk medication bottles.

Staff Development

The goal of staff development is to improve the knowledge and skills of pharmacy technicians by providing staff training materials, reading assignments, demonstrations, and written or practical tests. Other staff development opportunities may include discussion groups and seminars on topics pertaining to hospital pharmacy.

IV/Clean Room (IV admixtures)

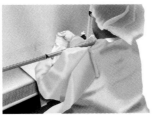

The main responsibility of the IV/clean room technician is to prepare intravenous medications for patients in the hospital. Special training is often required prior to working in the clean room. This role may also include preparation of chemotherapy and parenteral nutrition.

Inventory Control

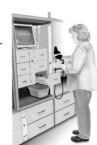

An inventory technician is responsible for maintaining the pharmacy stock. The duties include ordering medications and checking pharmacy invoices. Inventory technicians also assist in handling drug recalls, shortages and emergency drug procurement. In some hospitals, inventory technicians may also be responsible for filling automated dispensing cabinets in nursing and ancillary areas.

Pharmacy Technician Supervisor

This leadership role includes managing a team of hospital pharmacy technicians. The supervisor is often responsible for training technicians, creating work schedules, and completing annual evaluations for all technicians.

Satellite Pharmacies

Some hospitals have a main pharmacy along with smaller satellite pharmacies located in different areas of the hospital. Hospital pharmacy technicians need to complete more specific training to work in pharmacy satellites and may rotate through the different areas (e.g. pediatrics, oncology, operating room, etc).

Outpatient Pharmacy

The outpatient pharmacy technician assists the pharmacist in processing outpatient prescriptions for patients leaving the hospital or visiting their doctor.

Other Responsibilities

Complete other tasks or projects as assigned by supervising technician or pharmacist.

HOSPITAL PHARMACY AREAS

The *in-patient pharmacy* is the area of the hospital responsible for medication preparation and distribution.

Some hospitals may also have **pharmacy satellites** located in different areas of the hospital. A pharmacy satellite is a branch of the inpatient pharmacy dedicated to serving a particular group of hospitalized patients. Satellites are often located in the same area as the patient care units they are servicing (i.e., pediatrics, operating room). Satellites are responsible for providing first doses of new medications ordered, all emergency medications, and replacing any missing or lost doses. They have a limited supply of medications which are specific to the patient care areas they service. Satellite pharmacies may be open 24 hours a day or have limited hours (e.g. 7am–10pm).

In hospitals that have satellite pharmacies, the main in-patient pharmacy is called the *central pharmacy*.

The central pharmacy houses the bulk of the hospital's inventory of medications. The central pharmacy is generally responsible for preparation and delivery of unit-dose patient medication carts, **batching** of medications, and covers service areas not covered by pharmacy satellites. The central pharmacy also conducts a variety of packaging functions in order to keep other areas in the hospital supplied with the drugs they need.

In most hospitals, the central pharmacy is open 24 hours a day.

When a pharmacy satellite is closed, the central pharmacy will take over responsibility for servicing these areas as well.

The sterile product area or *clean room* is usually located in the central pharmacy.

Laminar flow hoods are located here since this is where the majority of intravenous medications are prepared.

USP 797

USP 797 is a set of regulations issued by the US Pharmacopoeia. These regulations must be followed by any pharmacy that prepares compounded sterile products. They

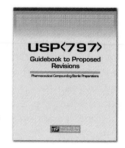

include a strict set of policies and practices for hospitals to use in sterile product preparation. The policies are intended to decrease infections transmitted to patients through drug preparation and better protect staff in their exposure to pharmaceuticals. All hospitals that are accredited by the Joint Commission of Health Care Organizations (JCAHO) must be compliant with USP 797 standards.

batching preparation of large quantities of unit-dose oral solutions/suspensions or small volume parenterals for future use.

clean room area designed for the preparation of sterile products.

in-patient pharmacy a pharmacy located in a hospital which services only those patients in the hospital and its ancillary areas.

pharmacy satellite a branch of the in-patient pharmacy responsible for preparing, dispensing, and monitoring medication for specific patient areas.

central pharmacy the main in-patient pharmacy in a hospital that has pharmacy satellites. It is the place where most of the hospital's medications are prepared and stored.

Many larger hospitals often have a separate drug information center with resources for answering drug-related questions. Other hospitals may set up a designated area in the pharmacy for drug references.

SOME PHARMACY SATELLITES

Pediatric satellite: Special considerations must be taken into account when dosing and preparing medications for pediatric patients. Pediatric doses are often individually calculated based on a patient's weight and frequently require special dilutions since they are much smaller doses than for adults. Pharmacists and pharmacy technicians in the pediatric satellite carefully review and monitor pediatric patient medications and prepare individualized doses of IV and oral medications.

Operating room (OR) satellite: The OR is a dynamic environment where it is difficult for physicians and nurses to track medications prepared and given to patients. Pharmacists and pharmacy technicians in an OR satellite help oversee and control drug distribution for all operating rooms, decrease controlled substance loss and waste, reduce inventory expenses, and improve documentation of patient medication charges.

Oncology satellite: Chemotherapy medications require special preparation and precautions since they can be toxic to the person preparing them if not managed appropriately. The oncology satellite reviews, prepares, and delivers antineoplastic agents (chemotherapy) for hospital patients. Pharmacy technicians in the oncology satellite require special training and chemotherapy certification from the pharmacy department.

 outpatient pharmacy a pharmacy attached to a hospital which services patients who have left the hospital or who are visiting doctors in a hospital outpatient clinic.

A centralized area for storage of drug product or "inventory" may also be a part of the pharmacy department.

In larger hospitals this area requires an entire staff of its own that deals only with the order and delivery of drug products for the other pharmacy areas. Technicians often make up a large portion of this staff and may be in charge of running the area.

A number of hospitals have an investigational drug service which is a specialized pharmacy subsection that deals solely with clinical drug trials.

These drug studies require a great deal of paperwork and special documentation of all doses of study medication. Technicians are frequently used in this area to assist the pharmacist with the large amount of documentation required and in preparing individual patient medication supplies and delivery. The investigational drug service may provide study drugs to both patients located in the hospital and those treated in outpatient clinics, but only patients who are enrolled in an investigational drug study or trial.

Quality assurance is another area in which pharmacy technicians are involved.

A pharmacy technician may be assigned to a specific area of the pharmacy to remove any outdated or "expired" medications. Another responsibility may be making sure refrigerators and freezers are maintained at correct temperatures and completing a daily log of temperatures. Pharmacy technicians may also be assigned to do unit inspections. A unit inspection is a review of a nursing unit to ensure compliance with hospital medication policies. This may include replacing expired medications, eliminating medications that should not be on the unit and citing the unit for not adhering to policies.

Doctor's offices or clinics along with an *outpatient pharmacy* are often located nearby hospitals.

These pharmacies provide prescription medications to patients visiting their doctor. They are run very similarly to a retail pharmacy, but hospital technicians may be required to staff in these areas in addition to their inpatient responsibilities. Although an outpatient pharmacy may be located within a hospital, it does not supply inpatient medications. It only provides medications for patients who have obtained prescriptions from their doctors at the clinic or upon leaving the hospital.

ORGANIZATION OF MEDICATIONS

In most hospital pharmacies, medications are organized according to a precise system.

First, medications are usually categorized and placed in defined areas of the pharmacy based on the specific route of administration such as intravenous, oral, ophthalmic, topical, etc. Intravenous medications may be further separated by vials, small volume parenterals and large volume parenterals. Oral drugs may be further divided into solid dosage forms (capsules, tablets) and liquids (suspensions, solutions) and placed in separate areas.

The second way medications are generally organized is in alphabetical order using the generic name of each drug.

This is different than most retail pharmacies which place drugs in order of brand name. Since both the generic and brand name may be on a medication label, it is important for the hospital pharmacy technician to have a good knowledge of brand vs. generic names. (See Chapter 18 for examples of common hospital drugs.)

Some medications require refrigeration or freezing.

It is imperative that the technician identify these items and promptly put them in the correct place so that the medications retain their stability. For example, most vaccines require refrigeration. If left at room temperature for too long, they may lose some of their effectiveness.

Narcotics and other controlled substances are often stored in a secure area of the pharmacy.

They may be stored in a locked cabinet or automated dispensing cabinet which requires a personal code and password. Some pharmacies will also have video surveillance of this area to decrease risk of diversion or mishandling of these medications. It is mandatory for hospital pharmacies to lock CII medications in a secure area. CIII-CV medications are stored according to each institution's policy. Other pharmacies choose to keep them all in a secure area.

EXTEMPORANEOUS COMPOUNDING

When required to prepare an extemporaneous oral compound, the pharmacy technician will need the recipe to follow in order to make the compound. All of the ingredients and supplies needed to make the drug solution should be collected and brought to the oral compounding area. Prior to preparing the medication, pharmacy technicians must first wash their hands and clean the surface to be used.

Once the medication is compounded, a record of the preparation and ingredients must be put in a **bulk compounding log**. Information must include a list of all the ingredients, amounts used, manufacturer, lot numbers and expiration dates of each specific ingredient. Also, the bulk bottle needs to be labeled with the name, concentration, lot number which will be specific to the hospital, expiration date, and initials of the pharmacist after he/she checks the preparation.

Examples of Refrigerated and Frozen Medications

Refrigerator: 2° to 8°C (36°–46°F)
➥ Alteplase (Activase®)
➥ Caspofungin (Cancidas®)
➥ Epoetin alfa (Epogen®, Procrit®)
➥ Filgrastim (Neupogen®)
➥ Fosphenytoin (Cerebyx®)
➥ Tobramycin for oral inhalation (Tobi®)
➥ Most vaccinations

Freezer: -10° to -20°C (Av -15°C, 5°F)
➥ Measles, Mumps, Rubella and Varicella combination vaccine (Proquad®)
➥ Varicella (chickenpox) vaccine (Varivax®)
➥ Zoster (shingles) vaccine (Zostavax®)

Most hospital pharmacies have an area for compounding oral solutions and suspensions.

In this area, bulk amounts of non-specific patient supplies are often compounded in advance for future needs of the hospitalized patients.

Some oral solutions and suspensions are available commercially, but need to be *reconstituted* prior to use.

These medications usually have a short stability (i.e., expire in 10–14 days) after they have been made. It is essential that the pharmacy technician labels the date of reconstitution and/or the date the reconstituted medication will expire, and places any other labels needed on the bottle (e.g., "Refrigerate," "Shake Well Before Using"). The pharmacist should then check the technician's procedure and initial the bottle. The technician can then draw specific doses of the medication in oral syringes or put the medication in the proper storage area.

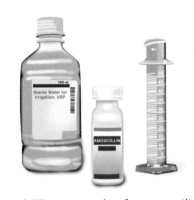

supplies gathered for preparation of an extemporaneous compound

If an oral medication is needed in liquid form but is not available commercially, it may be extemporaneously compounded.

"Recipes" or instructions on how to prepare **extemporaneous compounds** are usually stored in a binder or on a computer. The directions must be followed exactly since stability data is based on the precise preparation instructions that are listed. In the oral compounding area, the pharmacy technician should find the materials and ingredients commonly used in the preparation of extemporaneous compounds including mortar and pestles, calibrated measuring devices, and common ingredients (e.g., sterile water, simple syrup, glycerin).

amoxicillin suspension for reconstitution

bulk compounding log a record of medications that are compounded in the pharmacy for non-specific patients. Information must include a list of all the ingredients, amounts used, manufacturer, lot numbers and expiration dates of each specific ingredient.

reconstitute addition of water or other diluent to commercially made drug bottles or vials in order to make a solution or suspension from a pre-made powder form of the drug. This may include oral or parenteral products.

extemporaneous compounds medications which must be prepared following a specific recipe or formula, usually because they are not available commercially.

HOSPITAL FORMULARY

Because hospitals cannot afford to stock every medication that is available, many maintain a hospital *formulary*.

A **formulary** is a list of drugs that have been selected by health care professionals at the hospital based on therapeutic factors as well as cost. It is the responsibility of the Pharmacy and Therapeutics Committee to set up, add, remove and periodically evaluate medications listed on the hospital formulary. It is important, however, for anyone who orders, prepares, or dispenses medications to know the medications currently on the formulary.

A *"closed formulary"* means that the hospital carries only formulary medications and physicians must order from this list.

Of course, some exceptions apply and the pharmacy will have a section of "non-formulary" drugs. **Non-formulary** drugs may require a special form stating why the physician requires that specific medication. Since a non-formulary drug is not stocked by the pharmacy, there may be a delay in the patient receiving the drug. Once the non-formulary drug is approved by the pharmacist, the inventory technician must order the medication. Since it may take several days to arrive, it is important for the technician let the pharmacist know when the drug is scheduled to be delivered so the physician and patient can be made aware.

The Pharmacy and Therapeutics Committee (or "P&T Committee") consists of doctors, pharmacists, nurses, and other health care professionals.

They work as a team to review medications for the hospital formulary; evaluate medication use, adverse drug reactions, and drug-related errors in the hospital; and provide guidelines and protocols for medication use throughout the institution.

---

formulary a list of drugs stocked at the hospital which have been selected based on therapeutic factors as well as cost.

closed-formulary a type of formulary that requires physicians to order only those medications on the formulary list. (Some exceptions may apply.)

non-formulary drugs not on the formulary list which a physician can order; a physician may have to fill out a form stating why that specific medication is required.

COMMON HOSPITAL IV MEDICATIONS

Emergency Medications
➡ Adenosine (Adenocard®)
➡ Atropine (AtroPen®)
➡ Epinephrine (Adrenalin®, Epi-pen®)

Critical Care Medications
➡ Dopamine (generic)
➡ Dobutamine (Dobutrex®)
➡ Fentanyl (Sublimaze®)
➡ Fosphenytoin (Cerebyx®)
➡ Heparin (generic)
➡ Midazolam (Versed®)
➡ Milrinone (Primacor®)
➡ Nitroprusside (Nipride®, Nitropress®)
➡ Norepinephrine (Levophed®)
➡ Phenylephrine (Neo-synephrine®)
➡ Phenytoin (Dilantin®)
➡ Propofol (Diprivan®)
➡ Vecuronium (Nocuron®)

Intravenous Electrolytes
➡ Calcium gluconate
➡ Magnesium sulfate
➡ Potassium chloride
➡ Sodium phosphate

Intravenous Anti-infectives
➡ Acyclovir (Zovirax®)
➡ Ampicillin-sulbactam (Unasyn®)
➡ Cefazolin (Ancef®, Kefzol®)
➡ Ceftriaxone (Rocephin®)
➡ Clindamycin (Cleocin®)
➡ Fluconazole (Diflucan®)
➡ Ganciclovir (Cytovene®)
➡ Gentamicin (Geramycin®)
➡ Imipenem-cilastatin (Primaxin®)
➡ Metronidazole (Flagyl®)
➡ Piperacillin-sulbactam (Zosyn®)
➡ Vancomycin (Vancocin®)

THERAPEUTIC INTERCHANGE

sample therapeutic interchange protocol

Therapeutic Interchange Protocol
H-2 Receptor Antagonists

Background:
The purpose of this protocol is to optimize patient care while considering cost containment and cost-effectiveness. This protocol defines the equivalent doses of the H-2 Receptor Antagonists. This protocol has been approved by the Pharmacy and Therapeutics Committee (P&TC) and the Medical Executive Committee (MEC).

Statement:
The P&TC will establish which H-2 receptor antagonists will be on formulary. Pharmacists are permitted to convert orders according to the following protocol.

Protocol:
1) **Ranitidine (Zantac) is the <u>only</u> formulary agent.**
2) **Orders for nonformulary agents will be converted to the equivalent dose of ranitidine. The dosage regimens across each row are equivalent.**

Oral Conversion Table

Ranitidine (Zantac®)	Cimetidine (Tagamet®)	Famotidine (Pepcid®)	Nizatidine (Axid®)
150 mg PO BID	300 mg PO QID	20 mg PO BID	150 mg PO BID
150 mg PO BID	400 mg PO BID	20 mg PO BID	150 mg PO BID
150 mg PO BID	400 mg PO TID	20 mg PO BID	150 mg PO BID
300 mg PO HS	800 mg PO HS	40 mg PO HS	300 mg PO HS
150 mg PO QD	300 mg PO BID	20 mg PO QD	150 mg PO QD

Intravenous Conversion Table

Ranitidine (Zantac®)	Cimetidine (Tagamet®)	Famotidine (Pepcid®)
50 mg IV x 1	300 mg IV x 1	20 mg IV x 1
50 mg IV Q8H	300 mg IV Q6H	20 mg IV Q12H
50 mg IV Q12H	300 mg IV Q8H	20 mg IV Q24H
50 mg IV Q24H	300 mg IV Q12H	20 mg IV Q24H

*Nizatidine (Axid®) is not available IV.

Most hospital formularies include only a few medications in each specific class. This means that a patient who is admitted to the hospital may be taking a medication at home that is not included on the hospital formulary. In many of these cases there is another drug on the formulary that is in the same therapeutic class and works the same way but is a different drug entity (and usually of a different dose). The pharmacist is knowledgeable about therapeutic equivalence of drugs in the same class and can recommend the appropriate interchange for the doctor to order. Some hospitals have a formal therapeutic interchange program that allows the pharmacist to automatically change an order for a certain number of drugs without notifying the physician. In these cases a preset list of conditions must be fulfilled and the pharmacist must follow a strict protocol which includes entering into the computer an order for the formulary drug that was exchanged for the non-formulary drug.

UNIT DOSE SYSTEM

Oral medications are commonly provided to the nursing unit in medication carts containing 24 hour dosages for specific patients.

These carts have an individual drawer or tray for each patient on the nursing unit. Medications in the cart are packaged in individual containers holding the amount of drug required for one dose. This system is referred to as **unit dose** medication packaging. By preparing medication this way, nurses are not required to select medication from large bulk bottles, decreasing the chance of making an error.

Each individual drawer in a medication cart is filled daily to meet patient medication needs.

Technicians play a large role in this type of dispensing by either manually filling the carts or by operating equipment designed for that function. Computer generated drug profiles are prepared daily for each patient, and the appropriate amount of medications for the 24 hour period are placed manually or mechanically into each patient's tray. The trays are labeled with the patient's name and room number.

Some medications such as eye drops, creams and metered-dose inhalers cannot be divided into unit dose increments.

In these cases, the bulk item is filled only once and then used for the patient throughout the hospital admission.

Some nursing stations have automated dispensing systems that contain the most common unit-dose medications used in that patient care area.

This allows the nurse to obtain medication much more quickly. However, the nurse can access most of the medications only after a pharmacist reviews and verifies the order. A few emergency medications may be obtained without pharmacist verification, and this is governed by each hospital's policy.

The automated medication station may be used for the first dose of a new medication order or for all the doses during the length of the patient's stay in a hospital; hence, some hospitals do not have a 24 hour cart fill.

It is often the responsibility of the pharmacy technician to make sure these systems remain stocked.

PACKAGING

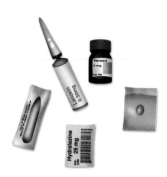

A number of different types of packages are used for unit dose medications.

Package Type	Used For
plastic blister	tablets/capsules
foil blister	tablets/capsules
packet	powder
tube	ointment/cream
foil/plastic cup	oral liquid
cartridge	syringe
vial	injection
ampule	injection
foil/plastic	suppository
IV syringe	injections
oral syringe	oral liquids

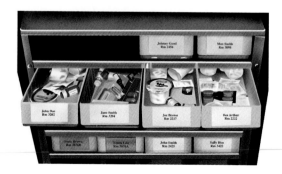

patient-specific trays

unit dose a package containing the amount of a drug required for one dose.

automated dispensing system a system in which medications are dispensed from an automated unit at the point of use.

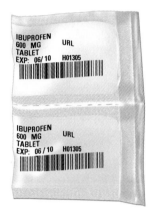

pre-pack label with bar code

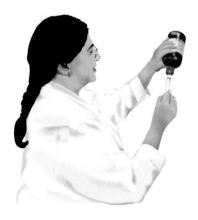

A technician prepares unit-doses of an oral solution.

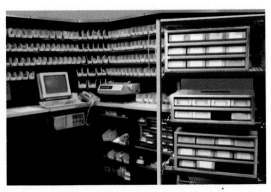

the cart filling area of a hospital pharmacy

Technicians often "pre-pack" medications that have been purchased in bulk into unit doses.

Many hospital pharmacies use machines to automate this process. The systems are generally used for pre-packing oral solid medications (tablets, capsules). They label each unit-dose package with the information required by the institution. The pharmacy technician is often responsible for keeping these machines stocked and for documenting all bulk bottles that are put into the system.

Separate technologies exist that can draw up oral unit dose syringes.

Otherwise, oral liquids need to be manually drawn into unit dose syringes and labeled by the technician. It is important for the pharmacy technician to always use "oral syringes" when drawing up oral liquids. Oral syringes differ from IV syringes because they are not able to accept a needle. This protects a patient from accidentally receiving an oral dosage form intravenously.

After a medication has been pre-packed, it is checked by a pharmacist.

Pharmacies keep documentation logs of pre-packed medications. The documentation logs have the medication name, manufacturer, dose, expiration date, lot number, and pharmacist's initials.

Unit dose labels may also contain bar codes for identification and control.

Bar-coded medications help to improve patient safety and can help with inventory management. Some computer systems require the nursing staff to scan a patient's arm band and then the medication before giving the medication to the patient. If the medication is not on the patient's profile, the computer will alarm.

Cart Filling Robots

Several machines referred to as robots have been developed to assist in the cart filling process. While this reduces the manual filling responsibilities of technicians, there is still a requirement for some medications, such as those stored in the refrigerator, to be hand filled. Additionally, there is a large amount of special packaging required to stock these robots, and technicians who would traditionally be hand filling trays often perform these duties. Cart-filling robots are very expensive and require a large amount of space within the pharmacy area; therefore, these machines are usually seen only in larger hospitals.

COMMUNICATION

In order to coordinate patient care, there must be communication between the various departments within the hospital.

Written and computer-generated medication orders are the routine method for letting the pharmacy know a medication is needed, but they are not the only ways pharmacy personnel interact with staff from other departments.

The pharmacy technician is often responsible for answering and directing phone calls.

When answering the phone, the technician should identify him/herself and use good etiquette. Any drug information questions that require the pharmacist's knowledge should be given to the pharmacist, but technicians should handle other phone calls related to their own job function.

Some information must be written or printed.

Fax machines and computer-generated print-outs are often used to quickly transmit written information such as drug orders from one area to another.

Some hospitals have advanced systems which allow for electronically transmitted communication.

Some systems can scan written medication orders into the computer system on the nursing unit and then transmit them as an electronic image to the pharmacy or other location. Computerized order entry systems allow medication orders to be put directly into the computer and transmitted to the pharmacy. They may also allow health care workers to send electronic messages to other areas of the hospital. For example, a nurse may send an electronic message to notify the pharmacy staff of a "missing medication," a new medication order that is needed right away, or that medication supplies that are low. The pharmacy technician is often responsible for checking these messages. In addition, electronic mail or "e-mail" has become an effective way of communicating information about new policies, medication recalls and shortages, changes in the formulary, or other administrative business.

pneumatic tube a system which shuttles objects through a tube using compressed air as the force.

PNEUMATIC TUBE SYSTEMS

A system that allows for the mechanical transfer of written communications and drugs is the **pneumatic tube**.

In the pneumatic tube system, medication orders and drugs are transferred via plastic capsules to and from stations in the pharmacy and other areas of the hospital. A destination is programmed into the tube station and in minutes the shuttle arrives at the desired location. Some limitations of the system are that it may not be used with unstable medications (e.g. albumin, insulin, IVIG), those that are too large for the tubes, and those restricted by hospital policy (e.g. narcotics).

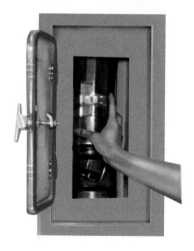
pneumatic tube and capsule

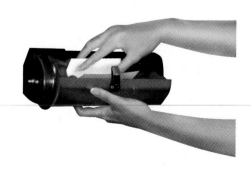
pneumatic capsule with document and medications

COMPUTER SYSTEMS

Most hospital information and documentation are computerized.

Information systems can integrate patient information, history of medications, laboratory data, general care of the patient, billing and many other types of information. However, each hospital system is customized to its own needs and therefore different. Individual systems may or may not integrate various areas of the hospital.

Hospital pharmacies rely heavily on computerized systems.

Knowledge of the hospital's pharmacy information system will be a large part of the initial training for a hospital pharmacy technician, since they must rely on it to perform many of their daily tasks including ordering pharmaceuticals, inventory control, and medication order processes.

An important responsibility for the pharmacist is to provide information on medications and their use to patients and other healthcare professionals.

Previously, much of this information was found in written form (e.g., Facts and Comparisons) or on disk. Newer hospital information systems link drug information directly with the pharmacy computer system allowing information on patients' specific medications to be viewed online. In addition, many drug references are available using a PDA (personal digital assistant), a small, hand-held electronic device that can store a large amount of information.

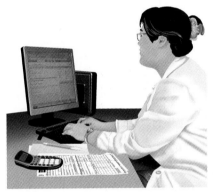

A technician using a hand held entry device for a computerized inventory system.

Among their many functions, hospital information systems provide the pharmacist with quick access to medication information.

Confidentiality and Security

The information contained on a hospital information system is *highly confidential.* In many cases (especially with patient information), it is illegal to give the information to anyone except those who are authorized to have it. As a result, access to the computer system is limited by password or other security measures. Passwords should never be shared and technicians should always sign off the system each time they leave the work station so no one else will have access to their sign-on.

The Health Insurance Portability and Accountability Act (HIPAA) is a federal privacy law enacted to safeguard a patient's protected information when it is spoken, written or transferred electronically. It includes regulations regarding privacy, confidentiality, assessing and releasing patient information, and complying with patients' rights. Technicians should never look at a patient's chart or computer profile unless specifically required to fulfill an assigned task. Likewise, technicians should not provide information to anyone unless specifically directed by the pharmacist.

MEDICAL RECORDS

Medical records or health records are detailed, chronological accounts of a patient's medical history and care. They provide information on the continuity of care which helps health care providers make the most appropriate, individualized decisions on the current care of a patient.

The medical record typically includes doctors' and other health care providers' notes.

It includes a detailed account of a patient's medical complaints and history, physical exams, current and past medications, laboratory results, diagnostic tests and procedures, and treatment plans. In a hospital setting, the medical record will also include daily progress notes and flow sheets which track the care of the patient while admitted to the hospital.

Medical records are traditionally compiled using paper charts and folders, but can also be created using paperless *electronic medical records (EMR)* or *electronic health records (EHR).*

Electronic medical records integrate patient medical records with billing as well as patient appointments and allow authorized health care providers to access a patient's medical information from any secure location. Most hospitals use a combination of both paper and electronic charts with some information located in a physical chart and other information stored in the computer record.

It is important for the pharmacy technician to know the components of a medical record since they may be asked to find information for the pharmacist.

It is just as important that a pharmacy technician views only the areas of the chart which are absolutely necessary; viewing other information would be breaking confidentiality rules set forth by HIPAA, and may lead to termination of their job.

electronic medical record (EMR) or electronic health record (EHR) a computerized patient medical record.

MILITARY TIME

Most hospitals use a 24-hour clock or "military time" to indicate when medications are due as well as when they expire. The day is divided into 24 hours: Midnight begins the clock at 00:00 and it goes until 23:59 before starting over.

12-hour clock	24-hour clock
Midnight	**00:00**
1 a.m.	01:00
2 a.m.	02:00
3 a.m.	03:00
4 a.m.	04:00
5 a.m.	05:00
6 a.m.	06:00
7 a.m.	07:00
8 a.m.	08:00
9 a.m.	09:00
10 a.m.	10:00
11 a.m.	11:00
Noon	**12:00**
1 p.m.	13:00
2 p.m.	14:00
3 p.m.	15:00
4 p.m.	16:00
5 p.m.	17:00
6 p.m.	18:00
7 p.m.	19:00
8 p.m.	20:00
9 p.m.	21:00
10 p.m.	22:00
11 p.m.	23:00

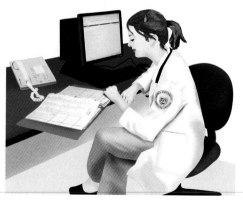

A physician reads a medical chart.

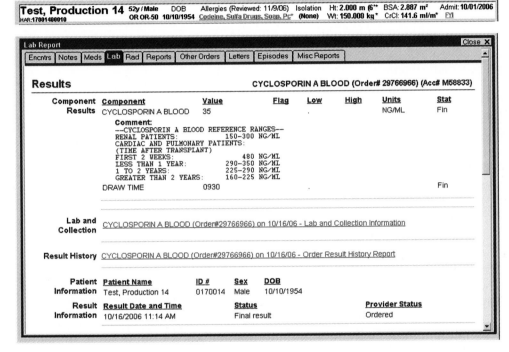

an example of an **electronic medical record**

A patient's medical chart and/or electronic medical record include many different sections:

➡ **Demographics:** personal identification information about the patient which is not medical. This includes the patient's phone numbers, addresses and emergency contact information but may also contain the patient's religion, race, occupation and insurance information.

➡ **Allergies:** list of drug and/or food allergies and the allergic response experienced (e.g., rash, anaphylaxis). NKA or NKDA are common abbreviations for "no known allergy" or "no known drug allergy."

➡ **Medical history:** list of present medical conditions or disease states as well as previous illnesses, surgeries, pregnancies, vaccinations, significant family and social history. A summary of prescription, over-the-counter and herbal medications taken at home may also be located here or in a separate section.

➡ **Medication orders:** orders written by a physician or agent of a physician for medication to be given to a patient. The order specifies the name of the drug, the dose, the route of administration, how often it is to be administered, and may include how long that order is to last.

➡ **Medication administration record:** a computerized or handwritten form that tracks the medications given to a patient, what time they were given, and who administered them.

➡ **Lab/test results:** Results for blood tests (e.g., blood sugar, drug levels), radiology exams (e.g., X-rays), microbiology (e.g., blood culture), and other specialized testing (e.g., biopsy).

➡ **Documentation flow sheet:** form filled out by nursing that tracks a patient's vitals on an hourly or scheduled basis, hourly rates of large volume IVs and medication drips, ventilator settings or other respiratory support, patient intake, urine output, pain scores, and other nursing notes.

➡ **Progress notes:** notes that detail the current progress of a patient and include any patient complaints, laboratory data, physical exam findings, overall assessment and plan for the patient. Usually written by physicians on a daily basis while the patient is in the hospital.

MEDICATION ORDERS

Several different professionals have the authority to write medication orders in the hospital setting.

The most obvious of these is the doctor. However, both nurses and pharmacists may write orders if they are directly instructed to do so by a doctor in person or over the telephone. These are referred to as verbal orders or telephone orders and must be co-signed by the physician who approved them. In some hospitals, specialized healthcare providers with advanced training can write orders without the signature of a physician. These people include physician's assistants and nurse practitioners.

In the hospital, all written orders for a patient are done so on a medication order form and not a prescription blank as seen in a community pharmacy.

Medication order forms are an all-purpose communication tool used by the various members of the healthcare team. Orders for various procedures, laboratory tests, and x-rays may be written on the form in addition to medication orders. Several medication orders may be written on one medication order form. These forms are traditionally prepared in duplicate or triplicate so that the original remains in the medical chart and only copies are sent to other areas of the hospital for processing.

An alternative to the traditional written order is computerized physician order entry (CPOE).

CPOE is a system in which the doctor or agent of the doctor enters orders directly into the hospital system. This helps to eliminate errors due to illegible handwriting and also expedites orders to the pharmacy, lab, radiology, etc. When a physician enters a medication order into the computer, a copy of the order is sent electronically to the pharmacy or generates a printout in the pharmacy for review by a pharmacist before the medication is dispensed.

There are several types of medication orders.

One is a standard medication order for patients to receive a certain drug at scheduled intervals throughout the day, sometimes called a **standing (or scheduled) order.** Orders for medications that are administered only on an as needed basis are called **PRN medication orders.** A third type of order is for a medication that is needed right away; these are referred to as **STAT orders.**

℞ Common abbreviations for medication orders can be found on pp. 77 and 86–87.

MEDICATION ORDER FORMS

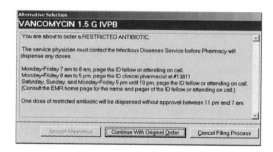

sample medication order form

Some medications are restricted and require approval from a specific hospital service before they can be dispensed from the pharmacy. (Copyright 1979–2010 Epic Systems Corporation. All rights reserved.)

ABCD *standing order* a standard medication order for patients to receive medication at scheduled intervals (e.g., 1 tablet every 8 hours).

PRN order an order for medication to be administered only on an as needed basis (e.g., 1 tablet every 4 to 6 hours as needed for pain).

STAT order an order for medication to be administered immediately.

MEDICATION ADMINISTRATION RECORDS

Nurses record and track medication orders using the **medication administration record (MAR)**. The MAR may be a written or computer generated form or may be electronic.

The MAR records every medication ordered for a patient over a 24 hour period, as well as the time the medications were administered and the person who gave each dose. Whether handwritten by the nursing staff or generated by the pharmacy computer system, the accuracy of this document is crucial.

In some hospitals, nurses may chart medications directly into the computer. Alternatively, the nurse may scan the medication bar code at the patients' bedside; this information will then be processed onto a computerized MAR.

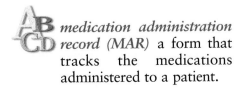

sample medication administration record

A **B** **C** **D** *medication administration record (MAR)* a form that tracks the medications administered to a patient.

O rder entry into a computer system may be performed by a unit clerk, pharmacy technician, pharmacist, nurse, or physician.

Before entering orders, technicians will require specialized training in the interpretation of medical orders as well as on how to use the pharmacy's computerized order-entry system. Each medication order must contain the medication name, dose, route and frequency. The order may also include the duration of therapy.

The technician must also be aware of any specialized protocols the hospital has in place such as "restricted" medications or automatic stop orders.

In order to ensure safety and appropriateness as well as contain costs, some medications may be restricted by certain services in the hospital (e.g., infectious diseases, hematology). Such restricted medications cannot be dispensed until the appropriate service approves the order. Other medications can only be ordered by a physician with a specialty in the area that the medication is used. For example, many hospitals will only allow an oncologist to order chemotherapy. Automatic stop orders are used for certain classes of medications, such as antibiotics or narcotics. These orders are active for only a limited period of time after which a new medication order is required to continue. Automatic stop orders help ensure that the patient's therapy is continually reassessed and monitored.

The hospital pharmacy technician plays an important role in assisting the pharmacist in making sure a medication and its dose are appropriate for each individual patient.

The pharmacist may ask the technician to get such information as weight, allergies or home medications from a patient's nurse or chart. The technician may also need to obtain laboratory or microbiology data from the hospital computer system.

The pharmacy technician may also screen medication orders for any that seem inappropriate.

For example, if a drug that is usually given once a day is ordered to be given four times a day, the technician should alert the pharmacist of the potential error. Although the pharmacist is required to review all orders before they are fully processed, the technician can serve as a valuable team member by flagging orders with potential problems.

ORDER PROCESSING

Once the medication order is approved by the pharmacist, the order needs to be filled.

There are several steps involved in this process.

1. Preparation: Since many medications look similar and the same drugs may come in several different doses, the technician must be vigilant in making sure the right medication and dose are being filled.

The technician should pay close attention to the following when preparing a medication for the final check by a pharmacist: drug, dosage form, concentration or strength, quantity, expiration date, base solution and volume.

2. Check: After the medication has been prepared, the technician must sign his/her initials on the medication label.

Some medications require special auxiliary labels (i.e., "Refrigeration," "High Risk Medication"), and should be affixed to the product by the pharmacy technician. Also, some intravenous medications (e.g., mannitol, phenytoin) require a **final filter** for the nursing staff to use upon administration. The pharmacy is usually responsible for providing the nursing staff with the filter.

In most states, medications are always required to be checked by a pharmacist before being sent to the nursing units.

However, nine states currently allows a process called tech-check-tech in hospital settings whereby a specially trained technician can check another technician's work before a medication is sent to the floor. Each state has specific training and auditing requirements in order for this process to occur.

3. Delivery: Delivery procedures vary depending on the hospital and the type of medication.

Medications may be delivered to patient care areas by pharmacy technicians, hospital delivery staff, or a pneumatic tube system. Often these deliveries, or rounds, are done on an hourly basis. While on rounds, the technician is often required to pick up medication returns and credit them to the patient.

℞ Controlled substances require someone to witness that the medication was received on the nursing unit. This can be done by using a paper or electronic signature log.

MANUAL ORDER PROCESSING

✔ Medication order is written in patient chart.

✔ Copy of medication order is removed from chart.

✔ Order is picked up at nursing station or faxed or tubed to the pharmacy.

✔ Medication order is entered into the pharmacy computer system.

✔ Pharmacist reviews and verifies medication order.

✔ Medication order is filled by a pharmacy technician and checked by pharmacist.

✔ Patient-specific medication is manually delivered or tubed to nursing unit.

AUTOMATED ORDER PROCESSING

✔ Physician or agent of the physician enters medication order directly into hospital computer system which automatically communicates order to the pharmacy.

✔ Pharmacist reviews and verifies medication order.

✔ RN retrieves medication from point-of-use automated medication station.

✔ Pharmacy technician fills inventory as medication supplies fall below par.

℞ Automated order processing may include only part of the above process. For instance, even though order processing may start with physician order entry directly into a computer, a hospital may not have point-of-use automated machines. In this case, the medication would still be manually delivered or tubed to the nursing station.

Missing doses: **Missing doses of medications for patients can be a challenge at hospitals.**

"Missing doses" refer to medications that should have already been delivered to the nursing unit but cannot be located. If a missing medication is requested, the technician should ask the following questions in order to ensure the patient receives the medication in a timely manner while minimizing duplication by the pharmacy staff:

➡ Is there a current order for the requested medication?

➡ Did the nurse check the correct area for the medication such as the refrigerator or automated dispensing cabinet?

➡ When was the medication last dispensed by pharmacy? (If a label was printed recently, the medication may still be in the pharmacy.)

➡ Was the patient transferred from a different unit in the hospital?

If the medication cannot be located, the technician should print another label and make sure the missing dose is sent to the nursing unit.

Drip Rounds: **Many hospitals have technicians perform drip rounds.**

This requires the pharmacy technician to go to specific nursing units (mainly intensive care units) and track what intravenous drips will be needed later that day. This may require the technician to communicate with the nursing staff to find out if an IV infusion (e.g., dopamine, fentanyl) will be discontinued, expire soon, or run out in a few hours. The purpose of drip rounds is to reduce the number of STAT medications and decrease the amount of work load on other pharmacy shifts.

final filter a device used to remove particulate matter. The filter should be placed at the end point of an IV line just before it enters a patient's vein.

drip rounds a process in which the pharmacy technician goes to specific nursing units to find out what IV drips will be needed later that day.

INVENTORY CONTROL

Another responsibility that may be assigned to the hospital pharmacy technician is inventory control.

Ensuring adequate supplies of medications are stocked throughout the hospital is the primary responsibility for staff in this area. This is especially important in the hospital setting where needing a medication may be a matter of life and death. Inventory duties may include ordering medication, storing medication in proper areas, checking the pharmacy order invoice, dealing with **drug recalls** and shortages, and **emergency drug procurement**.

The pharmacy inventory is usually ordered through a special computer program that communicates with the distributor/wholesaler.

One way the pharmacy technician knows what to order is by utilizing **par** levels for each drug product. "Par" is the quantity of drug that should be kept on the shelf. To make ordering inventory more accurate and cost-effective, many hospitals utilize bar coding technology for maintenance of the pharmacy inventory.

When a pharmacy shipment arrives, the pharmacy technician checks the order against the invoice.

If something is on the invoice but not in the shipment, the technician should notify his/her supervisor. When all items are accounted for, the technician places the medications in the appropriate location (e.g., refrigerator, overstock area, etc.).

A primary area of concern for inventory control is narcotics, or controlled substances.

Controlled substances require an exact record of the amount and location of every item, and must be ordered in a particular way according to state and federal laws. There are several systems for controlling narcotic inventory. Some are manual and others involve electronic equipment. Many hospitals require two people to count narcotic inventory before it is stored. Also, if a narcotic medication is damaged for any reason, two people must sign a form to witness the disposal.

 See Chapter 13 for more information on inventory systems.

INVENTORY

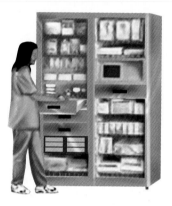

an automated Pyxis SupplyStation®

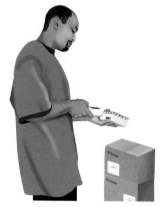

bar coding assists in inventory management

 drug recall the voluntary or involuntary removal of a drug product by the manufacturer. It usually only pertains to a particular shipment or lot number.

emergency drug procurement to quickly obtain a medication not currently in stock in the pharmacy in situations where the drug is urgently needed.

RESTRICTED DISTRIBUTION

Some medications have limitations on prescribing, dispensing, or distribution set forth by the FDA or manufacturer and require **restricted distribution**. Often, these requirements are due to safety concerns but may also be due to supply shortages.

The programs require the patient, doctor, and pharmacy to register with the company that makes the drug. They also often require the patient to follow a strict adherence to certain monitoring parameters such as pregnancy tests or specific blood tests. When a patient taking a restricted drug product is admitted to the hospital, the hospital pharmacy must call the company and make sure the patient is on the registry and in compliance with the monitoring parameters before dispensing the medication to the patient.

Examples of drugs which require restricted distribution include:

➡ Accutane® (isotretinoin)
➡ Thalomid® (thalidomide)
➡ Clozaril® (clozapine)
➡ Tikosyn® (dofetilide)
➡ Tracleer® (bosentan)
➡ Flolan® (epoprostenol)

Although there is usually a sufficient supply of drug products in the United States, shortages may occur due to problems in manufacturing, shortages of natural drug product, or discontinuation of one brand which may create a temporary shortage of another brand.

If not enough medication can be stocked, the inventory technician may have to go outside of their usual distributor. This may include using a secondary distributor, directly contacting the company that makes the drug product, or buying from a group purchasing organization. If it still is not possible to obtain enough drug product, the inventory technician notifies a pharmacist of the shortage and pharmacists work together in recommending alternatives to those medications. Sometimes, this alternative may not be on formulary. In these cases, the non-formulary drug will be stocked unrestricted until the formulary product is available again.

The pharmacy inventory staff is often responsible for removal of drug recalls from the pharmacy's inventory.

A drug may be recalled by the manufacturer for unknown reasons, or may be mandated by the FDA due to safety concerns.

Sometimes a medication that is not stocked by the pharmacy may be needed in an emergency.

In these cases the inventory technician may call other local hospitals to "borrow" a short-term supply of medication or the technician may be asked to order an emergency shipment from a wholesaler or drug manufacturer.

par amount of drug product that should be kept on the pharmacy shelf. Each drug product may have a different par value. Par levels may also be assigned to drug products in automated dispensing cabinets.

restricted distribution medications having limited availability due to cost, manufacturing problems, or safety concerns. Typically pharmacies must ensure enrollment before obtaining the restricted drug.

STERILE PRODUCTS

A large portion of the medication used in the hospital is administered intravenously.

The hospital pharmacy technician plays a large role in preparing these products. IV admixtures may include small and large volume parenterals, parenteral nutrition therapy, or chemotherapy. Preparation of these products requires special training and use of horizontal or vertical flow hoods. Most parenterals can be prepared in a horizontal hood. Chemotherapy and cytotoxic drugs, however, must be prepared in a biological safety cabinet or vertical flow hood which offers more protection.

There are several steps involved in preparing a parenteral medication correctly.

- The technician calculates the amount of drug needed to prepare the **IVPB**.
- The required equipment is gathered: medication vial, base solution bag, syringes, needles and alcohol swabs.
- Prior to preparation, hands should be washed, gloves and gown worn (if required), and laminar flow hood cleaned.
- The IVPB is prepared using proper aseptic technique to ensure sterility.
- A double check should always be completed: check for correct drug, concentration, volume, base solution and all calculations.
- The technician should write his initials on the label and add an expiration date and time prior to placing the label on the IVPB.
- Then the vial and syringes used in preparation are placed next to the IVPB for the pharmacist to check.
- All supplies used for product preparation should be disposed of in the proper bins as required by hospital pharmacy.

Advanced IV Preparation Technology

Robotics have been incorporated into some IV product preparation. Some products (e.g., IntelliFill™) utilize this technology to prepare patient specific small volume parenterals. Other robotics can fill patient specific IV syringes.

IVPB (intravenous piggyback) a small volume parenteral that will be added into or "piggybacked" into a large volume parenteral (LVP).

STERILE PRODUCTS

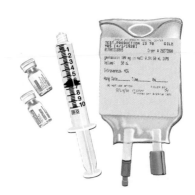

a small volume IVPB to be checked by a pharmacist

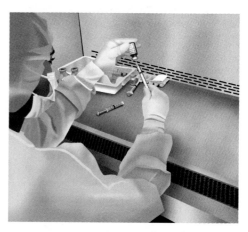

A pharmacy technician prepares IV products in a laminar flow hood.

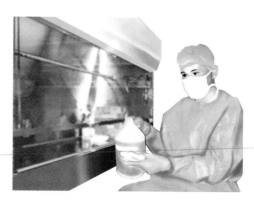

cleaning a vertical laminar flow hood

See Chapter 8 for more information on sterile techniques and preparing parenterals.

TPN PREPARATION

If a patient cannot eat or receive enteral feeds through an og or ng tube, he or she may need to receive nutrition intravenously. **Total parenteral nutrition (TPN)** contains protein, carbohydrates and essential nutrients to be given to the patient through an IV line. It may also contain fat-emulsion (3 in 1) or fat emulsion may be given separately (2 in 1). TPNs can be prepared by the inpatient pharmacy or can be outsourced to an outside facility for preparation.

TPNs are often prepared on a TPN compounder. The TPN compounder is a machine that pumps all the components of the TPN into a sterile empty bag. Often, pharmacy technicians are responsible for running the compounder.

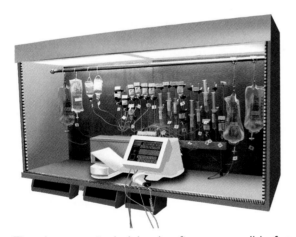

The pharmacy technician is often responsible for setting up the TPN compounder.

When selecting the medication vial to use for preparation of an IV product, it is important for the technician to pay attention to the type of vial.

Medication vials can be either single dose (one time use only) or multiple dose vials. Single dose vials are preservative-free but multi-dose vials contain preservatives that allow them to be drawn from multiple times. It is therefore important for the technician to visually inspect multi-dose vials for particulate matter prior to each use. Final preparation of medications should also be inspected for physical and chemical incompatibilities. Many medications are not compatible in certain solutions. For example, amphotericin B is an antifungal drug that is not compatible in sodium chloride solutions and will precipitate if mixed together. Other solutions may develop particulate matter for no known reason.

Some medications require special preparation.

Epidurals and intrathecal medications are to be administered into the epidural or intrathecal space of a patient's back (located near the spinal cord and backbone). Epidural and intrathecal medication cannot contain preservatives and must be sterile.

Certain IV medications have *short stability* or expire soon after preparation (e.g., sulfamethoxazole/trimethoprim, phenytoin).

Short stability medications are prepared right before the medication is due for the patient. Hospital IV rooms often have a box where they keep patient labels for medications with short stability. Often, it is the IV technician's responsibility to periodically check the short stability box and prepare the medications shortly before they are due.

Hospital pharmacies have policies in place for end product testing and validation.

The department will periodically take a sample of a prepared IVPB or LVP. The sample is sent to the laboratory and tested for contamination.

---

total parenteral nutrition (TPN) protein, carbohydrates and essential nutrients to be given to the patient through an IV line. It may also contain fat-emulsion (3 in 1).

epidural a sterile, preservative-free medication administered into a patient's epidural space (located near the spinal cord and backbone).

short stability medication that will expire soon after preparation (i.e., within 1–6 hours after preparation).

GENERAL HOSPITAL ISSUES

Hospital employees are required to meet some conditions of employment that may not be encountered in other pharmacy settings.

First, in addition to interviewing with the pharmacy department, prospective employees are usually required to interview with the Human Resources department. This department oversees the hiring process for the entire hospital.

All hospital employees are required to undergo a physical exam and often drug testing.

In addition, employees who may be exposed to blood products, which may or may not be the case for a pharmacy technician, are encouraged to receive the hepatitis B vaccination. Many hospitals provide this vaccine, as well as flu shots, free of charge to employees.

New employees are required to attend a hospital-wide orientation.

In this session, information is given about employee benefits, rules and regulations, and safety training for various situations such as fires, bomb threats, exposure to blood-borne pathogens, and chemical spills. This is in addition to the training that the pharmacy department provides.

Even if a technician has previous experience working in a hospital pharmacy he or she will go through training and a probationary period.

The probationary period gives the hospital time to assess whether the employee is actually suitable and qualified for the job. An employee may be terminated at any time during the probationary period. At the end of the probation, the employee's status may be changed to permanent, they may be terminated, or they may be placed on an additional three month probation.

All permanent employees receive an annual or semi-annual performance review.

Technicians are rated on technical skills and interpersonal skills, as well as issues such as tardiness, dress code, and ability to complete tasks on time.

REGULATORY AGENCIES

Several different regulatory bodies oversee all aspects of hospital operations including the pharmacy department.

➡ **The Joint Commission on Accreditation of Healthcare Organizations (JCAHO)**

JCAHO surveys and accredits healthcare organizations every 18 months to three years, laying out specific guidelines for every department within the hospital. Although this survey is not required, Medicare and several insurance providers require JCAHO accreditation for reimbursement.

➡ **Centers for Medicare and Medicaid Services (CMS)**

CMS inspects and approves hospitals to provide care for Medicaid patients. Approval by this organization is required to receive reimbursement for these patients.

➡ **The Department of Public Health (DPH)**

The DPH is a state run organization that oversees hospitals, including the pharmacy department, in order to assure compliance with hospital practice.

➡ **The State Board of Pharmacy (BOP)**

The BOP registers pharmacists and technicians. While they do not have the authority to govern hospital pharmacy departments, they do regulate the registration of the pharmacists and technicians that work there.

➡ **United States Pharmacopoeia (USP)**

The USP creates standards to assure the quality of medicines, dietary supplements and related products made available to the public.

➡ **Drug Enforcement Administration (DEA)**

A regulatory agency for controlled substances (CI–CV). The DEA ensures that hospitals follow controlled substances laws.

 code cart a locked cart of medications and other medical equipment designed for emergency use only.

SAFETY

All patient care areas are required to have **code carts** which are used in the case of a medical emergency on the floor.

These carts contain different medications and equipment commonly used in emergency situations. Each code cart has a special lock that can be broken when the cart needs to be used. Once a lock is broken, it cannot be reused and the medication drawer must be replaced. The pharmacy is responsible for maintaining these medication drawers. The technician refills the medication trays in the cart and charges the missing medications to the appropriate patient.

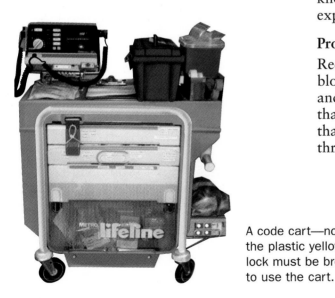

A code cart—note that the plastic yellow tie-lock must be broken to use the cart.

The Policy and Procedure Manual

All departments within the hospital are required to maintain a policy and procedures manual from regulating agencies. This document contains information about every aspect of the job from dress codes to disciplinary actions as well as step-by-step directions on how to perform various tasks. It is absolutely essential that technicians know what they must and must not do in their job, as outlined in their institution's policy and procedure manual.

During safety training employees learn "universal precautions" and how to handle hazardous substance spills.

Universal precautions are practices and guidelines that reduce the probability of exposure to bloodborne pathogens and explain what to do if an exposure occurs. These precautions include the use of protective barriers (gloves, gowns, masks, and protective eyewear) and how to prevent injuries from needlesticks. Even employees who may not have direct contact with blood products must be trained in universal precautions.

Some medications can be hazardous to healthcare personnel.

In cases of hazardous substance spills (e.g., cytotoxic drugs, harmful chemicals or drugs), special procedures are required which involve identifying the hazardous substance, containing the spill, and disposing of the waste. The Material Safety Data Sheets (MSDS) contain information regarding safe handling procedures, signs and symptoms of exposure, and exposure limits. The technician should know where the MSDS are located since these will explain how to proceed if a spill occurs.

Proper waste disposal is extremely important.

Red bags are usually used for items containing blood or other body linens. Soiled linen, scrubs, and items such as cleaning rags are cleaned rather than disposed in red bags. Needles or other items that may cut or puncture the skin should always be thrown away in designated "sharps" containers.

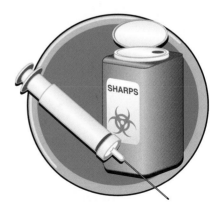

sharps container

CALCULATIONS

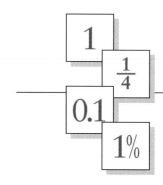

Many different types of calculations are performed by hospital pharmacy technicians on a daily basis. Some hospitals require technicians to pass a calculations test prior to completing their training.

EXAMPLE CALCULATION

When pharmacy technicians have to manually draw up unit-dose oral syringes, there are usually important calculations involved.

For example, a medication order reads: Gabapentin 300 mg ng tid

Question 1: How many mL(s) of drug should be drawn up per dose?

Answer: Gabapentin is available in a 50 mg/mL concentration. Calculate the volume needed:

$$300 \text{ mg} \div 50 \text{ mg/mL} = 6 \text{ mL} \qquad \textbf{OR} \qquad \text{solve for X:} \quad \frac{300 \text{ mg}}{X} = \frac{50 \text{ mg}}{1 \text{ mL}} \qquad X = 6 \text{ mL}$$

Question 2: How many syringes are needed for a 24 hour supply?

Answer: Since t.i.d. stands for three times daily, you would need 3 syringes.

FLOW RATE CALCULATIONS

It is important for the technician to be able to perform flow rate calculations. Calculating flow rates can help prevent errors, decrease pharmacy waste, and help keep IV drips from running out before a new one arrives.

Example Flow Rate Calculation

A medication order reads: Milrinone 0.75 mcg/kg/min; patient wt = 154 lbs. Milrinone is available as a pre-made IVPB with a concentration of 200 mcg/mL. Remember: 1kg = 2.2 lbs. (wt = 154 lbs = 70 kg).

Question: How long will a 100 mL vs. a 200 mL ready-to-use (RTU) IVPB last?

Step 1: Calculate rate in mL/hr:

$$\frac{0.75 \text{ mcg}}{\text{kg} \times \text{min}} \times 70 \text{ kg} \times \frac{60 \text{ min}}{1 \text{ hr}} \times \frac{1 \text{ mL}}{200 \text{ mcg}} = 15.75 \text{ mL / hr}$$

Step 2: Calculate how long the 100 mL vs. 200 mL bag will last:

100 mL IVPB   200 mL IVPB

$$\frac{100 \text{ mL}}{15.75 \text{ mL/hr}} = 6.3 \text{hrs} \qquad\qquad \frac{200 \text{ mL}}{15.75 \text{ mL/hr}} = 12.6 \text{ hrs}$$

Answer: In this case it may be more advantageous to use a 200 mL bag since that will need to be replaced only every 12 hours instead of every 6 hours.

SMALL VOLUME PARENTERALS

Several calculations are required when preparing small volume parenterals. If the calculations are not performed correctly, this could lead to an overdose (if too much is given) or underdose (if too little is given).

Example Calculation for a Small Volume Parenteral

Medication label reads: Cefazolin (Ancef®)   750 mg
in NaCl 0.9%   50 mL

Problem: Cefazolin is available as a 1 gram powder vial. The directions on the vial state to add 4.5 ml sterile water to give a final product of 1 gram/5 ml. Reconstitute vial as directed. Remember: 1 g = 1000 mg.

Step 1: Calculate the amount of mL's needed to make 750 mg:

First, set up the ratio:

$$\frac{750 \text{ mg}}{X} = \frac{1000 \text{ mg}}{5 \text{ mL}}$$

Second, solve for X:

$$X = 3.75 \text{ mL}$$

OR

First, figure out the concentration of drug per mL:

$$\frac{1000 \text{ mg}}{5 \text{ mL}} = 200 \text{ mg/mL}$$

Second, calculate mL's needed:

$$750 \text{ mg} \div 200 \text{ mg/mL} = 3.75 \text{ mL drug}$$

Step 2: Add 3.75 mL of the reconstituted drug to a 50 mL bag of NaCl 0.9%.

Step 3: Initial the medication label and write the expiration date/time.

TIMING OF MEDICATIONS

Technicians need to know how to calculate the timing of medications.

Example Calculation for Timing of Medications

A nurse calls at 4 pm (military time 16:00) regarding a missing dose of Gentamicin for a patient. The patient has an active medication order for Gentamicin 100 mg IV q 8H. The last dose was given at noon. IV batch deliveries are made daily at 06:00 and 18:00.

Question: How should the pharmacy technician handle this phone call?

Step 1: Check to see when the last dose was given: 12:00 (noon).

Step 2: Verify the dose interval: every 8 hours.

Step 3: Calculate when the next dose is due: 12:00 + 8 hrs = 20:00 (8 p.m.).

Answer: The medication is actually not missing since it is not due until 20:00 (8 p.m). The technician should let the nurse know that the medication will arrive with IV batch delivery at 18:00 (6 p.m.).

CALCULATIONS (cont'd)

DRIP RATE CALCULATION

While on drip rounds in the Pediatric ICU, a technician notices that a drip containing insulin 100 units in 100 mL and is running at 13.5 mL/hr. The technician thinks that this rate seems high. The patient is 12 years old and weighs 198 pounds. The technician knows that the usual dose of an insulin drip is between 0.05–0.2 units/kg/hr.

Question: What dose of insulin (in units/kg/hr) is the patient receiving?

Step 1: Convert the patient's weight from pounds to kg. (Remember: 1 kg = 2.2 pounds):

$$198 \text{ pounds } \times \frac{1 \text{ kg}}{2.2 \text{ pounds}} = 90 \text{ kg}$$

Step 2: Calculate how much the insulin drip is delivering in units/kg/hr:

$$\frac{13.5 \text{ mL}}{\text{hr}} \times \frac{100 \text{ units}}{100 \text{ mL}} = 13.5 \text{ units/hr} \div 90 \text{ kg} = 0.15 \text{ units/kg/hr}$$

After calculating the rate of infusion, the technician realizes the dose is within normal limits. (However, insulin is titrated based on glucose levels and they should be monitored closely).

INTRAVENOUS ORDER AND CALCULATIONS

The pharmacy receives a written order for "potassium chloride (KCl) 20 mEq IV rider over 3 hours" for a patient in the Cardiac Care Unit (CCU). It is part of the technician's job to type the order into the pharmacy computer system.

Question 1: How should the technician proceed?

Step 1: The technician should check the patient's potassium (K+) level so the pharmacist can evaluate if the order is appropriate.

Step 2: The technician must enter the order in the computer system with the dose of the drug AND the volume of the IV solution. The technician will be utilizing the potassium chloride solution that contains 0.4 mEq/mL. From this information, he can calculate how much fluid should be ordered:

First, set up the ratio:

$$\frac{20 \text{ mEq}}{X} = \frac{0.4 \text{ mEq}}{\text{mL}}$$

Second, solve for X:

$$X = 50 \text{ mL}$$

OR

Calculate the volume needed as follows:

$$20 \text{ mEq} \div 0.4 \text{ mEq/mL} = 50 \text{ mL}$$

Question 2: At what rate should the KCl rider be infused (in mL/hr)?

Answer: 50 mL ÷ 3 hours = 16.7 mL/hr

PERCENT CALCULATION

The IV technician receives an order for 500 mL of dextrose 12.5%. The pharmacy has a stock solution of dextrose 70% and sterile water to prepare the fluid. How many mL of dextrose 70% and how many mL of sterile water should the technician use to prepare the solution properly?

Step 1: Calculate the number of grams dextrose needed to prepare 500 ml of D12.5W (dextrose 12.5% in water). Remember: weight to volume % = grams/100ml (g/100ml):

$$\frac{12.5 \text{ g dextrose}}{100 \text{ mL}} = \frac{X}{500 \text{ mL}} \qquad X = 62.5 \text{ g dextrose}$$

Step 2: Calculate how many mL of dextrose 70% needed to give 62.5 g dextrose:

$$\frac{62.5 \text{ g dextrose}}{X} \quad x \quad \frac{70 \text{ g dextrose}}{100 \text{ mL}} \qquad X = 89.3 \text{ mL of D70W}$$

Step 3: Calculate the volume of sterile water needed. Remember: the total volume of solution will be 500 mL.

500 mL − 89.3 mL = 410.7 mL of sterile water

Step 4: Double check your calculations:

$$\frac{62.5 \text{ g dextrose}}{89.3 \text{ mL (D70W)} + 410.7 \text{ mL (Sterile Water)}} = \frac{62.5 \text{ g}}{500 \text{ mL}} = \frac{12.5 \text{ g}}{100 \text{ mL}} = 12.5\%$$

DILUTION CALCULATION

The pharmacy needs to prepare a furosemide IV dilution of 1 mg/mL. Furosemide is commercially available as 10 mg/mL. How many mL of drug is needed to prepare 20 mL of injection dilution at a concentration of 1 mg/mL? How many mL of diluent is needed?

Step 1: Calculate the amount of drug (in mg) needed for 20 mL of 1 mg/mL concentration:

$$\frac{X}{20 \text{ mL}} = \frac{1 \text{ mg}}{\text{mL}} \qquad X = 20 \qquad \text{OR} \qquad 20 \text{ mL} \div 1 \text{ mg/mL} = 20 \text{ mg}$$

Step 2: Calculate the volume (in mL) of the commercially available drug needed for 20 mg:

$$\frac{10 \text{ mg}}{\text{mL}} = \frac{20 \text{ mg}}{X} \qquad \text{OR} \qquad 20 \text{ mg} \div 10 \text{ mg/mL} = 2 \text{ mL}$$

Step 3: Subtract volume of drug from total volume to calculate diluent volume:

20 mL (total volume) − 2 mL (drug volume) = 18 mL diluent

So, to make 20 mL of this dilution, the technician would draw up 2 mL of commercially available furosemide and add it to 18 mL of diluent to make 20 mg/20 mL (which = 1 mg/mL).

REVIEW

KEY CONCEPTS

HOSPITAL PHARMACY

✔ Patient rooms are divided into groups called nursing units or patient care units; patients with similar problems are often located on the same unit.

HOSPITAL TECHNICIAN ROLES

✔ Hospital pharmacy technicians have many roles and responsibilities and are often cross-trained to work in different areas of the pharmacy.

HOSPITAL PHARMACY AREAS

✔ The in-patient pharmacy is responsible for medication preparation and distribution.

ORGANIZATION OF MEDICATIONS

✔ In hospital pharmacies, medications are organized in alphabetical order using generic names.

HOSPITAL FORMULARY

✔ Since hospitals cannot stock every medication available, most have a hospital formulary which is a list of medications the pharmacy keeps on its shelves and from which doctors can order.

UNIT DOSE SYSTEM

✔ In the hospital, medications are often packed in individual packets which contain the amount of medication needed for each individual dose, called a unit dose.

✔ When medications are packaged from multi-dose containers, the unit dose container must be labeled with the drug dose, manufacturer, lot or pharmacy number, and expiration date.

COMMUNICATION AND COMPUTER SYSTEMS

✔ There are several ways the pharmacy communicates with other areas of the hospital including telephones, fax machines, computerized printouts, pneumatic tubes, and in person.

MEDICAL RECORDS

✔ Medical records are detailed chronological accounts of a patient's medical history and care received. The medical record may be in the form of a paper chart or electronic system.

MEDICATION ORDERS

✔ In the hospital, all drugs ordered for a patient are written on a medication order form or are electronically entered through a computerized physician order entry (CPOE) system.

ORDER PROCESSING

✔ When preparing a medication, the technician must pay close attention to the drug name, dosage form, concentration or strength, quantity and expiration date; and for IV's, solution and volume.

INVENTORY CONTROL

✔ To assist in the process of ordering inventory, par levels are assigned to each drug. Par is the quantity of drug that should be kept on the pharmacy shelf or in automated dispensing systems.

STERILE PRODUCTS

✔ Technicians may be responsible for preparing small and large volume parenterals, parenteral nutrition therapy, and chemotherapy.

GENERAL HOSPITAL ISSUES

✔ Needles or other items that may cut or puncture the skin should always be thrown away in designated "sharps" containers.

HOSPITAL PHARMACY CALCULATIONS

✔ Hospital pharmacy technicians perform many calculations on a daily basis, all of which are critically important to a patient's health and safety. Some examples include calculations for preparing small volume parenterals, calculations for timing medications, and flow rate calculations.

SELF TEST

MATCH THE TERMS: I *the answer key begins on page 511*

1. automated dispensing system ____

2. batching ____

3. bulk compounding log ____

4. central pharmacy ____

5. clean room ____

6. closed formulary ____

7. code cart ____

8. drip rounds ____

9. drug recall ____

10. electronic medical record (EMR) ____

11. emergency drug procurement ____

12. epidural ____

13. extemporaneous compounds ____

14. final filter ____

15. formulary ____

16. in-patient pharmacy ____

17. intravenous piggyback (IVPB) ____

18. medication administration record ____

a. the process of quickly obtaining an out-of-stock medication in an urgent situation.

b. area designed for the preparation of sterile products.

c. voluntary or involuntary removal of a drug product by the manufacturer, usually pertaining to a particular shipment or lot number.

d. a system in which medications are dispensed from an automated unit at the point of use.

e. a list of drugs stocked at the hospital which have been selected based on therapeutic factors as well as cost.

f. a pharmacy located in a hospital that services only those patients in the hospital and its ancillary areas.

g. the main in-patient pharmacy in a hospital that has pharmacy satellites.

h. advance preparation of large quantities of unit-dose oral solutions/suspensions or small volume parenterals for future use.

i. a record of medications compounded in the pharmacy.

j. medications which must be prepared by following a specific recipe or formula, usually because they are not available commercially.

k. a type of formulary that requires physicians to order only the medications on the formulary list.

l. a computerized patient medical record; also known as an electronic health record (EHR).

m. a device placed at the end of an IV line that is used to remove particulate matter.

n. a process in which the pharmacy technician goes to specific nursing units to find out what IV drips will be needed later that day.

o. a small volume parenteral added into or "piggybacked" on to a large volume parenteral (LVP).

p. a sterile, preservative-free medication administered into a patient's epidural space (located near the spinal cord and backbone).

q. a locked cart of medications and other medical equipment for emergency use only.

r. a form that tracks the medications administered to a patient.

REVIEW

MATCH THE TERMS: II   *the answer key begins on page 511*

1. non-formulary drugs ____

2. outpatient pharmacy ____

3. par ____

4. pharmacy satellite ____

5. pneumatic tube ____

6. PRN order ____

7. reconstitute ____

8. restricted distribution ____

9. short stability ____

10. standing order ____

11. STAT order ____

12. total parenteral nutrition (TPN) ____

13. unit dose ____

a. medications having limited availability due to cost, manufacturing problems, or safety concerns.

b. the amount of a drug product that should be kept on the pharmacy shelf.

c. protein, carbohydrates and essential nutrients given to the patient through an IV line.

d. a branch of the in-patient pharmacy responsible for preparing, dispensing, and monitoring medications for specific patient areas.

e. a system that shuttles objects through a tube using compressed air as the force.

f. an order for medication to be administered only on an as-needed basis.

g. a hospital pharmacy that services patients who have left the hospital or who are visiting doctors in a hospital out patient clinic.

h. making a solution or suspension by adding water or other diluent to a pre-made powder form of a drug in a drug bottle or vial.

i. medication that will expire soon after preparation (i.e., within 1–6 hours after preparation).

j. an order to give medication to at scheduled intervals.

k. an order to administer medication immediately.

l. a package containing the amount of a drug required for one dose.

m. drugs not on the formulary list which a physician can special order; a physician may have to fill out a form stating why that specific medication is required.

CHOOSE THE BEST ANSWER   *the answer key begins on page 511*

1. The main responsibilities of a pharmacy technician may include all of the following EXCEPT:
   a. preparing medications orders.
   b. conducting unit inspections.
   c. administering medications to patients.
   d. monitoring patients drug therapy.

2. Which of the following health care workers is NOT allowed to prescribe medications for patients?
   a. MD
   b. NP
   c. DO
   d. PCT

3. A quality assurance pharmacy technician:
   a. transports medications from the pharmacy to patient care areas.
   b. prepares intravenous medications.
   c. conducts unit inspections.
   d. prepares extemporaneous compounds.

4. Hepatitis B Vaccine requires refrigeration. This means it must be kept between:
   a. 2 to 8 degrees Celsius.
   b. 8 to 15 degrees Celsius.
   c. 15 to 25 degrees Celsius.
   d. 25 to 30 degrees Celsius.

5. Automated dispensing systems
   a. contain unit dose medications.
   b. are often restocked by technicians.
   c. allow nurses to quickly obtain medications.
   d. all of the above

6. Bulk bottles used for extemporaneous oral compounding MUST be labeled with the name of drug, expiration date, and:
   a. concentration, lot number specific to the hospital, and pharmacist initials.
   b. concentration, lot numbers for all ingredients used in the preparation of the product, and pharmacist initials.
   c. manufacturer for all ingredients used in the preparation of the product, and pharmacy technician initials.
   d. manufacturer for all ingredients used in the preparation of the product, and pharmacist initials.

7. When the pharmacy technician pre-packs oral liquids the syringes MUST be:
   a. amber colored.
   b. at least 5 mL in volume.
   c. able to accept a needle.
   d. unable to accept a needle.

8. HIPAA is a federal law that protects a patient's private information when it is
   a. spoken.
   b. written.
   c. electronically transferred.
   d. all of the above

9. An IVPB is due at 2 p.m. What time would that be using military time?
   a. 0200
   b. 1200
   c. 1400
   d. 2000

10. In a medical chart, notes that detail the current progress of a patient are located in which section?
    a. documentation flow sheet
    b. demographics
    c. medication administration record
    d. progress notes

11. Which of the following allows a patient to receive medications "as needed"?
    a. STAT order
    b. standing order
    c. parenteral
    d. PRN order

12. Nurses track medication administration on a(an)
    a. PCU.
    b. PRN.
    c. STAT.
    d. MAR.

13. A medication order reads, "Ciprofloxacin 400 mg q 12 hours X 7 days." What essential information missing from this order?
    a. dose
    b. route
    c. drug interactions
    d. timing

REVIEW

14. When "restricted" medications are ordered, according to hospital policy they must be:
    a. prepared by the lead technician.
    b. dispensed by the pharmacist in charge.
    c. non-formulary medications.
    d. approved by the appropriate service before they can be dispensed.

15. When addressing a missing dose phone call, the technician should ask all of the following EXCEPT:
    a. Is there a current order for the medication?
    b. When was the medication last dispensed?
    c. Did the nurse check the correct area for the medication?
    d. Why was the medication ordered?

16. A single dose vial
    a. can be used for 30 days after opening.
    b. should never be used in a hospital.
    c. contains no preservative.
    d. must always be reconstituted.

17. An IV infusion order calls for dopamine 800 mg in 250 mL of D5W to be infused at 10 mcg/kg/min. The patient weighs 55 kg. What will the flow rate be in mL/hr?
    a. 0.2 mL/hr
    b. 10.3 mL/hr
    c. 22.7 mL/hr
    d. 105.6 mL/hr

18. If a patient's current rate of NaCl 0.9% is 125 mL/hr, how long will a 1 L bag last?
    a. 6 hours
    b. 8 hours
    c. 12 hours
    d. 24 hours

19. A medication order is received for milrinone 40 mg in 200 mL of D5W to be infused at 0.3 mcg/kg/min. The patient weighs 70 kg. What will the flow rate be in mL/hr?
    a. 6.3 ml/hr
    b. 0.1ml/hr
    c. 630ml/hr
    d. 5ml/hr

20. A medication order reads: lansoprazole 15 mg po bid. Lansoprazole 3 mg/mL is extemporaneously compounded to fill this order. How many milliliters of lansoprazole suspension are required for each dose?
    a. 3 mL
    b. 5 mL
    c. 10 mL
    d. 15 mL

21. A medication order reads: gentamicin 120 mg iv 8 hours. The last dose was given to the patient at 1600. When is the next dose due?
    a. 1400
    b. 1800
    c. 1200
    d. 0000

22. How many doses of amoxicillin 500 mg can be drawn up from a 250 mL bottle of amoxicillin 250 mg/5 mL oral suspension?
    a. 10
    b. 50
    c. 25
    d. 20

23. Ampicillin/Sulbactam (Unasyn®) 3 grams is reconstituted with 6.4 mL to give a final concentration of 375 mg/mL. How many mL are required to give a dose of 2 grams?
    a. 4.3 mL
    b. 5.3 mL
    c. 6.4 mL
    d. 7.5 mL

17

OTHER ENVIRONMENTS

LEARNING OBJECTIVES

At the completion of study, the student will:

➡ know what kind of prescriptions mail order pharmacy is most commonly used for.

➡ understand the importance of automated systems in mail order pharmacy.

➡ be aware of how state and federal laws apply to mail order pharmacy.

➡ understand how long-term care organizations typically handle pharmacy services.

➡ be aware of the different types of home infusion therapies and what rules govern preparing home infusion admixtures.

MAIL ORDER PHARMACY

Chain community pharmacies are the largest segment of the retail pharmacy market, but mail order pharmacy is the fastest growing.

A mail order pharmacy sends medications to patients through mail or other delivery services. They have staffs of pharmacists, registered nurses, and technicians and can offer all the services of a community pharmacy, including compounding.

Because mail order medications involve a delivery time of at least 24–48 hours, they are used in situations where the need for the medication is known in advance.

This is true of **chronic conditions** like diabetes, high blood pressure, or depression, where the need for medication can be predicted and the supply can be easily maintained by mail delivery. This type of medication is called a **maintenance medication,** because it is used to maintain the patient with a chronic condition. By comparison, if a patient has an **acute condition,** such as a sudden infection, they would go to their community pharmacy to obtain the prescribed medication immediately after diagnosis.

Because they use the mail, mail order pharmacies can serve broad geographic areas.

In the U.S., for example, they can provide services to all states. This means that they can operate at a high volume. In addition to high volume discounts, this provides mail order pharmacies with economies of scale. These and other factors allow them to sell their medications at lower costs than community pharmacies. For this reason, mail order pharmacies are increasingly popular with third party insurers, a major source of their growth.

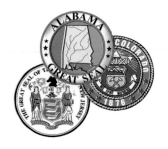

Regulation and Licensing

Though mail order pharmacies must follow federal and state requirements in processing prescriptions, they are not necessarily licensed in each state to which they send medications. As a condition for doing business there, some states now require that mail order pharmacies employ pharmacists licensed to practice in that state. However, not all do.

Online Drugstores

Online drugstores are a type of mail order pharmacy that use the Internet to advertise and take orders for drugs which are then mailed to the customer. Some online drugstores also use traditional mail order marketing methods and like mail order pharmacies they have a full staff of pharmacists, technicians and doctors employed to ensure proper filling of prescriptions as well as provide patient counseling regarding medications.

Drugs cost less in Canada and U.S. cross-border regulations allow Canadian pharmacies to fill individual prescriptions from U.S. consumers for small amounts of drugs. Because of this, the Canadian online drugstore industry has grown rapidly, and has been the subject of much consumer and political debate.

chronic condition a continuing condition that requires ongoing treatment for a prolonged period.

maintenance medication a medication that is required on a continuing basis for the treatment of a chronic condition.

acute condition a sudden condition requiring immediate treatment.

Automation and Quality Control

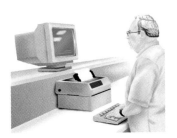

Mail order pharmacies are generally large scale operations that are highly automated. They use assembly line processing in which each step in the prescription fill process is completed or managed by a person who specializes in that step. For example, one technician may be responsible for entering prescriptions into the system, another for running an automated dispensing machine to fill prescriptions, and another for preparing the prescription for shipping. There are also steps for pharmacists to review the prescription before and after filling. Bar-coding of each prescription is used so that the prescription may be checked continually throughout the process against the information in the system. This ensures a high level of quality control. In fact, the increasing ability of automated systems to deliver a high quality product is one of the key contributing factors in the growth of mail order pharmacy.

Counseling and Information

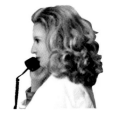

Mail order pharmacies have help desk or customer service numbers that patients can call when in need of counseling. Since calls may be related to medications, billing or other issues, these areas can be staffed with a mix of pharmacists, nurses, and technicians. As in the community pharmacy, technicians may not answer any questions related to medications, but of course can answer questions regarding forms, claims, and other non-medication issues.

Mail Order and Community Pharmacy

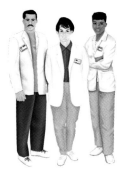

Much of the growth of mail order pharmacy has come at the expense of community pharmacy, which has historically served all patients, including those with chronic conditions. The large scale and sophistication of mail order pharmacies gives them many advantages (price being an extremely important one) which will undoubtedly help them to continue growing. At the same time, the personal availability of the pharmacist and the face-to-face interaction between pharmacist and patient in the community pharmacy are advantages that are likely to ensure the continuation of their vital role in the health of their communities. Both areas offer excellent career opportunities to pharmacy technicians.

LONG-TERM CARE

Long-term care facilities provide care for people unable to care for themselves because of mental or physical impairment.

Patients may be of any age and include chronically ill elderly, impaired children, and permanently disabled adults whose families can no longer care for their needs. Nursing homes make up the majority of long-term care facilities, but others include psychiatric institutions, chronic disease and rehabilitation facilities. The amount of time a patient may need long-term care can extend from months to years or even a lifetime.

Because of limited resources, most long-term care facilities will contract out dispensing and clinical pharmacy services.

This means that they will pay for another company to take care of the majority of patient medicines. The licensed professional pharmacy or practice that provides medications and/or clinical services to long-term care facilities and their residents is called a long-term care pharmacy organization. Although a pharmacist or pharmacy technician does not have to physically be present at the facility during all hours, pharmacy services must be made available 24 hours a day (i.e., by phone pager).

Pharmacists perform two types of functions for long-term care: distributive and consultant.

The **distributive pharmacist** is responsible for making sure the patients are receiving the correct medicines that were ordered. This job is mainly done outside of the long-term care facility itself.

The *consultant pharmacist* is responsible for developing and maintaining an individualized pharmaceutical plan for every long-term care resident.

This is done by reviewing patient charts, assessing how a patient may receive optimal benefits from their medicines, and monitoring for drug-related problems. They interact with doctors, nurses, and other health professionals. An individual consultant pharmacist is usually responsible for several different nursing homes or other facilities and so may only visit each on certain weekly or monthly intervals. It is important to make the distinction between these types of responsibilities because the pharmacy technician working for a long-term care pharmacy organization may be assisting in these different tasks.

ENVIRONMENT

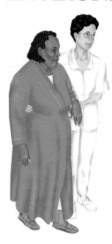

Nursing Homes

Most long-term care facilities are nursing homes that provide daily nursing care. Patients in this setting are generally referred to as residents.

Residents' Rights

Because residents of nursing homes were often victimized by people who were supposed to provide their care, federal and state laws were enacted in the U.S. designed to ensure residents' basic quality of life. These laws guarantee residents' rights to the following:

➡ safe and adequate care in a decent environment.
➡ privacy and confidentiality.
➡ personal property and clothing.
➡ personal privacy.
➡ freedom from abuse.

distributive pharmacist makes sure long-term care patients receive the correct medications ordered.

consultant pharmacist develops and maintains an individual pharmaceutical plan for each long-term care patient.

Training

The orientation process at a long-term care pharmacy organization is comparable to the hospital setting. There is an initial orientation and training regarding performance of assigned functions and special requirements in the long-term care setting. Also, there is a written job description of the functions the pharmacy technicians may perform in accordance with specific regulations in the state. It is important to be aware of what the pharmacy technician is able to do or not do according to the law.

Changing Responsibilities

In addition to typical duties such as preparing, packaging, stocking, and delivering medications, new opportunities are emerging for pharmacy technicians in the long-term care environment. These include working closer with the consultant pharmacist to assist in the collection of data for patient assessment, compiling quality improvement data, maintaining computerized information between dispensing and consultant pharmacists, performing reviews of drug use in individual long-term care facilities, and preparing pharmacy reports.

Automated Dispensing Systems

When a medication is needed suddenly, the time it takes for delivery from an outside supplier can present problems. Because of this, many nursing homes are turning to point-of-use automated dispensing systems. The medication order is communicated by computer to a central pharmacy system which then sends a confirmation of the order to the unit at the point of use. As soon as the unit receives this confirmation, a nurse can get the medication from the unit.

Many of the duties of pharmacy technicians in the long-term care pharmacy organization are similar to those in the hospital.

These include filling medication carts, packaging prescriptions, mixing intravenous solutions, ordering medication stock, maintaining **automated dispensing systems** and emergency medication carts, and crediting returned medications. As in the hospital environment, the technician works under supervision of the pharmacist and must understand the limitations set forth by law.

In some facilities, the medication cart may be filled with enough medications to last for a week.

This is different from the hospital setting as there is much less medication and patients' drug therapies are not changed as frequently. However, if a patient receives a new medication order, there must be a system in place to make sure the appropriate drugs are received. To handle this, the pharmacy organization in charge of the facility may make arrangements with an alternative pharmacy or use an automated dispensing system. Copies of new medication orders may be faxed to an alternative pharmacy that will deliver the appropriate drugs. Some facilities may have a limited drug inventory stored in a secured location where only authorized personnel may obtain access, and pharmacy technicians may be required to keep track of inventory in these locations.

Emergency kits, or code carts, similar to those in hospitals are also located in long-term care facilities for emergency situations.

As in hospitals, if these emergency kits are opened, the appropriate patient must be charged for the medications used and the cart must be refilled. The technician is responsible for these duties and the pharmacist makes a final check before the cart is resealed. A pharmacy technician working with the pharmacist may also be responsible for the inventory of controlled substances stored in the long-term care facility.

automated dispensing system a system in which medications are dispensed from an automated unit at the point of use upon confirmation of an order communicated by computer from a central system.

HOME INFUSION

Home care provides health care in a patient's home that might otherwise be provided in an institutional setting or physician's office. The primary providers of such care are home care agencies. Care is supervised by a registered nurse who works with a physician, pharmacist, and others to administer a care plan that involves the patient or another care giver. The primary advantage of home care over institutional care is a better quality of life, though in many cases it may also be less expensive.

The fastest growing area of home health care is home infusion.

Advances in infusion pump technology have made the infusion process more accurate and easier to administer and have been a major factor in the growth of home infusion. Pumps are available for specific therapies or multiple therapies. There are ambulatory pumps that can be worn by patients and allow freedom of movement compared to being restricted to an infusion pump attached to an administration pole.

Pumps are chosen for therapy based on various factors.

These include the type of therapy or therapies, the ambulatory status of the patient, the involvement of care givers, and so on. The supervising nurse and the pharmacist consult on the patient's care plan and choose the appropriate pump.

One of the fundamental activities of home care is patient education.

That is, the patient is educated about their therapy: how to self-administer, monitor, report problems, and so on. The supervising nurse is the primary person responsible for personally educating the patient or their care giver about therapy. However, the pharmacist is responsible for providing medication information to the supervising nurse and the patient or care giver. Patients or care givers are generally required by law to sign a form indicating that they have received the appropriate information.

Primary Providers

The primary providers of home infusion services are:

➡ **Home Care Agencies:** These are essentially home nursing care businesses that provide a range of home health care services, which can include infusion.

➡ **Home Infusion Pharmacies:** These are specialized pharmacies that prepare admixtures, provide infusion pumps, and are involved in various aspects of the patient's care plan.

➡ **Hospitals:** Many hospitals offer home infusion therapies as a way to ensure continued therapy outside the hospital after patients are released.

Primary Home Infusion Therapies

The primary therapies provided by home infusion services are:

➡ **Antibiotic Therapy:** Antibiotic therapy is a common home infusion service used in treating AIDS related and other infections.

➡ **Parenteral Nutrition:** Parenteral nutrition is often required for patients with various intestinal disorders or AIDS.

➡ **Pain Management:** This generally applies to the infusion of narcotics for patients with painful terminal illnesses or other types of severe chronic pain.

➡ **Chemotherapy:** In certain situations, chemotherapy is provided in the home, generally in conjunction with an oncology program at a hospital or clinic.

home care agencies home nursing care businesses that provide a range of health care services, including infusion.

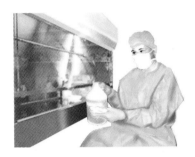

Compounding

The same rules apply to preparing parenteral admixtures in the home infusion setting as in the hospital. Compounding such admixtures requires the use of clean rooms, special equipment such as laminar flow hoods, and the use of aseptic practices. As with other parenteral admixtures, stability of the admixture for its intended use is a primary issue and storage a major concern. A complicating factor is that storage cannot be monitored as closely in a patient's home as an institutional setting. This results in short stability time limits that along with storage conditions require special attention. It also sometimes results in the on site preparation of certain therapies by the patient or care giver. In addition, automated devices that mix parenteral nutrition formulations at the time of administration are sometimes used.

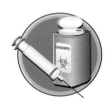

Hazardous Waste

Chemotherapy, the treatment of AIDS patients, and other infusion therapies involve the transportation, storage, and disposal of hazardous materials and is a primary area of concern. Home infusion personnel, patients and care givers must comply with all regulations governing such material. Compliance is a fundamental responsibility of home infusion personnel and is monitored by various regulatory agencies.

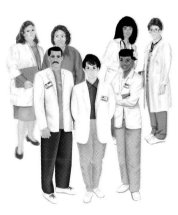

Home Care Team

The team that provides home health care includes the following:

Physician: The patient's physician orders the infusion therapy.

Registered Nurse: The nurse is responsible for coordinating and monitoring the care plan and the home care team, and for educating the patient.

Pharmacist: The pharmacist works with the supervising nurse to develop a pharmaceutical care plan which includes selection of the infusion device, identification of potential adverse reactions and interventions, and monitoring practices.

Pharmacy Technician: The technician works under the pharmacist's supervision and may be involved with compounding, labeling, delivery, and other non-consulting activities.

Home Care Aide: Aides are non-professional staff employed by the home care agency who work under the supervision of the registered nurse. They assist in various aspects of a patient's care, but generally not in medication therapy.

REVIEW

KEY CONCEPTS

MAIL ORDER PHARMACY

✔ Mail order pharmacy is used for maintenance therapy for such chronic conditions as depression, gastrointestinal disorders, heart disease, hypertension, and diabetes.

✔ Mail order pharmacies must follow federal and state requirements in processing prescriptions, but are not necessarily licensed in each state to which they send medications.

✔ Mail order pharmacies are generally large scale operations that are highly automated.

✔ Pharmacists review mail order prescriptions before and after filling.

LONG-TERM CARE

✔ Because of limited resources, most long-term care facilities will contract out dispensing and clinical pharmacy services.

HOME INFUSION

✔ Home care is supervised by a registered nurse who works with a physician, pharmacist, and others to administer a care plan that involves the patient or another care giver.

✔ The fastest growing area of home health care is home infusion.

✔ Infusion pumps are available for specific therapies or multiple therapies, and include ambulatory pumps that can be worn by patients.

✔ In home infusion, the patient or their care giver is educated about their therapy: how to self administer, monitor, report problems, and so on.

✔ The primary therapies provided by home infusion services are: antibiotic therapy, parenteral nutrition, pain management, and chemotherapy.

✔ The same rules apply to preparing parenteral admixtures in the home setting as in the hospital.

SELF TEST

the answer key begins on page 511

MATCH THE TERMS

1. acute condition ____

2. antibiotic therapy ____

3. automated dispensing system ____

4. chronic condition ____

5. consultant pharmacist ____

6. distributive pharmacist ___

7. home care agencies ____

8. maintenance medication __

a. a continuing condition that requires ongoing treatment for a prolonged period.

b. develops and maintains an individual pharmaceutical plan for each long-term care patient.

c. a medication that is required on a continuing basis for the treatment of a chronic condition.

d. a sudden condition requiring immediate treatment.

e. a common home infusion service used in treating AIDS related and other infections.

f. businesses that provide a range of home nursing care services, including infusion.

g. makes sure long-term care patients receive the correct medications ordered.

h. a system in which medications are dispensed from an automated unit at the point of use upon confirmation of an order communicated by computer from a central system.

the answer key begins on page 511

CHOOSE THE BEST ANSWER

1. Mail order pharmacies are used for maintenance medications, for chronic conditions. Which of the following conditions would NOT be likely to require maintenance medication?
   a. root canal
   b. HIV/AIDS
   c. depression
   d. hypertension

2. The delivery time for mail order medications is at least
   a. 24 to 48 hours.
   b. 2 weeks.
   c. 4 weeks.
   d. 6 weeks.

3. A sudden condition requiring immediate treatment is a(an)
   a. chronic condition.
   b. PRN condition.
   c. acute condition.
   d. maintenance condition.

4. A continuing condition that requires ongoing treatment for a prolonged period is called a(an)
   a. chronic condition.
   b. acute condition.
   c. infectious condition.
   d. maintenance condition.

5. Mail order pharmacies must follow _____ requirements.
   a. only state
   b. federal and state
   c. international
   d. only federal

6. The type of order processing used by mail order pharmacies in which each step in the prescription fill process is completed or managed by a person who specializes in that step is called
   a. extemporaneous processing.
   b. assembly line processing.
   c. bin fill processing.
   d. automated processing.

7. The fastest growing area of home health care is
   a. CCU.
   b. ICU.
   c. home infusion.
   d. ambulatory care.

8. Home infusion pharmacies are involved in
   a. dispensing unit doses of tablets and capsules.
   b. providing maintenance medications.
   c. mail order pharmacy.
   d. preparing admixtures and providing infusion pumps.

9. Many hospitals offer home infusion services.
   a. True
   b. False

10. The type of infusion therapy used to treat infections is called
    a. antibiotic therapy
    b. PO
    c. admixture therapy
    d. TPNs

11. The type of infusion therapy associated with patients with digestive disorders or AIDS is called
    a. admixture therapy.
    b. PO.
    c. NPO.
    d. parenteral nutrition therapy.

REVIEW

12. The type of infusion therapy generally associated with an oncology program at a hospital or clinic is called
    a. chemotherapy.
    b. antibiotic therapy.
    c. PO.
    d. NPO.

13. Compounding parenteral admixtures for home infusion requires all of the following EXCEPT:
    a. aseptic practices.
    b. laminar flow hoods.
    c. ointment tiles.
    d. use of clean rooms.

14. Which member of the home care team orders the infusion therapy?
    a. R.Ph.
    b. physician
    c. Pharm.D.
    d. pharmacy technician

15. Which member of the home care team coordinates and monitors the care plan?
    a. home care aide
    b. registered nurse
    c. R.Ph.
    d. Pharm.D.

16. Which member of the home care team works with the supervising nurse to select the appropriate infusion device?
    a. home care aide
    b. physician
    c. pharmacy technician
    d. pharmacist

17. Which member of the home care team may be involved with compounding, labeling, delivery, and other non-consulting activities?
    a. R.Ph.
    b. home care aide
    c. pharmacy technician
    d. Pharm.D.

18. Which member of the home care team works under the supervision of the registered nurse?
    a. home care aide
    b. pharmacy technician
    c. R.Ph.
    d. Pharm.D.

19. Which member of the home care team is not involved in medication therapy?
    a. pharmacy technician
    b. nurse
    c. home care aide
    d. physician

20. The person who develops and maintains an individual pharmaceutical plan for each patient in a long-term care facility is a
    a. consultant pharmacist.
    b. community pharmacist.
    c. distributive pharmacist.
    d. pharmacy technician.

COMMON DRUGS & THEIR USES

DRUG NAMES & CLASSES

When a drug compound is first synthesized or isolated, it is known by its atomic composition: the types and numbers of atoms contained in it. For example, the compound $C_{14}H_{19}Cl_2NO_2$ has 14 carbon atoms, 19 hydrogen atoms, 2 chlorine atoms, 1 nitrogen atom, and 2 oxygen atoms. Besides being awkward to pronounce, this kind of identification does not really describe the structure of the molecule.

A drug's name begins with a chemical name that describes its structure and its components.

These names identify a specific compound, but they are long and complicated and not useful for general communication. As a result, highly specific chemical names are shortened to less descriptive but more easily pronounceable ones.

While a potential drug is under development, the developer gives it a code number or a "suggested nonproprietary name."

Once a suggested nonproprietary name is officially approved, it becomes the generic name of the drug compound. Many pharmaceutical companies will assign code numbers to their compounds in the earliest development stages, and then a suggested nonproprietary name if the compound shows promise of being effective as a drug. At that point, the sponsor will apply for a proprietary or trademark name from both the U.S. Patent Office and foreign agencies. If approved, the proprietary name will have the ® symbol next to it when used in interstate commerce.

When a drug is under patent protection, it has one nonproprietary name and one proprietary or brand name, but the proprietary name belongs to the sponsor.

When a drug goes off-patent, other companies may market the same compound under their own brand names. For example, amoxicillin is a generic drug that has been off patent for many years. It is available as Amoxil® and Trimox®. Both Amoxil® and Trimox® are brand names used by different companies. But Viagra® (which has the generic name sildenafil) is available only under one brand name because the compound is still under patent protection. The point to remember is that there is only one nonproprietary (generic) name for a drug, but it may be sold under many different brand names once its patent protection has expired.

WHAT'S IN A NAME

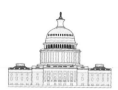

USAN

The United States Adopted Names Council (USAN) designates nonproprietary names for drugs. This council was organized in the early 1960s at the joint recommendation of the American Medical Association and the United States Pharmacopeia (USP) Convention. Other organizations, the American Pharmaceutical Association (now the American Pharmacists Association) and the FDA, were included in the Council during the latter part of the 1960s. There are publications that list "official" nonproprietary and proprietary names, as well as drug code designations, empirical names, chemical names, and show the molecular structures. The USP Dictionary of USAN and International Drug Names is such a reference.

Applying for a Name

To apply for a name, the sponsoring company initiates a request for a name. The USAN and the sponsor will arrive at a "Proposed USAN" that is suitable to both. This proposed name is then submitted for consideration to US and foreign drug regulatory agencies. When approved by these different agencies, the name becomes the "official" name of the drug. The USAN guidelines for the recommendation of names include that the name should:

➡ be short and distinctive in sound and spelling and not be such that it is easily confused with existing names;

➡ indicate the general pharmacological or therapeutic class into which the substance falls or the general chemical nature of the substance if the latter is associated with the specific pharmacological activity;

➡ and embody the syllable or syllables characteristic of a related group of compounds.

STEMS & CLASSES

Following are the USAN approved stems and the drug classes associated with them.

Stem	Drug Class
-alol	Combined alpha and beta blockers
-andr-	Androgens
-anserin	Serotonin 5-HT$_2$ receptor antagonists
-arabine	Antineoplastics (arabinofuranosyl derivatives)
-ase	Enzymes
-azepam	Antianxiety agents (diazepam type)
-azosin	Antihypertensives (prazosin type)
-bactam	Beta-lactamase inhibitors
-bamate	Tranquilizers/antiepileptics
-barb	Barbituric acid derivatives
-butazone	Anti-inflammatory analgesics (phenylbutazone type)
-caine	Local anesthetics
-cef	Cephalosporins
-cillin	Penicillins
-conazole	Anti-fungals (miconazole type)
-cort-	Cortisone derivatives
-curium	Neuromuscular blocking agents
-cycline	Antibiotics (tetracycline type)
-dralazine	Antihypertensives (hydrazine-phthalazines)
-erg-	Ergot alkaloid derivatives
estr-	Estrogens
-fibrate	Antihyperlipidemics
-flurane	Inhalation anesthetics
-gest-	Progestins
-irudin	Anticoagulants (hirudin type)
-leukin	Interleukin-2 derivatives
-lukast	Leukotriene antagonists
-mab	Monoclonal antibodies
-mantadine	Antivirals
-monam	Monobactam antibiotics
-mustine	Antineoplastics
-mycin	Antibiotics
-olol	Beta-blockers (propranolol type)
-olone	Steroids
-oxacin	Antibiotics (quinolone derivatives)
-pamide	Diuretics (sulfamoylbenzoic acid derivatives)

Drug classes are group names for drugs that have similar activities or are used for the same type of diseases and disorders. The assignment of a drug to a drug class is proposed when the sponsor makes an application to the USAN Council for an adopted name. The USAN Council and the sponsor then agree to a pharmacological or therapeutic classification. Unlike the generic and brand names, this classification is not an "official" one, however, and the drug may be listed in different classifications by different sources. For example, drugs classified one way in this chapter may appear in other classifications in other reference works.

There are common stems or syllables that are used to identify the different drug classes.

The USAN Council approves the stems and syllables and recommends using them in making new nonproprietary names. There are always new stems and syllables being approved by the Council, so the list is ever changing. On this page is a list of some common stems and syllables and the drug class associated with them.

Stem	Drug Class
-pamil	Coronary vasodilators
-parin	Heparin derivatives
-peridol	Antipsychotics (haloperidol type)
-poetin	Erythropoietins
-pramine	Antidepressants (imipramine type)
-pred	Prednisone derivatives
-pril	Antihypertensives (ACE inhibitors)
-profen	Anti-inflammatory/analgesic agents (ibuprofen type)
-rubicin	Antineoplastic antibiotics (daunorubicin type)
-sartan	Angiotensin II receptor antagonists
-sertron	Serotonin 5-HT$_3$ receptor antagonists
-sulfa	Antibiotics (sulfonamide derivatives)
-terol	Bronchodilators (phenethylamine derivatives)
-thiazide	Diuretics (thiazide derivatives)
-tiazem	Calcium channel blockers (diltiazem derivatives)
-tocin	Oxytocin derivatives
-trexate	Antimetabolites (folic acid derivatives)
-triptyline	Antidepressants
-vastatin	Antihyperlipidemics (HMG-CoA inhibitors)

CLASSIFICATION SCHEMES

There are various systems for classifying drugs: by disorder, body system affected, type of receptor acted on, type of action, etc. This text uses common classifications, but it is important to recognize that there is no standard classification system used in medicine.

A number of classifications are based on whether they influence the parasympathetic or sympathetic nervous system.

Most organs in the body are influenced by both the parasympathetic and sympathetic nervous systems. These systems generally stimulate opposing responses, which balances their effects and results in a normal state of **homeostasis**. Drugs that act on the parasympathetic system are called cholinergic because acetylcholine is the **neurotransmitter** of this system. Drugs that act on the sympathetic nervous system are called adrenergic, because the neurotransmitters for this system (norepinephrine and epinephrine) are secreted from the adrenal glands.

Many classifications are also named for the type of interaction with the receptor.

Agonist or antagonist interaction is the primary basis for classification (i.e., cholinergic antagonist, etc.), but drugs may be classified based on specific receptor characteristics. For example, adrenergic receptor responses may be categorized as alpha (α) and beta (β).

Classification schemes have grown significantly as different types of receptors have been discovered.

Each new type of receptor has been found to be responsible for a specific pharmacological effect. As drugs designed to interact with these receptors are developed the complexity of classifications increases.

There are also other factors that complicate classification schemes.

One factor for drugs that affect the autonomic nervous system is the use of prefixes or suffixes such as **blocker**, -lytic, or anti- to mean antagonist, and **mimetic** to mean agonist. Another factor is the presence of neurotransmitters other than acetylcholine, norepinephrine, and epinephrine. These include serotonin, dopamine, histamine, gamma-amino butyric acid (GABA), etc. Each has subtypes, and each has agonists and antagonists that act by a variety of mechanisms.

CLASSIFICATIONS

Classification schemes for drugs can be highly complex. They can also vary greatly and any combination of terms or nomenclature schemes might be used. The classifications used in this text should provide insight into how and why the drugs in them are used, but are not the only way to classify these drugs.

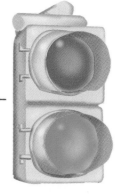

antagonists block action

———

agonists activate receptors

blocker another term for an antagonist drug, because antagonists block the action of neurotransmitters.

homeostasis the state of equilibrium of the body.

mimetic another term for an agonist, because agonists imitate or "mimic" the action of the neurotransmitter.

neurotransmitter substances that carry the impulses from one neuron to another.

Note: Throughout this chapter, drugs highlighted in green are parenteral drugs that are commonly found in hospitals and other institutional settings.

The Primary Classifications Used in this Text

Analgesics
    Salicylates
    NSAIDs
    Non-aspirin, non-NSAID
    Opiates
Anesthetic Agents
    Local
    General
Anti-infectives
    Antibiotics (antimicrobials)
    Antivirals
    Antifungals
    Antimycobacterials
    Antiprotozoals
    Anthelmintics
Antineoplastics
    Antimetabolites
    Alkylating agents
    Plant alkaloids
    Hormones
    Anti-tumor antibiotics
    Radioactive isotopes
Cardiovascular Agents
    Beta blockers
    Calcium channel blockers
    Diuretics
    ACE inhibitors
    Vasodilators
    Antianginals
    Antiarrhythmics
    Antihyperlipidemics
    Antihypertensives
    Thrombolytics/Anticoagulants
    Vasopressors
Dermatologicals
Electrolytic Agents
Gastrointestinal & Urinary Tract Agents
    Enzymes
    Antidiarrheals
    Antiemetics
    Antacid/antiulcer agents
    Laxatives and stool softeners
    Urinary tract agents

Hematological Agents
    Hematopoietic agents
    Hemostatic agents
Hormones & Modifiers
    Thyroid & Parathyroid agents
    Pituitary agents
    Adrenal agents
    Insulins
    Oral antidiabetics
    Androgens
    Phosphodiesterase inhibitors
    Progestins
    Estrogens
    Contraceptives
Immunobiologic Agents
    Immune globulins
    Vaccines
Musculoskeletal Agents
    Anti-gout agents
    Osteoporitics
    Muscle relaxants
    Antispasmodics
Neurological Agents
    Antiparkinsonian agents
    Anti-Alzheimer's agents
    Anti-epileptics
    Anti-migraine agents
Ophthalmic and Otic Agents
    Antiglaucoma agents
    Other ophthalmics
    Otics
Psychotropic Agents
    Antipsychotics
    Sedatives & hypnotics
    Antianxiety agents
    Antidepressants
    Drug dependency
Respiratory Agents
    Antihistamines
    Decongestants
    Antitussives
    Expectorants and mucolytics
    Bronchodilators

ANALGESICS

Analgesic drugs create a state in which the pain from a painful medical condition is reduced or not felt.

Once pain has signaled the presence of a medical condition, its usefulness is generally complete and in most cases it can be safely blocked with the use of an analgesic.

There are several types of analgesics.

Two groups are used for mild to moderate pain, the non-steroidal anti-inflammatory drugs (NSAIDs) and the salicylates. Acetaminophen is also a popular agent for treating mild to moderate pain that some consider an NSAID but others do not.

Opiate-type narcotic analgesics are used for severe pain.

The naturally occurring opiates (morphine and codeine) and the synthetic opioids such as meperidine and propoxyphene are called "narcotic analgesics" and have a high abuse potential. In this section, we'll explore the types of analgesics and identify and describe common drug examples of each group.

Opiate-type Drugs & the Brain

Three specific receptors in the brain have been identified to react to opiate and opioid drugs:

- Mu (μ): produces euphoria, respiratory depression and physical dependence.
- Kappa (κ): produces analgesia,
- Sigma (σ): produces dysphoria and hallucinations.

The Transmission of Pain

Nerve fibers carry pain impulses from the body's receptor sites through the spinal cord and up to the thalamus and cerebral cortex. The cerebral cortex is the ridge-like neural tissue that covers the brain's hemispheres. Analgesics are thought to depress the thalamus and interfere with the transmission of pain impulses. In addition, the brain's interpretation of pain may be altered with the use of these drugs.

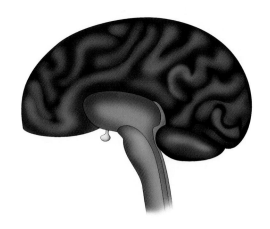

Some Common Analgesic Drugs		
Type	Brand Name	Generic Name
Salicylates	Bayer	acetlsalicylic acid (aspirin)
Non-aspirin, non-NSAID	Tylenol	acetaminophen
NSAID	Motrin, Advil	ibuprofen
NSAID	Naprosyn	naproxen
Opiates	MS Contin	morphine
Opiates	Demerol	meperidine
Opiates	Darvon	propoxyphene

See Additional Common Drugs by Classification on pp 473–477 for more drugs in this class.

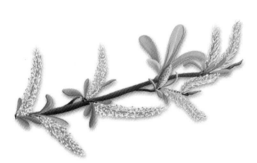

the white willow, a source of salicylic acid

Salicylates

� Relieve mild to moderate pain.

� Anti-inflammatory.

� Anti-pyretic.

Acetaminophen

� Relieves mild to moderate pain.

� Anti-pyretic.

NSAIDs

� More potent than salicylates.

� Relieve mild to moderate pain.

� Anti-inflammatory.

� Anti-pyretic.

Opiate-type

� For severe pain.

� Addicting.

analgesia a state in which pain is not felt even though a painful condition exists.

anti-pyretic reduces fever.

An extract of willow bark, salicylic acid has been used to relieve pain for thousands of years.

Hippocrates and other ancient physicians used plants such as gaultheria and the poplar tree to obtain natural salicylates. Today, non-addicting analgesic products such as aspirin (acetylsalicylic acid) and methyl salicylate are widely used. Salicylates, acting both centrally and peripherally, are found effective as mild to moderate pain relievers, anti-inflammatory medications and fever reducers (**anti-pyretics**).

The action of non-steroidal anti-inflammatory drugs (NSAIDs) is both analgesic and anti-inflammatory.

They are generally more potent than the salicylates and serve to relieve mild to moderate pain, reduce fever and treat rheumatic symptoms. At higher doses, NSAIDs inhibit the synthesis of prostaglandins, a chief contributor to the inflammation process. As a result, inflammation is slowed or reduced. The effect of lower doses is analgesic. The selection and dosing of these drugs is very patient specific as one NSAID may be more effective than another for any given patient. NSAIDs may also have an anti-pyretic quality by which they reduce fever. The temperature regulating brain center is the hypothalamus and it is believed that some NSAIDs affect select areas of the hypothalamus to increase vasodilation, sweating, and encourage excess heat loss. Common drugs in this category include ibuprofen (Motrin®) and naproxen (Naprosyn®).

Taken from the poppy plant, Papaver Somniferum, opium was also used in ancient times to relieve pain.

Opiate-type and opioid narcotics of today have been found to affect the CNS by reducing the awareness and perception of pain. They mimic the actions of the body's natural narcotic-like substances called endorphins. The narcotic analgesics do not eradicate the pain, but rather alter the patient's perception of it. Therefore, these drugs are thought to be most helpful if given before the severe pain is present. Common naturally occurring opiate-type drugs include morphine and codeine, while common opioid drugs include meperidine (Demerol®) and propoxyphene (Darvon®).

ANESTHETIC AGENTS

Anesthetics cause an absence of sensation or pain.

They are classified into two groups: local and general.

Local anesthetics block pain conduction from peripheral nerves to the central nervous system without causing a loss of consciousness.

They do this by allowing the nerve's membrane to stabilize in a resting position and not respond to painful stimuli. Cocaine is credited by some sources as the first recognized local anesthetic, but it has a limited use today (i.e., topical application in eye and nasal surgery) and is a Schedule II substance.

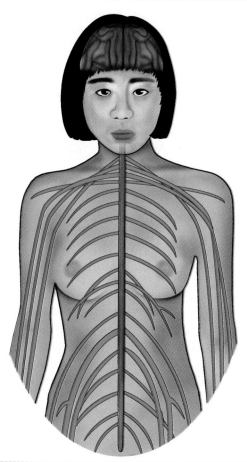

LOCAL ANESTHETICS

Indications

Common indications for local anesthetics include:

➥ dental work or discomfort (topical or injection);

➥ birth pain (spinal, epidural or caudal IV);

➥ sunburn, hemorrhoids and skin irritations (topical).

Groups

Local anesthetics can be grouped by chemical structure as follows:

➥ **Esters**—metabolized by enzymes found in the blood or skin, short to moderate duration of effectiveness.

➥ **Amides**—metabolized in the liver and therefore longer acting.

➥ **Others**—those agents suitable for patients with allergies to esthers or amides.

Blocking Pain

Pain is conducted from its local site through the Peripheral Nervous System (blue) to the Central Nervous System (red). Local anesthetics block pain conduction to the CNS, but do not affect the CNS, so the patient remains conscious. General anesthetics block pain sensation by depressing the CNS, causing unconsciousness.

Some Common Local Anesthetics		
Type	**Brand Name**	**Generic Name**
Ester	Novocain	procaine
Ester	Pontocaine	tetracaine
Amide	Xylocaine	lidocaine
Amide	Marcaine	bupivacaine
Other	Cepacol	dyclonine

See Additional Common Drugs by Classification on pp 473–477 for more drugs in this class.

surgical anesthesia the stage of anesthesia in which surgery can be safely conducted.

medullary paralysis an overdose of anesthesia that paralyzes the respiratory and heart centers of the medulla, leading to death.

GENERAL ANESTHESIA

The Four Stages

There are four stages of general anesthesia:

Stage I—Analgesia Euphoria with loss of pain and consciousness.

Stage II—Excitement Increase in sympathetic nervous system effects such as blood pressure, heart and respiratory rate.

Stage III—*Surgical Anesthesia* The stage in which surgery can safely be conducted. There are four levels of surgical anesthesia, with the higher numbered levels producing deeper anesthesia and more serious systemic effects.

Stage IV—Medullary Paralysis An overdose of anesthesia can compromise the respiratory and heart centers of the brain's medulla and cause death.

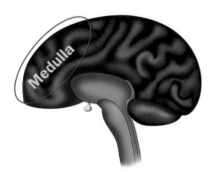

℞ Drugs highlighted in green in the text and tables are parenteral drugs commonly found in hospitals and other institutional settings.

General anesthetics depress the CNS (central nervous system) to the level of unconsciousness.

The first general anesthetic, nitrous oxide (laughing gas), was developed about 150 years ago. The vapors ethyl ether and chloroform followed soon after. However, these products were found to have many safety concerns and less hazardous agents have been subsequently developed.

General anesthetics are generally classified according to their route of administration: inhalation or intravenous (IV).

IV anesthesia often produces a more pleasant, smoother and quicker onset than the inhaled anesthetics. A combination of various agents is widely used to avoid undesired side effects and produce the best effects of general anesthesia.

General anesthesia is administered by a medical doctor called an anesthesiologist.

The desired level of general anesthesia can be controlled by balancing the amount of anesthesia the patient receives with the amount their lungs eliminate through exhalation. In ceasing the administration of anesthesia, the process will reverse and the level of anesthesia lighten.

In addition to the anesthetic drug choice, adjunctive drugs such as analgesics, atropine-like drugs, and anti-infectives may also be used.

This is to prevent certain negative side effects (those that occur from too much of one anesthetic), potentiate other desired effects (such as pain relief and reduced amount of anesthesia), cause the drying of secretions (preventing aspiration during surgery), or act to prevent infections (post-op). The safety, comfort, and general well being of the patient are of utmost concern when an anesthesiologist chooses the anesthetic or combination of anesthetics that are the most appropriately indicated for a particular case.

Some Common General Anesthetics		
Type	**Brand Name**	**Generic Name**
Inhalation	Forane	isoflurane
Inhalation	Ultane	sevoflurane
Inhalation	Suprane	desflurane
IV	Diprivan	propofol
IV	Valium	diazepam
IV	Amidate	etomidate

ANTI-INFECTIVES

Anti-infectives treat disease produced by microorganisms such as bacteria, viruses, fungi, protozoa, and parasitic worms. Historically, natural chemicals from the earth such as mercury and molds have been used to treat infections, but it wasn't until Paul Ehrlich synthesized hundreds of chemicals in the 1930's, that a chemotherapeutic approach was widely used. There are now a large number of naturally occurring, semi-synthetic, and synthetic drugs and vaccines available for treatments of infectious diseases.

In this section, antibiotics (antimicrobials), antivirals, and antifungals will be discussed and explored.

Other forms of anti-infectives include: antimycobacterials (agents that treat tuberculosis, leprosy and the MAC complex in AIDS); antiprotozoals (agents that treat malaria, vaginitis, and sleeping sickness); and **anthelmintics** (agents that treat parasitic worms in the GI tract)·

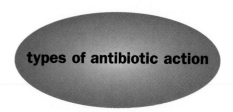

types of antibiotic action

➡ **damage bacterial cell wall**
(e.g., penicillins and cephalosporins)

➡ **modify protein synthesis**
(e.g., erythromycin and tetracycline)

➡ **modify energy metabolism**
(e.g., sulfonamides)

➡ **modify DNA synthesis**
(e.g., ofloxacin and ciprofloxacin)

Some Common Anti-infectives

Type	Brand Name	Generic Name
Antibiotic	Zithromax	azithromycin
Antibiotic/natural penicillin	Veetids	penicillin
Antibiotic/synthetic penicillin	Principen	ampicillin
Antibiotic/synthetic penicillin	Augmentin	amoxicillin w/potassium clavulanate
Antibiotic/semi-synthetic	Geocillin	carbenicillin
Antibiotic/cephalosprin	Ceclor	cefaclor
Antibiotic/tetracycline	Sumycin	tetracycline
Antibiotic/sulfonamide	Bactrim DS	sulfamethoxazole/trimethoprim
Antiviral	Valtrex	valacyclovir
Antiviral/protease inhibitor	Viracept	nelfinavir
Antifungal	Mycostatin	nystatin
Antimycobacterial	Nydrazid	isoniazid
Antiprotozoal	Flagyl	metronidazole
Anthelmintic	Vermox	mebendazole

See Additional Common Drugs by Classification on pp 473–477 for more drugs in this class.

anthelmintics drugs that destroy worms.
bactericidal bacteria killing.
bacteriostatic bacteria inhibiting.

protease inhibitor an antiviral used for HIV and Hepatitis C that blocks the enzyme responsible for viral replication.

426

CLASSES

Antibiotics (Antimicrobials)

The term antibiotic (or antimicrobial) refers to chemicals of bacterial microorganisms which suppress the growth of other microorganisms. Early discovery of antibiotics came from Sir Alexander Fleming and his work isolating the naturally occurring penicillin. Later, a team from Oxford reinvestigated this research and developed potent extracts which were important in fighting infections during WWII. Since that time, synthetic penicillins such as ampicillin and the first semisynthetic penicillin (carbenicillin), have been introduced. Other forms of antibiotics include: cephalosporins (cefazolin, cefoxitin, ceftibuten, cefepime, etc.); tetracyclines (tetracycline, doxycycline, etc.); sulfonamides or "sulfa drugs" (sulfamethoxazole, etc.). Some common other antibiotics are azithromycin (Zithromax®) and amoxicillin with potassium clavulanate (Augmentin®).

Antimicrobials can be either **bacteriostatic** (inhibiting bacterial growth) or **bactericidal** (bacteria killing). Different antibiotics have different types of action such as modifying protein synthesis, modifying energy metabolism, modifying DNA metabolism, or damaging the bacteria's cell wall.

Antivirals

Antivirals inhibit the replication of viruses (and so are virustatic). The viral microorganism will invade the host cell and proliferate using the cell's DNA and RNA. To effectively treat viral infections, the drug needs to stop the viral replication without destroying the patient's healthy cells. Mutations and resistance are common setbacks with this therapy. Antimicrobials are not effective with viral infections, but may be used in cases of accompanying secondary bacterial infection. **Protease inhibitors** such as nelfinavir (Viracept®) are a class of medications used to treat HIV and Hepatitis C. by blocking the enzyme responsible for viral replication. Other common antiviral agents include: valacyclovir (Valtrex®) and acyclovir (Zovirax®).

Antifungals

Antifungals are used to treat fungal infections. Fungi are plant-like microorganisms commonly found in molds and yeast. The drugs chosen to treat these mycosis or mycotic infections are usually fungicidal. The fungal cell is destroyed as the drug prevents cell permeability and nutrition. Common fungal infections include: candidiasis (vaginal yeast infection), ringworm, and athlete's foot. Nystatin (Mycostatin®) and fluconazole (Diflucan®) are popular antifungal drugs.

℞ safety you should know

➥ Do NOT refrigerate Biaxin® suspension.

➥ Erythromycins and Biaxin® have many serious drug interactions.

➥ Many antibiotics can decrease the effectiveness of oral contraceptives.

➥ Tetracyclines should not be used during pregnancy.

➥ Tetracyclines should not be used in children under eight years old.

➥ Tetracyclines and some other antibiotics can cause photosensitivity.

➥ Avoid dairy products, vitamins, or antacids within two hours of taking tetracyclines.

➥ Many antibiotics have serious interactions with warfarin (Coumadin®).

➥ Alcohol should be avoided until one day after therapy with metronidazole.

➥ Patients taking sulfa drugs should drink plenty of water.

ANTINEOPLASTICS

Oncology is the branch of medicine that deals with the study and treatment of cancer.

Antineoplastics inhibit the new growth of cancer cells or **neoplasms**. Typically, cancer cells are abnormal in structure and growth rate. They offer no useful function, have unusual genetic content, and often reproduce quickly and uncontrollably. Antineoplastics present a chemotherapeutic approach to the treatment of cancer and together with surgery, radiation and perhaps alternative medicine, comprise an often hopeful and successful treatment protocol.

Malignancy means a life-threatening, cancerous group of cells or tumor is present.

If this original (primary) cell group spreads to other areas, often via the lymphatic or circulatory systems, it is said to have **metastasized**. Treatment to **remission** (state of cancer inactivity) or cure is more successful if little or no metastasis has occurred. However, current chemotherapeutic research and development is offering encouragement for cancers in later stages of growth.

The side effects caused by many of these drugs are often uncomfortable and serious.

They include immunosuppression, anemia (decreased count of red blood cells), alopecia (hair loss), GI ulceration, and dehydration/weight loss from nausea and vomiting.

The Lymphatic System

The lymphatic system is the center of the body's immune system. It collects plasma water from the blood vessels, filters it for impurities through the lymph nodes, and returns the lymph fluid back to the general circulation. Carried in the lymph are **lymphocytes**, a type of white blood cell that releases antibodies that attack and destroy antigens like bacteria and disease cells (including cancer). This is the body's immune response to antigens. T-cells and B-cells are the primary lymphocytes. Maintenance of the body's lymphocyte supply is largely performed by the bone marrow.

Antineoplastic drugs are targeted at cells with fast growth rates, which not only includes cancer cells but bone marrow as well. As a result, a serious side effect of antineoplastics is that they depress the immune system (immunosuppression), leaving chemotherapy patients prone to infections.

lymphocyte a type of white blood cell that releases antibodies that destroy disease cells.

metastasis when cancer cells spread beyond their original site.

neoplasm a new and abnormal tissue growth, often referring to cancer cells.

remission a state in which cancer cells are inactive.

Controlling Cell Growth

Normal cell growth (shown below) is highly structured and steady, but cancer cells often reproduce quickly and uncontrollably. Antineoplastic drugs act on various stages of the cell replication process to stop the growth of cancerous cells.

Since cancer cells can mutate in many ways, different chemicals are used to stop their growth. This results in the "cocktail" approach to chemotherapy, in which a number of drugs are administered to a patient. Because these cocktails also affect normal cells, they are administered in cycles to allow patients to recover from adverse effects before the next round of administration.

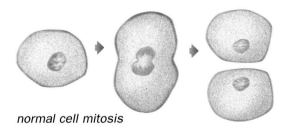

normal cell mitosis

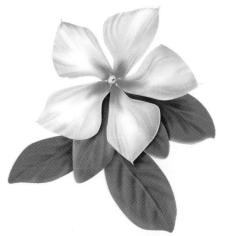

The rosy periwinkle of Madagascar is the source of the antineoplastic vincristine.

Due to the toxicity of many antineoplastics, normal healthy cells are destroyed along with the cancerous cells.

Rapidly replicating cells such as those of the GI tract, bone marrow, and hair follicles are most often affected by selected antineoplastics, causing nausea/vomiting, bone marrow suppression, and hair loss.

Current widely-used antineoplastic drugs include alkylating agents (nitrogen mustards), antimetabolites, and plant alkaloids.

They are usually given in cycles (e.g., 3–4 weeks between treatments), allowing rest and recovery periods for the patient. In theory, during the healthy cells recovery, neoplastic cells are entering a rapid division phase and are destroyed in greater numbers when chemotherapy is again begun. Drug resistance to a particular antineoplastic agent may occur, however, so a combination of these drugs may be given at one time to assure effectiveness. This "cocktail," as it is sometimes called, offers drugs of different actions and structure to address whatever type of cancerous cell group is suspected to be present.

Hormones, anti-tumor antibiotics, and radioactive isotopes are also classified as antineoplastic agents, generally for specific site treatment.

For example, if a tumor is found to be hormone dependent, surgical removal of the affected organ is often indicated (e.g., prostate, breast, or uterus), thus eliminating the chance for hormonal support. In addition, the synthetic antiestrogen agent, tamoxifen, is often used for the treatment of breast cancer in post-menopausal women. Certain antibiotics such as bleomycin and doxorubicin will be ordered to treat skin cancers, lymphomas, and leukemias. The radioactive isotopes, such as gold (AU198) and iodine (I131), are also generally organ specific, but are radioactive and special caution is needed during their use.

ANTINEOPLASTICS (cont'd)

CLASSES

Antimetabolites

Classified in accordance with the substances they interfere with, these antineoplastic drugs inhibit cell growth and replication by mimicking natural metabolites and taking their place within the cells. These fake metabolites inhibit the synthesis of important cellular enzymes, including DNA.

Alkylating Agents

These drugs interfere with mitosis or cell division by binding with DNA and preventing cellular replication. The early alkylating drugs were developed in World War I to introduce chemical warfare. Known as nitrogen mustard gases, these chemicals possessed properties which inhibited cellular growth and sperm counts while depressing bone marrow and damaging intestinal mucosa. Although these agents will adversely affect all cells, those that are growing at a more rapid rate (presumably cancerous) will be more affected. Nitrosureas, a more recent type of alkylating agent, are lipid soluble and pass easily into the brain where they are effective in treating brain cancers.

Plant Alkaloids

Derived from natural products or semisynthetically produced using natural products, some of these drugs inhibit the enzyme topoisomerase.

Topoisomerase is required for molecular cell growth or mitosis and therefore certain plant alkaloids interfere with cellular DNA replication. Other mechanisms of growth inhibition are not clearly understood.

Some Common Antineoplastics

Type	Brand Name	Generic Name
Antimetabolite	Adrucil	fluorouracil
Antimetabolite	Rheumatrex	methotrexate
Alkylating agent/nitrogen mustard	Mustargen	mechlorethamine
Alkylating agent/nitrosurea	BiCNU	carmustine
Plant alkaloid	Oncovin	vincristine
Plant alkaloid	Velban	vinblastine
Hormone agonist	Lupron	leuprolide
Hormone/antiestrogen	Nolvadex	tamoxifen
Anti-tumor antibiotic	Blenoxane	bleomycin
Anti-tumor antibiotic	Adriamycin	doxorubicin
Anti-tumor antibiotic	Cerubidine	daunorubicin
Radioactive isotope	Bexxar	tositumomab and iodine I 131

See Additional Common Drugs by Classification on pp 473–477 for more drugs in this class.

Hormones

Hormone therapy can be used to treat certain cancers that require hormones to grow. Hormone therapy works by preventing cancer cells from using the hormones they need to grow. Examples include tamoxifen (Nolvadex®) and leuprolide (Lupron®).

Anti-tumor Antibiotics

Anti-tumor antibiotics are drugs that interact directly with cancer cells to prevent the DNA from functioning normally. This can sometimes result in killing the cancer cells. Examples include bleomycin (Blenoxane®), daunorubicin (Cerubidine®), and doxorubicin (Adriamycin®).

Radioactive Isotopes

Radioactive substances can be used to kill cancer cells in a targeted area. Radiation treatments can be given by a machine that directs radiation at the tumor area. Treatments can otherwise be given internally using needles, seeds, wires, or catheters that contain a radioactive substance and are placed directly in or near the tumor. Radioactive isotopes are sometimes given in combination with other therapeutic approaches. For example, Bexxar® contains tositumomab and iodine I 131 and is used to treat some types of non-Hodgkins lymphoma. It attaches to cancer cells and releases radiation that damages the cancer cells.

℞ safety you should know

➥ Drugs that are used to treat cancer may cause very serious side effects.

➥ Pharmacists and pharmacy technicians must be very careful with all calculations associated with drugs that are used to treat cancer.

➥ Some of the drugs that are used to treat cancer are also used to treat other conditions besides cancer.

℞ Note: Drugs highlighted in green in the text and tables are parenteral drugs commonly found in hospitals and other institutional settings.

CARDIOVASCULAR AGENTS

Some of the most widely used medications available are used to treat diseases and conditions of the cardiovascular system.

Cardiovascular agents include antianginals, antiarrhythmics, antihypertensives, vasopressors, antihyperlipidemics, thrombolytics and anticoagulants. They are used in treating myocardial infarction (heart attack), angina, cerebral vascular accident (CVA) or stroke, hyper/hypotension (high/low blood pressure), congestive heart failure (CHF), coronary artery disease (CAD), arrhythmias, high cholesterol, unwanted blood clots, and arteriosclerosis.

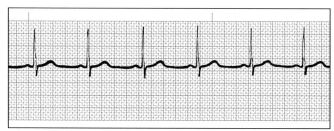

An EKG strip for a normal heart rhythm—variations from this pattern indicate an arrhythmia. The type of arrhythmia can be determined by the nature of the variation.

Arrhythmias

Normally, the electrical system of the heart causes it to contract (or beat) in a regular and organized rhythm that can be graphed by an **electrocardiogram** (**EKG** or **ECG**). An **arrhythmia** is an abnormal heart rhythm that can interfere with the heart's ability to pump in an effective, organized manner. Arrhythmias range from minor to life-threatening. They are classified by degree of seriousness, site of origin (where the electrical impulse causing the rhythm came from), and rate or speed. Familiar arrhythmias include:

➥ tachycardia;

➥ bradycardia;

➥ premature or ectopic beats;

➥ flutter and fibrillation.

THE HEART

Conduction

The heart is a pump that uses complex chemical and electrical processes to function. Chemically charged particles (ions) stimulate heart muscle to contract and relax systematically, pumping blood through the cardiovascular system. This contraction and relaxation is referred to as the **cardiac cycle**.

The SA node is the fastest generating electrical impulse area of the heart and it sets the pace. The atria and ventricles follow the conduction signal while the AV node together with the fine fibers (Purkinje Fibers) at the base of the heart transmit the impulse.

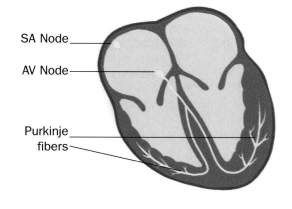

arrhythmia an abnormal heart rhythm.

electrocardiogram (EKG or ECG) a graph of the heart's rhythms.

cardiac cycle the contraction and relaxation of the heart that pumps blood through the cardiovascular system.

The Heart and Circulation

The heart is a muscular organ which powers blood circulation for the entire body. Divided into four chambers, the right and left atria (top chambers) and the right and left ventricles (bottom chambers), the heart receives deoxygenated blood into the right side (referred to as pulmonary circulation) and oxygenated blood into the left side (referred to as systemic circulation).

The right ventricle pumps blood to the lungs where it will mix with oxygen. The left ventricle pumps oxygenated blood to the body. The **myocardium** (heart muscle) is supplied fresh oxygen-rich blood by the coronary arteries, which branch from the aorta and circle back to the heart.

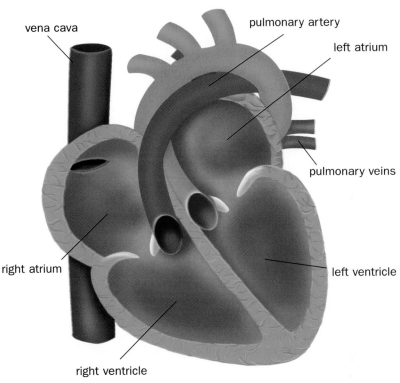

vena cava

pulmonary artery

left atrium

pulmonary veins

right atrium

left ventricle

right ventricle

Blood Clotting

Clotting is an essential function of blood that prevents excessive blood loss from injuries. Though clotting factors are the primary influence on clotting, adequate platelets and healthy blood vessel walls are also important. Too much clotting can be dangerous, however. If a clot (**thrombus**) is formed in the bloodstream, it can be carried to a location where it blocks a blood vessel and blood flow. Such blockages are called **embolisms**, and they can cause strokes and death.

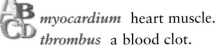
myocardium heart muscle.

thrombus a blood clot.

embolism, embolus a clot that has traveled in the bloodstream to a point where it obstructs flow.

Blood Pressure

Blood pressure is the outward pressure of the blood against the arteries as it is pumped through the body by the heart. Current literature recommends a blood pressure no higher than 126/76 for 40% of a normal healthy adult's day. The first number is the **systolic** value that represents the maximum pressure as the heart contracts to pump blood out. The second number is the **diastolic** value that represents the minimum pressure in the artery as the heart relaxes.

systolic pressure the maximum blood pressure when the heart contracts; the first number in a blood pressure reading.

diastolic pressure the minimum blood pressure when the heart relaxes; the second number in a blood pressure reading.

CARDIOVASCULAR AGENTS (cont'd)

CLASSES BY MECHANISM OF ACTION

In addition to classifying cardiovascular drugs by the conditions they treat, some of these drugs are also grouped by their mechanisms of action or how they work in the body. There are five main groupings of cardiovascular drugs by mechanism of action: beta blockers, calcium channel blockers, diuretics, ace inhibitors, and vasodilators.

As you learn about the drugs you will find that some beta blockers or calcium channel blockers can be used to treat a variety of conditions including hypertension, arrhythmias, and angina. You will also find that different ACE inhibitors have indications for different conditions.

Beta Blockers

Beta blockers are drugs that reduce the oxygen demands of the heart muscle. They are often used to treat high blood pressure or arrhythmias. Some examples include propranolol (Inderal®), nadolol (Corgard®), metoprolol (Lopressor®), and atenolol (Tenormin®).

Calcium Channel Blockers

Calcium channel blockers are drugs that relax the heart by reducing heart conduction. They are also often used to treat high blood pressure or arrhythmias. Some examples include verapamil (Calan®), diltiazem (Cardizem®), nifedipine (Procardia®), and amlodipine (Norvasc®).

Diuretics

Diuretics decrease blood pressure by decreasing blood volume. They decrease volume by increasing the elimination of salts and water through urination. Some examples include hydrochlorothiazide (Hydrodiuril®), furosemide (Lasix®), and bumetanide (Bumex®).

ACE Inhibitors

The "-pril" drugs, ace inhibitors relax the blood vessels. They are often used to treat high blood pressure. Note: the "-sartan" drugs are considered a subgroup of ACE inhibitors. Some examples include captopril (Capoten®), enalapril (Vasotec®), and lisinopril (Zestril®).

Vasodilators

Vasodilators relax and expand the blood vessels. Some examples include hydralazine (Apresoline®), and minoxidil (Loniten®).

℞ safety you should know

- Beta blockers and calcium channel blockers should not be discontinued abruptly without medical supervision.
- Some calcium channel blockers have important drug interactions. Check with your pharmacist when drug interactions are detected by the computer.
- Some diuretics cause sun sensitivity.
- Most diuretics can cause hypokalemia (low levels of potassium). Exceptions are triamterene and spironolactone which can cause hyperkalemia (high potassium levels).
- ACE inhibitors have special warnings in pregnancy.
- Some ACE inhibitors may cause hyperkalemia (high levels of potassium).
- Some ACE inhibitors may cause coughing.

Some Common Cardiovascular Drugs by Mechanism of Action

Type	Brand Name	Generic Name
Beta blocker	Inderal	propranolol
Beta blocker	Tenormin	atenolol
Beta blocker	Corgard	nadolol
Beta blocker	Lopressor	metoprolol
Calcium channel blocker	Calan	verapamil
Calcium channel blocker	Norvasc	amlodipine
Calcium channel blocker	Procardia	nifedipine
Calcium channel blocker	Cardizem	diltiazem
Diuretics	Lasix	furosemide
Diuretics	Hydrodiuril	hydrochlorothiazide
Diuretics	Aldactone	spironolactone
ACE inhibitor	Capoten	captopril
ACE inhibitor	Vasotec	enalapril
ACE inhibitor	Zestril	lisinopril
Vasodilator	Apresoline	hydralazine
Vasodilator	Loniten	minoxidil

CLASSES BY CONDITION

Antianginals

Antianginals are used to treat cardiac related chest pain (angina) resulting from ischemic heart disease. Patients with this condition suffer a lack of oxygen and blood flow to the myocardium. Nitrates, beta-blockers, and calcium channel blockers such as nitroglycerin (Nitrostat®) and nifedipine (Procardia®), are examples of antianginals.

Antiarrhythmics

Antiarrhythmics are used to treat irregular heart rhythms. They regulate the conduction activity of the heart by inhibiting abnormal pacemaker cells or recurring abnormal impulses and restoring a normal rhythm. Antiarrhythmics such as digoxin (Lanoxin®) and sotalol (Betapace®) include beta blockers and drugs that block sodium, potassium ion, and calcium channels.

℞ safety you should know
➡ Some cardiovascular drugs have significant interactions with grapefruit juice.

CARDIOVASCULAR AGENTS (cont'd)

CLASSES BY CONDITION, CONT'D

Antihyperlipidemics

Antihyperlipidemics are used to lower high levels of cholesterol that can lead to blocked blood vessels. Cholesterol is a lipid normally present in the body that is essential for healthy cell function. Proteins and carbohydrates, as well as fat are responsible for natural cholesterol production. Cholesterol levels are measured as total cholesterol, LDL (low-density lipoprotein), and HDL (high-density lipoprotein). Excess amounts of LDL can lead to blocked blood vessels and cardiovascular problems. HMG-CoA Reductase inhibitors are used to treat high LDL levels. Examples are simvastatin (Zocor®), ezetimibe with simvastatin (Vytorin®), and pravastatin (Pravachol®).

Antihypertensives

Antihypertensives are used to reduce a sustained elevation in blood pressure. Factors affecting blood pressure include stress, blood volume, arterial narrowing, age, gender and general condition of health. Common antihypertensives include beta-blockers to reduce cardiac output, diuretics to decrease fluid volume, ACE inhibitors to reduce salt and water retention and inhibit vascular constriction, and calcium channel blockers to relax blood vessels. Examples of diuretics are furosemide (Lasix®) and ramipril (Altace®). An example of a potassium sparing diuretic is spironolactone (Aldactone®). (Note that some antihypertensive agents also have other such as treating heart conditions and preventing migraine headaches.)

Thrombolytics/Anticoagulants

Thrombolytics dissolve blood clots and anticoagulants prevent their formation. Thrombolytics can be dangerous since blood clotting can be disturbed, resulting in profuse bleeding and even bleeding to death. However, in cases of impending myocardial infarction or stroke, a travelling blood clot (embolus) can be dissolved and the stroke prevented. There has been much success with this group of drugs in recent years. A common thrombolytic agent is alteplase. Common anticoagulants include warfarin (Coumadin®) and heparin (Hep-Lock®).

Vasopressors

Vasopressors act to increase blood pressure. If a patient is in a state of shock due to decreased blood volume, inadequate cardiac output or severe infection, fluids may be introduced to provide adequate blood volume. In addition to fluid replacement, vasopressors may be used to help supply blood to the brain and kidney. The patient may for example be given an intravenous solution made up of containing dobutamine (Dobutrex®).

℞ **safety you should know**

➡ Many antianginal drugs cause headaches, dizziness and/or flushing.

➡ Nitroglycerin products should be kept in the container they came in, tightly closed, and out of reach of children.

➡ Nitroglycerin tablets that are more than 12 months old should not be used.

➡ Digoxin (Lanoxin®) is associated with several serious drug interactions.

➡ Many antihypertensive drugs can cause dizziness and can cause orthostatic hypotension (dizziness associated with standing up quickly).

Some Common Cardiovascular Drugs by Condition

Type	Brand Name	Generic Name
Antianginal	Nitrostat	nitroglycerin
Antianginal	Procardia	nifedipine
Antiarryhthmic	Lanoxin	digoxin
Antiarryhthmic	Betapace	sotalol
Antihyperlipidemic	Vytorin	ezetimibe w/simvastatin
Antihyperlipidemic	Zocor	simvastatin
Antihyperlipidemic	Pravachol	pravastatin
Antihypertensive/diuretic	Lasix	furosemide
Antihypertensive/ACE inhibitor	Altace	ramipril
Antihypertensive/diuretic	Aldactone	spironolactone
Thrombolytic	Cathflo Activase	alteplase
Anticoagulant	Coumadin	warfarin
Anticoagulant	Hep-Lock	heparin
Vasopressor	Dobutrex	dobutamine

See Additional Common Drugs by Classification on pp 473–477 for more drugs in this class.

Rx safety you should know: warfarin (Coumadin®)

➥ Warfarin (Coumadin®) has many significant drug interactions.

➥ There is a serious drug interaction with aspirin and warfarin. Patients taking warfarin should carefully check all OTC products to be sure they are not inadvertently taking aspirin.

➥ Dosing for warfarin is individualized and is carefully adjusted according to blood tests.

➥ Overdosing with warfarin can cause life-threatening conditions. Special care is needed with the many different strengths that are available.

Rx Note: Drugs highlighted in green in the text and tables are parenteral drugs commonly found in hospitals and other institutional settings.

DERMATOLOGICALS

The skin is the body's protective barrier.

It is the largest of the body's organs and protects the other organs against microorganisms, trauma, extreme temperature, and other harmful elements. It is comprised of several layers: the epidermis (top layer), dermis (middle layer), and subcutaneous tissue (bottom layer). Within these layers, structures such as hair follicles and shafts, sebaceous and sweat glands, veins, arteries, and sensory nerves are found.

Dermatological **refers to a drug used to treat a condition or disease related to the skin.**

Medical conditions and diseases which occur on or in the skin can be caused by inflammation, infection, growth rate changes, trauma, or structural dysfunction. Examples of skin conditions are burns, cuts, rashes, dandruff, eczema, and skin cancer.

THE SKIN

The skin, also called the **Integumentary System,** is generally 3–5 millimeters thick, though it is thicker in the palms of the hands and soles of the feet and thinner in the eyelids and genitals.

The outer layer of the epidermis (called the stratum corneum) is constantly replenished with new cells from underneath. The turnover time from cell development to shedding (sloughing) is about 21 days.

Contained within the skin are accessory structures: hair follicles, sweat glands, sebaceous glands, and nails.

Note also that the subcutaneous layer is not always considered a part of the skin but simply loose connective tissue that separates the skin from the underlying organs. It is, however, so closely interconnected that it is generally described with the integumentary system.

} epidermis

} dermis

} subcutaneous

} muscle

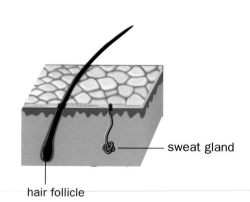

sweat gland

hair follicle

dermatological a product used to treat a skin condition.
integumentary system the skin.

Skin Conditions

The following are examples of skin reactions that selected dermatologicals address:

- trauma (burns, cuts, abrasions, bruises).
- fluid accumulation (edema, cellulitis, blisters).
- discoloration and pigmentation, rashes, freckles, drug or allergy related photosensitivity.
- hyper- or hypo-melanin (skin pigment).
- dry skin or scaling (dandruff).
- cancers (basal cell, squamous cell, or melanoma).
- non-malignant growths (keratoses).

In addition, the following common skin diseases are often treated with both prescription and non-prescription medications:

- eczema.
- psoriasis.
- acne.
- fungal infections (athlete's foot, ringworm).
- viral infections (herpes simplex).
- general dermatitis, hives or other allergic reactions caused by food, plants, insects, or sunburn.

Some Common Dermatologicals

Type	Brand Name	Generic Name
Steroid	Westcort	hydrocortisone cream
Antihistamine	Benadryl	diphenhydramine
Anti-infective	Silvadene	silver sulfadiazine cream
Anti-infective	Vibramycin	doxycycline hyclate
Anti-infective	Floxin	ofloxacin
Antimetabolite	Efudex	fluorouracil cream

See Additional Common Drugs by Classification on pp 473-477 for more drugs in this class.

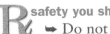 **safety you should know**
- Do not apply fluorouracil to tender skin areas such as the eyelids or the eyes, nose, or mouth.
- Topical products are for external use.
- Wash hands before and after use of topical products.

 Note: The drying agent zinc oxide is often seen in a combination product with the local anesthetic camphor, moisture absorbing agent kaolin, and an anti-infective such as triclosan when treating diaper rash.

ELECTROLYTIC AGENTS

Maintaining the proper balance of body fluids is essential to health and body function.

Water is the primary element in the body, accounting for more than half of body weight. It is found inside cells (**intracellular fluid**) and outside them (**extracellular fluid**) in plasma and tissue (**interstitial fluid**).

Electrolytes are water soluble substances that are contained in our body fluids as salts.

They form electrically charged particles called **ions**, which attract water. They have both positive (**cations**) and negative (**anions**) charges and are responsible for fluid movement into and out of cells. Changes in the body's normal electrolyte count affect fluid movement and balance and consequently various body functions.

Examples of common electrolytes include sodium (Na^+), potassium (K^+), calcium (Ca^{++}), chloride (Cl^-) and bicarbonate (HCO_3^-).

The plus and minus signs indicate their electrical charges. Functions these electrolytes affect include blood pressure, blood coagulation, muscle contractions, myocardial conduction, energy levels and enzyme production. Electrolytic therapy is aimed at restoring normal sodium, potassium, calcium and magnesium balances.

COMMON ELECTROLYTES

Sodium

Sodium is the major cation in fluid outside of cells and sodium regulates the amount of water in the body. Excess sodium is normally excreted in the urine.

Potassium

Potassium is the major cation found inside of cells. Proper potassium balance is important for normal cell function and is especially important for heart and muscle functions. Hypokalemia is the term for low potassium and hyperkalemia is the term for abnormally high potassium. Extreme hypokalemia can be fatal.

Chloride

Chloride is the major anion in the fluid outside of cells.

Bicarbonate

Bicarbonate is an ion that works as a buffer to maintain a proper acid-base balance.

Opposites Attract

Water molecules (H_2O) are polarized. That is, they have positively and negatively charged sides. For this reason, many compounds **dissociate** (come apart) in water to form ions and the ions in turn associate with the water molecules.

The dissociation of sodium chloride (NaCl) into Na^+ and Cl^- ions followed by their association with water molecules is depicted at right. H_2O is attracted at its negative pole to the positive sodium ion and at its positive pole to the negative chloride ion.

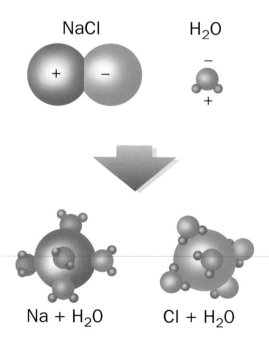

NaCl H_2O

Na + H_2O Cl + H_2O

SOME ELECTROLYTE SOLUTIONS

Lactated Ringer's™ Solution is a balanced and isotonic solution. Balanced means the electrolyte concentration is similar to serum and isotonic means the osmolarity is similar to serum. Lactated Ringer's™ Solution contains sodium, potassium calcium, and lactate.

Polyionic R-148 is a balanced and isotonic solution and contains sodium, potassium, magnesium, chloride, acetate, and gluconate.

Polyionic R-148D5 is a balanced and hypertonic solution and contains sodium, potassium, magnesium, chloride, acetate, gluconate, and dextrose.

D5LR is a balanced and hypertonic solution and contains sodium, potassium calcium, lactate, and dextrose.

Normal saline is an isotonic solution of sodium chloride.

Electrolyte balance is important for healthy body function.

Electrolytes are especially important in the regulation of heart function, as well as fluid balance, acid-base balance and neurological function. The most common cause of electrolyte disturbances is kidney failure. Additionally, dehydration can lead to electrolyte imbalance. Severe diarrhea or vomiting, along with other causes can also lead to electrolyte disturbances. Serious problems can arise when electrolyte imbalances involve potassium, sodium and/or calcium.

℞ **safety you should know**
➡ Oral potassium supplements may cause gastrointestinal upset.
➡ Appropriate potassium balance is important for cardiac function.

dissociation when a compound breaks down and separates into smaller components.

electrolytes a substance that in solution forms ions that conduct an electrical current.

extracellular fluid the fluid outside the body's individual cells found in plasma and tissue fluid.

interstitial fluid tissue fluid.

intracellular fluid cell fluid.

ions electrically charged particles.

anions negatively charged particles.

cations positively charged particles.

Some Common Electrolytic Agents

Type	Brand Name	Generic Name
Potassium supplement	K-Dur Tablets, Klor-Con	potassium chloride
Electrolyte replacement	Rehydralyte Solution	sodium, potassium, chloride, citrate
Electrolyte replacement	Infalyte Oral Solution	sodium, potassium, chloride, citrate
Electrolyte replacement	Resol Solution	sodium, potassium, chloride, citrate, calcium, magnesium, phosphate
Electrolyte replacement	Naturalyte Solution	sodium, potassium, chloride, citrate
Electrolyte replacement	Pedialyte Solution	sodium, potassium, chloride, citrate

GASTROINTESTINAL & URINARY TRACT AGENTS

Gastrointestinal agents are used to treat disorders of the stomach and/or the intestines.

The drugs that address and treat various stomach and intestinal disorders include enzymes, antidiarrheals, antiemetics (anti-vomiting), antiulcer agents, laxatives, and stool softeners.

The GI organs are intimately related to the digestive system as a whole.

The other alimentary tract organs (mouth and esophagus), the accessory organs of digestion (salivary, gastric, and intestinal glands, liver, gall bladder, and pancreas), and the organs of elimination (rectum and anus) are often affected by direct GI disorders. For example, it is not uncommon for a colon cancer to metastasize not only to the stomach, but to the pancreas, liver, and rectum as well. As a result, although specific site antineoplastic drugs and treatments are available, agents may be used that treat more than one site and cell type at a time. Gastric reflux is another example. Gastric hyperacidity will often travel toward the chest and throat area via the esophagus. Antacid drugs that inhibit acidity of the stomach will provide for rest and healing of the esophagus when this happens.

THE DIGESTIVE SYSTEM

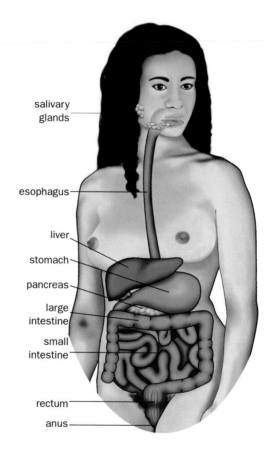

salivary glands

esophagus

liver

stomach

pancreas

large intestine

small intestine

rectum

anus

The stomach lies in the upper left quadrant of the abdomen between the lower end of the esophagus and the beginning of the small intestine (duodenum). This organ serves to store and chemically break down food using hydrochloric acid and pepsinogen. **Chyme** is the semi-liquid form of food as it enters the duodenum. **Peristalsis** is the wave-like motion which moves the food products along the intestinal tract.

Together, the small intestine and the large intestine make up about 28 feet of bowel (intestine). Most food absorption takes place in the small intestine. The large intestine absorbs water and connects to the rectum and anus for stool evacuation.

The GI organs are large in mass compared to other systems' organs and play a major role in normal body function. As a result, dysfunction, abnormality or other pathologic medical conditions of the GI tract may require serious and immediate drug therapy as well as other forms of medical or surgical intervention. Similar to other organ systems, preventive care and early detection of pathology is suggested and encouraged.

The urinary system produces, stores, and eliminates urine and consists of the kidneys, ureters, bladder, urethra, and the penis in males. It is sometimes called the genitourinary system.

chyme the semi-liquid form of food as it enters the intestinal tract.

peristalsis the wave-like motion of the intestines that moves food through them.

CLASSES

Enzymes

Pepsin is a normally present gastric enzyme that breaks down proteins. However, in the absence of pepsin, it is still possible for the digestive system to break down protein molecules into amino acids using proteolytic enzymes from the pancreas that are found in the small intestine. These enzymes are capable of attacking starches and fats. If a patient's condition warrants treatment using enzyme therapy (as with cystic fibrosis and chronic pancreatitis), products that contain pancreatin, an agent prepared from hog pancreas, or pancrelipase may be indicated. Malabsorption conditions such as steatorrhea, where fat is inadequately digested and is excreted in large amounts in feces, may be treated with pancrelipase.

Antidiarrheals

Diarrhea is a condition of frequent watery stools which results from microorganism invasion, drug or stress reaction, and/or other circumstances causing a decrease in intestinal absorption of water, an increased secretion of electrolytes into the intestines or an excessive amount of mucus production. Antiperistalsis drugs slow the movement of the intestinal contents to allow for greater water and electrolyte absorption. Loperamide (Imodium®) is a common antiperistalsis agent and diphenoxylate plus atropine (Lomotil®) is another popular antidiarrheal agent. Bismuth subsalicylate (Pepto-Bismol®) is a secretion inhibitor that acts to prevent organisms from attaching to the intestinal mucosa and may deactivate certain toxins as well. In cases of infectious diarrhea, antibiotics such as metronidazole and vancomycin may also be indicated and ordered in conjunction with other therapies. Note: Some antibiotics can kill normal bacterial flora or facilitate regrowth of resistant microorganisms, and so lead to diarrhea.

Antiemetics

This class of drugs treats the condition of nausea and vomiting. There are many causes for this condition which is usually a symptom or side effect as opposed to being the actual condition itself: food or drug reaction or allergy, pregnancy, anxiety, exhaustion, dehydration, and a large number of diseases or illnesses such as cancer, or a microorganism related infectious process such as a middle ear infection. Often, antiemetics are ordered concurrently with other drug therapies used to treat the underlying condition. Examples are trimethobenzamide (Tigan®) and prochlorperazine (Compazine®). Vomiting is a reflex that occurs from a variety of stimuli. The treatment is to reduce the hyperactivity of stimuli receptors and lower the impulse rate. Also, decreasing the sensitivity to emetic chemicals found in the blood will inhibit the vomiting reflex. Dehydration and electrolyte imbalance are of major concern with prolonged vomiting.

Some Common Gastrointestinal Tract Drugs: Enzymes, Antidiarrheals, and Antiemetics		
Type	**Brand Name**	**Generic Name**
Enzyme	Creon	pancrelipase
Enzyme	Pancrease	pancrelipase
Enzyme	Ultrace	pancrelipase
Antidiarrheal	Imodium	loperamide
Antidiarrheal	Lomotil	diphenoxylate plus atropine
Antidiarrheal	Pepto-Bismol	bismuth subsalicylate
Antiemetic	Tigan	trimethobenzamide
Antiemetic	Compazine	prochlorperazine

See Additional Common Drugs by Classification on pp 473-477 for more drugs in this class.

GASTROINTESTINAL & URINARY TRACT AGENTS

Antacid/Antiulcer Agents

Antacids, generally composed of inorganic salts such as calcium carbonate, aluminum hydroxide, and magnesium hydroxide are popular antiulcer agents that act to neutralize existing acid, as opposed to inhibiting its production. Antacids are most indicated at the onset of hypergastric activity, are pain relieving yet short acting, and not strong enough for a diagnosed ulcer condition. Caution should be exercised to not rely on antacids alone or for a prolonged time. If ulcer symptoms persist, the physician should be notified. Maalox® Advanced Liquid is an example of a common antacid.

Cimetidine is a histamine receptor antagonist. It inhibits the secretion of gastric acid by blocking the effects of histamine. This type of agent was first approved for use in 1977 and revolutionized standard antacid therapy. Cimetidine has a history of drug interactions, however, and improved histamine antagonists such as ranitidine (Zantac®), famotidine (Pepcid®), and nizatidine (Axid®) have since been developed.

Omeprazole (Prilosec®) is a proton-pump inhibitor. It works by decreasing the amount of acid made in the stomach. Omeprazole is available a delayed-release capsule (Prilosec®), a non-prescription delayed-release tablet (Prilosec OTC®), a powder for suspension (Zegerid®), and a regular capsule (Zegerid®).

Peptic ulcer is caused by hypergastric acidity that erodes tissue in localized areas of the stomach and intestines. While these lesions are normally benign, they may produce symptoms that are mild and of minor discomfort or they may be more serious and extend to underlying layers of connective tissue and smooth muscle. In these cases, blood vessels can be affected and bleeding can occur. A special dietary regime (i.e., frequent, small, bland, non-acid containing meals) together with selected drug therapy is commonly recommended for treatment of this condition.

Gastric reflux is a more serious gastric acid condition that is often treated with a strong antacid.

Laxatives and Stool Softeners

These agents are commonly prescribed to treat constipation, the condition of dehydrated stool in which bowel movements are infrequent, hard, and often painful and difficult. Aside from changing a patient's diet, fluid intake and activity level, drug therapy may be suggested. Laxatives promote defecation without stress or pain and are often suggested for use prior to certain medical procedures related to the bowel (e.g., colonoscopy, barium enema), for constipation, and for patients who have hemorrhoids, recent hernia surgery, or a heart attack.

There are several types of laxatives available: bulk forming, that swell as they mix with intestinal contents; stimulant, that irritate the lining and nerves of the intestine; saline, that rapidly promote watery stool by drawing water into the intestine; and osmotic, that increase the stool's water content using osmosis. The osmotic laxative is often used as a retention enema, although it can be powerful and cause cramping. Lactulose (Kristalose®) is an example of a commonly prescribed saline laxative.

Docusate sodium (Colace®) is a commonly ordered stool softener, or emollient laxative. It promotes the mixing of fatty and watery intestinal substances to soften the stool's contents and ease the evacuation of feces.

Enemas may be placed into this category since they are indicated in cases of constipation, pre-medical treatment, and to ease the stress of bowel movements. Fleets®, sodium biphosphate and sodium phosphate, is a popular saline enema.

R̸ safety you should know

➡ Phenazopyridine may discolor urine reddish orange and an auxiliary label about urine discoloration may be helpful to the patient.

Urinary Tract Agents

Urinary agents are used to treat conditions affecting the flow of urine. Symptoms can include difficulty urinating, painful urination, and urinary frequency and urgency. One common condition that affects urination in males is benign prostatic hyperplasia (BPH). Examples of drugs that are used include drugs to treat BPH include tamsulosin (Flomax®), alfuzosin (Uroxatral®), finasteride (Proscar®), and dutasteride (Avodart®). Other urinary drugs are used to treat urinary frequency and include tolterodine (Detrol LA®), darifenacin (Enablex®), and solifenacin (Vesicare®).

Some Common Gastrointestinal Tract Drugs: Antacid/Antiulcer and Laxatives & Stool Softeners

Type	Brand Name	Generic Name
Antacid/antiulcer	Maalox Advanced Liquid	magnesium hydroxide, aluminum hydroxide, simethicone
Antacid/antiulcer	Tagamet	cimetidine
Antacid/antiulcer	Zantac	ranitidine
Antacid/antiulcer	Pepcid	famotidine
Antacid/antiulcer	Axid	nizatidine
Antacid/antiulcer; proton pump inhibitor	Prilosec	omeprazole
Laxative	Kristalose	lactulose
Stool softener	Colace	docusate sodium

See Additional Common Drugs by Classification on pp 473–477 for more drugs in this class.

Some Common Urinary Tract Agents

Type	Brand Name	Generic Name
Urinary tract agent	Flomax	tamsulosin
Urinary tract agent	Uroxatral	alfuzosin
Urinary tract agent	Proscar	finasteride
Urinary tract agent	Avodart	dutasteride
Urinary tract agent	Detrol LA	tolterodine
Urinary tract agent	Enablex	darifenacin
Urinary tract agent	Vesicare	solifenacin
Urinary tract agent	Pyridium	phenazopyridine

R̸ safety you should know

➡ Cimetidine has several significant drug interactions. You should check with the pharmacist when alerted to drug interactions with cimetidine.

➡ Misoprostol is contraindicated during pregnancy.

➡ Some antacids have significant drug interactions with tetracyclines.

➡ Most antispasmodics can cause dizziness, drowsiness or blurred vision.

➡ Sulfasalazine is contraindicated in patients who are hypersensitive to sulfasalazine, its metabolites, sulfonamides, or salicylates.

➡ Women who are, could become, or may be pregnant should not touch broken or crushed finasteride tablets. If taken by pregnant women, finasteride can harm the male fetus.

HEMATOLOGICAL AGENTS

Blood coagulation or clotting is a complex process in which the protein *fibrinogen* is transformed to an insoluble fiber called *fibrin.* The enzyme thrombin, which comes from prothrombin, acts on fibrinogen in the blood to cause the transformation. Prothrombin and fibrinogen are **clotting factors** or coagulation factors. Other clotting factors, adequate platelets, and healthy blood vessel walls are also essential components to balanced coagulation.

Each stage of clot development can be affected by clotting factors as well as drugs.

For example, patients with hemophilia A have a genetic deficiency in factor VIII (*most clotting factors are denoted by Roman Numerals*) and can be successfully treated with concentrates of Antihemophilic Factor (AHF) that are commercially available. Factor VIII concentrate or cryoprecipitate and desmopressin acetate (DDAVP®) are other agents that will act to shorten bleeding time. Von Willebrand's disease, a very common congenital coagulation disorder, is also caused by a deficiency in factor VIII. Factor IX concentrates (Christmas factor) are available for patients with hemophilia B, a condition marked by a deficiency in clotting factor IX.

Phytonadione (Mephyton®) , or Vitamin K$_1$, is a drug that stimulates the liver to produce several clotting factors and mimics the action of Vitamin K (a natural clotting promoter).

Patients who may develop Vitamin K deficiency and require coagulation enhancer therapy include "at risk" infants whose liver and intestines are not fully developed, users of antibiotics that "sterilize" the intestines and prevent vitamin K synthesis, and those with malabsorption disorders such as Whipple's Disease and obstructive jaundice. In addition, patients with liver disease may suffer with bleeding disorders since the liver is responsible for the synthesizing of many clotting factors.

Clotting

The main stages of natural clot formation and dissolution are:

Thromboplastin is formed from blood and tissue (platelet aggregation at injury site).

Thrombin is formed from prothrombin and thromboplastin.

The fiber fibrin is formed from thrombin acting on fibrinogen (clot formation).

Fibrinolysin breaks down fibrin (clot breakdown).

R̶ safety you should know

➡ Accidental overdose of products containing iron is a leading cause of fatal poisoning in children under the age of six.

➡ Although symptoms of iron deficiency usually improve within a few days, patients may have to take ferrous sulfate for several months.

Some Common Hematological Drugs		
Type	**Brand Name**	**Generic Name**
Hematopoietic	Slow Fe	ferrous sulfate
Hematopoietic	Rubramin	cyanocobalamin
Hemostatic	Amicar	aminocaproic acid
Hemostatic	Cyklokapron	tranexamic acid
Hemostatic/topical	Surgicel	oxidized cellulose

See Additional Common Drugs by Classification on pp 473-477 for more drugs in this class.

Hematopoietics are drugs that treat various forms of anemias by stimulating or helping to stimulate blood cell growth.

Anemias are generally characterized by a decrease in hemoglobin or red blood cells which leads to a series of other disorders manifested by oxygen deficiency. The classifications of anemias include cell shape and structure, cause, and the pathophysiology or disease tract the particular anemia will take.

Most commonly, anemias develop in the elderly from iron deficiency, as a result of genetic predisposition (e.g., Sickle Cell anemia), or due to vitamin B_{12} deficiency (pernicious anemia).

An additional type of anemia is associated with chronic disease. Correction of the underlying illness will improve this anemia. Anemias may also occur as a result of cancer or other diseases and treatments that cause bone marrow suppression and decrease of erythropoietin (which stimulates red blood cell production). In addition, a decrease in the granulocyte colony stimulating factor (G-CSF) and granulocyte macrophage colony stimulating factor (GM-CSF), excessive blood loss, infections, and inflammatory processes contribute to anemia. Common drug therapies for anemias include ferrous sulfate (Slow Fe®) for iron-deficiency anemia and cyanocobalamin (Crystamine®) for vitamin B_{12} deficiency anemia.

Hemostatic drugs are used to treat or prevent excessive bleeding.

Patients who have hemophilia or thrombocytic purpura may receive hemostatic medications. They suffer from a lack of platelets and/or blood clotting factors found in the first stage of clotting. Systemic hemostatic agents include aminocaproic acid and tranexamic acid. Their indications range from preventing hemorrhages during dental procedures to prevention of blood loss in cardiopulmonary bypass surgery. Their primary action is to inhibit the activation of plasminogen. **Topical hemostatics** are used for minor bleeding of small blood vessels when sutures are not appropriate. An example of a topical hemostatic is oxidized cellulose.

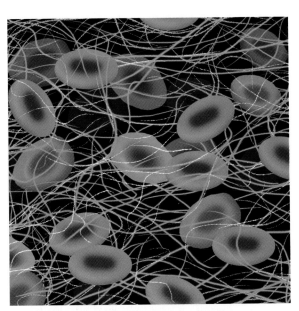

Strands of fibrin interweave and trap red blood cells to form a blood clot.

ABCD *clotting factors* factors in the blood coagulation process.

fibrinogen Factor I.

fibrin the fiber that serves as the structure for clot formation.

anemia a decrease in hemoglobin or red blood cells.

hematopoietics drugs used to treat anemia.

hemostatic drugs drugs that prevent excessive bleeding.

topical hemostatics drugs used for minor bleeding when sutures are not appropriate.

R Note: Drugs highlighted in green in the text and tables are parenteral drugs commonly found in hospitals and other institutional settings.

R Aside from drug therapy, patients with excessive bleeding may receive whole blood and blood products such as packed cells, platelets, and plasma to treat this serious situation.

HORMONES & MODIFIERS

Hormones are secretions of the *endocrine system's* ductless glands.

These substances control or influence a selected organ or set of organs to produce an effect. If a patient does not naturally produce enough or produces too much of a particular hormone, selected drugs can be given to stimulate or inhibit hormone secretion. These hormones and hormone modifiers can either be extracted from animals or reproduced synthetically.

The pituitary gland is also known as the "master gland" because it regulates the activities of the entire endocrine system.

This pea-sized organ is located deep within the cranium, at the base of the brain. In turn, another major system, the nervous system, greatly controls the pituitary gland and together these two systems are responsible for a large number of our body's regulatory processes.

The thyroid gland is located in front of the trachea and secretes hormones that affect metabolism, growth, and central nervous system development.

Thyroxine (T_4) and triiodothyronine (T_3) are thyroid hormones. Their normal secretion is dependent on appropriate amounts of iodine and TSH (thyroid stimulating hormone) in the circulating blood. **Hyperthyroidism** is a disorder of overproduction of thyroid hormones that increases the metabolism. Symptoms include increased nervousness and heart rate. Treatment includes surgery and antithyroid medications. **Hypothyroidism** is a disorder of underproduction of thyroid hormone, resulting in a lower metabolism. Symptoms include tiredness, low blood pressure, slow heart rate, and weight gain. Treatment includes thyroid hormone and increased dietary intake of iodine.

 endocrine system the system of hormone secreting glands.

hormone a chemical secretion that influences or controls an organ or organs in the body.

hyperthyroidism overproduction of thyroid hormone.

hypothyroidism underproduction of thyroid hormone.

THE ENDOCRINE SYSTEM

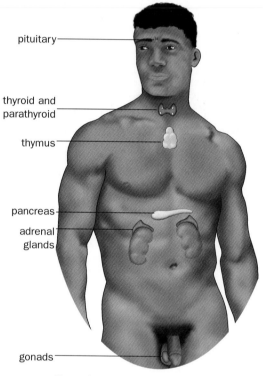

pituitary

thyroid and parathyroid

thymus

pancreas

adrenal glands

gonads

Note: the gonads of males are called testes and of females, ovaries.

Pituitary Gland
➥ Regulation of endocrine system and growth.

Thyroid and Parathyroid
➥ Metabolic and calcium regulation.

Thymus
➥ Lymphatic regulation.

Pancreas
➥ Blood sugar regulation.

Adrenal Glands
➥ Metabolism and energy regulation.

Gonads
➥ Sexual characteristics.

Divided into posterior and anterior lobes, the pituitary gland controls metabolism, growth, water loss and retention, electrolyte balance, and the reproductive cycle.

An example of a hormone secreted by the posterior lobe is ADH or antidiuretic hormone. Also known as vasopressin, this hormone acts to help the kidneys conserve water and prevent dehydration. Diabetes Insipidus is caused by a deficiency in this hormone and marked by excretion of large amounts of urine (polyuria) and excessive thirst (polydipsia).

Oxytocin is another posterior lobe hormone.

It helps stimulate uterine contraction and promote birth or inhibit uterine bleeding post birth.

FSH or follicle stimulating hormone is an anterior lobe hormone called a gonadatropin (stimulator of reproductive organ function).

It acts to stimulate the egg follicle to produce eggs. Clomiphene is a popular synthetic nonsteroidal agent used to induce ovulation and establish fertility in otherwise unfertile women.

The Parathyroid Glands

PTH (parathyroid hormone) and calcitonin are the hormones secreted by the parathyroid glands.

These hormones regulate the body's serum calcium and phosphorus levels which are integral to normal muscle contraction, bone formation, blood coagulation, milk production in the lactating mother, and nerve impulse conduction. These four small round organs are located behind the thyroid gland and reduction of their function can cause low calcium levels, convulsions, and possible death. Calcitonin-salmon is a common parathyroid gland synthetic hormone.

℞ safety you should know
➥ Brands of drugs used for thyroid hormone replacement are not generally interchangeable. Take special care to check with your pharmacist before substituting.

℞ Note: Drugs highlighted in green in the text and tables are parenteral drugs commonly found in hospitals and other institutional settings.

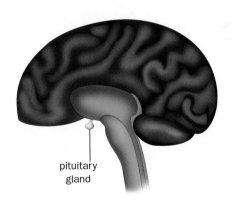

pituitary gland

Some Common Hormones & Modifiers: Thyroid, Parathyroid, and Pituitary Drugs		
Type	Brand Name	Generic Name
Thyroid	Armour Thyroid	thyroid desiccated
Thyroid	Synthroid	levothyroxine
Parathyroid	Miacalcin	calcitonin-salmon
Pituitary/ovulatory stimulant	Clomid	clomiphene
Pituitary/hypothalamus	Pitocin	oxytocin

See Additional Common Drugs by Classification on pp 473–477 for more drugs in this class.

HORMONES & MODIFIERS

Located above each kidney, the adrenal glands consist of an outer section, the cortex, and an inner section, the medulla.

The cortex secretes **corticosteroids** which regulate the body's ability to handle stress, resist infection, affect glucose, fat, protein and carbohydrate metabolism and maintain salt and water balance. The adrenal medulla secretes the neurotransmitter epinephrine which acts as a stimulator to the sympathetic nervous system.

This hormone, referred to as a catecholamine, is generally released during stress or activities of "fight or flight."

Epinephrine will generally cause a rise in blood pressure, strength and rate of heart beat, blood glucose, metabolic rate, a relaxation of bronchi muscles, coronary and uterine muscles, and dilation of the eye's pupil. Epinephrine is commercially available and used often in serious or medical emergency situations.

Adrenal Glands

The adrenal glands sit atop the kidneys. They secrete corticosteroids and epinephrine, which influence many aspects of metabolism and energy regulation.

Corticosteroids

Hydrocortisone and methylprednisolone are two adrenal cortex corticosteroids that act to control anti-inflammatory response and the immune response system. In the 1940's cortisone was recognized as having anti-inflammatory properties. Since then, many synthetic corticosteroids such as prednisone (Sterapred®) and triamcinolone (Kenalog®) have been developed and indicated for a number of inflammatory conditions (e.g., arthritis, intestinal disorders, and various respiratory pathologies).

The corticosteroid aldosterone helps maintain an adequate supply of serum sodium which accommodates sufficient extracellular fluid or blood volume. A severe deficiency in aldosterone could lead to low blood pressure and circulatory collapse.

R **safety you should know**
➥ Corticosteroids should not be abruptly discontinued.

Some Common Hormones & Modifiers: Adrenal Drugs		
Type	**Brand Name**	**Generic Name**
Adrenal/sympathomimetic	Adrenalin	epinephrine
Adrenal/corticosteroid	Cortef	hydrocortisone
Adrenal/corticosteroid	Medrol	methylprednisolone
Adrenal/corticosteroid	Sterapred	prednisone
Adrenal/corticosteroid	Kenalog	triamcinolone

See Additional Common Drugs by Classification on pp 473–477 for more drugs in this class.

ABCD *corticosteroid* hormonal steroid substances produced by the cortex of the adrenal gland.

insulin a hormone that controls the body's use of glucose.

glucagon a hormone that helps convert amino acids to glucose.

diabetes mellitus a condition in which the body does not produce enough insulin or is unable to use it efficiently.

serum glucose blood sugar.

Islands (or Islets) of Langerhans specialized cells of the pancreas that secrete insulin.

℞ Note: Drugs highlighted in green in the text and tables are parenteral drugs commonly found in hospitals and other institutional settings.

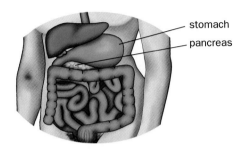

The pancreas is located behind the stomach.

stomach
pancreas

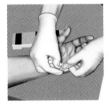 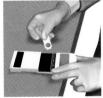

Glucose Monitoring

Patients with diabetes mellitus routinely monitor their blood glucose levels with a glucometer. This involves taking a small blood sample, usually from a fingertip, and inserting the sample into the glucometer for analysis. Newer systems are being developed that read glucose levels through the skin and do not require blood specimens.

The pancreas secretes the hormones *insulin* and *glucagon*.

The pancreas is an irregularly shaped organ located between the adrenal glands and behind the stomach. A specialized cluster of pancreatic beta cells called the **Islands (or Islets) of Langerhans** produce insulin, a hormone that controls the body's use of glucose, its normal source of energy. The alpha cells of the pancreas secrete the hormone glucagon which helps convert amino acids (by products of protein digestion) to glucose and raise the level of **serum glucose** (blood sugar). As the serum glucose level increases in a healthy individual, insulin secretion is stimulated. Glucagon and insulin ideally work together to strike a delicate balance and maintain homeostasis. Glucagon is available commercially and given to release glucose into the blood stream for severely hypoglycemic patients.

Without adequate insulin levels, serum glucose is not reabsorbed into the intestine, and it spills into the urine for excretion.

Instead of using glucose as it should, the body uses fat and protein as energy sources. This condition, **diabetes mellitus**, is marked by frequent urination, excessive thirst, elevated blood glucose levels, and positive urine glucose and acetone levels. In the early 1920's, Canadian researchers noted a link between the absence of a pancreas and diabetic symptoms. Insulin (i.e., Humulin® N, Humulin® R, Humulin® 70/30, and Lantus®) is given to treat diabetes mellitus. Several oral diabetic agents are also available (i.e., glyburide and glipizide). Note that insulin does not cure diabetes. It is merely a treatment for it.

℞ safety you should know
➡ Diabetic patients using insulin should consistently use the same type and brand of syringe.

Some Common Hormones & Modifiers: Insulin and Oral Antidiabetic Drugs		
Type	**Brand Name**	**Generic Name**
Insulin	Humulin N	NPH
Insulin	Humulin R	regular
Insulin	Humulin L	lente
Insulin	Lantus	glargine
Oral antidiabetic	Diabeta	glyburide
Oral antidiabetic	Glucotrol	glipizide

See Additional Common Drugs by Classification on pp 473–477 for more drugs in this class.

HORMONES & MODIFIERS

The ovaries are almond shaped organs found on either side of the uterus within the female pelvis.

Under control of the anterior pituitary gland, the ovaries are responsible for the production of ova (eggs) as well as the secretion of the hormones **estrogen** and **progesterone**. These hormones are essential for primary and secondary sex characteristic development, menstruation, healthy pregnancies (gestation), and milk production (lactation).

The testes secretes the male hormone *testosterone*.

Male hormones are called **androgens**. The development and maintenance of the male reproductive tract includes enhancement of secondary sexual characteristics, muscle development, sex organ growth, and body fat distribution. In addition, testosterone also contributes to the building of tissues and prevention of their breakdown. Commercially available testosterone products are often indicated in cases of male hypogonadism or in females for certain breast cancers or engorgement. Methyltestosterone is a common example of this androgen.

Besides androgens, another class of drugs called phosphodiesterase inhibitors is used to treat erectile dysfunction.

Popular erectile dysfunction medications include Cialis® and Viagra®.

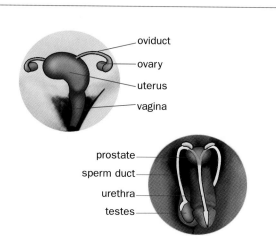

- oviduct
- ovary
- uterus
- vagina

- prostate
- sperm duct
- urethra
- testes

Estrogen

First produced in large quantities at puberty, women secrete estrogens until menopause. Due to their adjunctive role in calcium and phosphorus conservation, many women receive replacement estrogen therapy in their post menopausal years.

Women who experience a lack of these hormones during their child bearing years and/or post menopause, may receive them as natural and synthetic products.

Synthetic estrogen may also be indicated in cases of breast engorgement, to stunt female growth in height, and for men with prostate cancer.

Estradiol and Premarin are examples of an estrogen mix/replacement. Estrogens are generally contraindicated in cases of breast and/or genital cancer history or if there has been unexplained uterine bleeding.

Progesterone

Progesterone, which is naturally responsible for placenta development and prevention of ovulation, may be indicated in cases of amenorrhea (absence of menstruation), endometreosis (sloughing off of uterine tissue with subsequent attachment to other pelvic organs), dysfunctional uterine bleeding, and for oral contraceptive use.

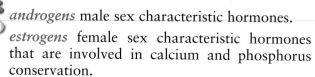

androgens male sex characteristic hormones.

estrogens female sex characteristic hormones that are involved in calcium and phosphorus conservation.

progestins female sex characteristic hormones that are involved in ovulation prevention.

testosterone the primary androgen.

Oral Contraceptives

There are three types of oral contraceptives:

- monophasic,
- biphasic, and
- triphasic.

Monophasic contraceptives offer a fixed dose of estrogen and progestin (progesterone) while the biphasic and triphasic types deliver the hormones more as they would be naturally secreted by the ovaries.

Ortho Novum®, depending on its estrogen/progestin mix, is an example of an oral contraceptive available as any one of the three above mentioned types.

Other oral contraceptives include Trinessa®, Yasmin 28®, Ortho Tricyclen Lo®, and Ortho Evra®, a contraceptive patch.

Some Common Hormones & Modifiers: Reproductive System Drugs

Type	Brand Name	Generic Name
Androgen	Android	methyltestosterone
Phosphodiesterase inhibitor	Cialis	tadalafil
Phosphodiesterase inhibitor	Viagra	sildenafil
Oral contraceptive	Ortho Novum	norethindrone and ethinyl estradiol
Oral contraceptive	Trinessa	norgestimate and ethinyl estradiol
Oral contraceptive	Yasmin 28	drospirenone and ethinyl estradiol
Oral contraceptive	Ortho Tricyclen Lo	norgestimate and ethinyl estradiol
Contraceptive patch	Ortho Evra Patch	norelgestromin and ethinyl estradiol
Estrogen replacement	Vagifem	estradiol
Estrogen replacement	Premarin	conjugated estrogens
Progestin	Provera	medroxyprogesterone

See Additional Common Drugs by Classification on pp 473–477 for more drugs in this class.

R safety you should know

- Antibiotics, especially penicillins, tetracyclines, and griseofulvin, can have significant interactions with oral contraceptives.
- Anticonvulsants (especially Tegretol®, Dilantin®, and Topamax®) can have significant interactions with oral contraceptives.
- St. John's Wort can have a significant interaction with oral contraceptives.
- Cigarette smoking can increase the risk of serious side effects from oral contraceptives; the risk is higher for women over 35 years old and heavy smokers.
- Some oral contraceptives have other uses including menstrual cycle regularity, dysmenorrhea, and acne vulgaris.

IMMUNOBIOLOGIC AGENTS & VACCINES

Immunity against pathogens is either passive or active.

Passive immunity occurs when a patient is given a pre-formed antibody from another source, such as with immune globulins. Active immunity occurs when the body is exposed to a pathogen, develops the disease, and manufactures its own antibodies against a future invasion, such as with vaccines.

Immune globulins are specialized proteins that provide passive immunity.

The antibodies used in immune globulins are produced by other humans or animals and are recovered through high tech purification processes. Injections of immune globulins are not as common in contemporary medical practice as they were in the past, but the FDA has approved immune globulins for tetanus, diphtheria, measles, mumps, Hepatitis A and B, and chicken pox. Candidates for immune globulin injections include patients who have been exposed to these diseases but have not been previously vaccinated for them, as well as people who have contracted diseases such as botulism and rabies. Immunoglobulins can also address issues associated with blood type and tissue compatibility between kidney donors and recipients.

One negative aspect of passive immunity is that it generally offers a shorter period of protection than does active immunity.

Another concern is the possibility of allergic reaction that may occur in some individuals. Further, hypersensitization may follow the receipt of passive immunity and render the host more prone to allergic response with each subsequent exposure. Severe anaphylactic reactions are possible.

Most vaccines provide an active form of immunity.

Vaccines are suspensions containing infectious agents used to boost the body's own immune system response. Toxoids are sometimes used in some vaccines to cause an immune response. The toxoids of diphtheria and tetanus provide two examples of toxoids that are used in vaccines.

IMMUNE GLOBULINS

Pathogens for which animals antibodies may be used for immune globulins:

➥ Diphtheria (using Antitoxin, USP)
➥ Rabies (using Antirabies serum)
➥ Botulism
➥ Black Widow Spider Venom

Human antibodies are used in immune globulins in the treatment of:

➥ Measles (using Measles Immune Globulin, USP)
➥ Pertussis (using Pertussis Immune Globulin, USP)
➥ Mumps (using Mumps Immune Globulin, USP)
➥ Tetanus (using Tetanus Immune Globulin, USP)
➥ Hepatitis A and B.

Note: Diphtheria, Tetanus, Hepatitis B, Measles, Mumps, and Rabies may also be treated with vaccines.

Some Common Immune Globulins	
Brand Name	**Type**
Flebogamma	immune globulin (human)
Octagam	immune globulin (human)
Gammagard	immune globulin (human)
Gamunex	immune globulin (human)
Carimune NF	immune globulin (human)
Iveegam EN	immune globulin (human)
Privigen	immune globulin (human)

Rx In 1999 the U.S. Public Health Service and the American Academy of Pediatrics as a precautionary measure issued a joint statement urging vaccine manufacturers to eliminate thimerosal, a preservative, from vaccines routinely administered to children age 6 and under. However, some versions of the inactivated influenza vaccine do still use it, and other vaccines may still contain trace amounts, as indicated on package inserts. Source: FDA.gov.

℞ Note: Drugs highlighted in green in the text and tables are parenteral drugs commonly found in hospitals and other institutional settings.

INFLUENZA & H1N1 VACCINES

Because influenza viruses are always changing, the content of the seasonal influenza vaccine changes each year. Protection for three different viruses is included in typical influenza vaccines.

Influenza vaccines are available as an intramuscular injection or nasal spray. The nasal spray contains a live attenuated virus and has been approved only for patients between the ages of 2–49; it is contraindicated for pregnant women and there are restrictions for individuals within the eligible age group who have asthma or wheezing conditions, have experienced Guillain-Barré syndrome, or have a weakened immune system, heart disease, kidney disease, or diabetes.

In June, 2009, the World Health Organization (WHO) issued a worldwide pandemic alert for the H1N1 or "Swine Flu" virus, which is different from the seasonal flu virus. An H1N1 vaccine was developed in addition to the seasonal flu vaccine for the 2009–2010 flu season. Like the seasonal flu vaccine, the H1N1 vaccine is available both as an intramuscular injection and nasal spray.

In the last half of the 20th century many new vaccines were developed.

These include DPT (diphtheria, pertussis and tetanus), MMR (measles, mumps and rubella), Polio, Typhoid, Rabies, Hepatitis A and B, BCG (an antitubercular agent), Haemophilus Influenzae Type B (Hib), and Chicken Pox. Today, state laws require most children to have a certification of immunization against most of these diseases, and others, prior to attending school. This has resulted in both a dramatic decrease in the incidence of these diseases and also in the average child receiving 32 doses of 13 different viral and bacterial vaccines by age six.

Vaccine Information Statements (VIS) prepared by the Centers for Disease Control and Prevention (CDC) provide information about the risks and benefits of each vaccine.

The National Childhood Vaccine Injury Act (NCVIA) requires healthcare providers to provide a copy of the VIS to either the adult recipient or a child's parent/legal representative before administering the following vaccines: diphtheria, tetanus, pertussis, measles, mumps, rubella, polio, hepatitis A, hepatitis B, Haemophilus influenzae type b (Hib), influenza, and pneumococcal conjugate. The vaccine information statements are available at http://www.immunize.org/vis/. Adverse reactions to vaccines should be reported through the Vaccine Adverse Event Reporting System (VAERS) maintained by the CDC.

Some Common Vaccines	
Brand Name	**Vaccine**
Daptacel, Infanrix, Tripedia	Diphtheria, Tetanus, Pertussis (DTaP, DT, Tdap, Td)
Liquid Pedvax HIB, ActHIB, HibTITER	Haemophilus influenzae type b (Hib)
Havrix, VAQTA	Hepatitis A (HepA)
Engerix-B, Recombivax HB, Twinrix	Hepatitis B (HepB)
FluMist	Influenza, live attenuated (LAIV)
Afluria, Fluarix, FluLaval, Fluvirin, Fluzone	Influenza, trivalent inactivated (TIV)
Attenuvax, M-M-R II, Mumpsvax, Meruvax II	Measles, mumps, rubella (MMR)
Menomune	Meningococcal, conjugated (MCV4)
Prevnar	Pneumococcal conjugate (PCV)
Pneumovax 23	Pneumococcal polysaccharide (PPV)
Varivax	Varicella (Var)
Comvax	Hib+HepB (combination)
Pediarix	DTaP+HepB+IPV (combination)
ProQuad	MMR+Var (combination)
TriHIBit	DTaP+Hib (combination)

MUSCULOSKELETAL AGENTS

Rheumatoid arthritis is a chronic and often progressive inflammatory condition linked to the dysfunction of the immune system. Antibodies called rheumatoid factors contribute to the course of the disease. Inflammation caused by the release of histamine and prostaglandins leads to swelling, feelings of warmth, and pain in joints (especially in the hands, wrists, feet, hips, knees, and ankles). As the disease progresses, a decrease in range of motion and an increase in bony fusion and muscle deformity may occur. Patients often show fatigue, low-grade fever, stiffness, and joint pain, especially in the morning.

There is no known cure or method of prevention for rheumatoid arthritis.

Treatment may include drug therapy, physical therapy, occupational therapy, weight reduction, rest, and the use of adaptive or assistive devices. Drug therapy primarily consists of NSAIDs that inhibit prostaglandins synthesis and reduce inflammation. They are also the first line drug of choice due to their analgesic properties. However, as the condition progresses, disease modifying antirheumatic drugs (DMARD's) such as methotrexate (Rheumatrex®) as well as gold preparations such as aurothioglucose (suspended in oil) are indicated.

Gout **is an inflammatory condition in which an excess of uric acid and urate crystals accumulate in synovial fluids of the joints.**

This leads to joint swelling, redness, warmth, and pain. The cause of the gout may be dietary or due to a metabolism dysfunction. A patient may experience an acute attack of gouty arthritis with severe pain, fever, swelling of joints, and inflammation. Stress, diet (e.g., foods high in iodine such as shellfish), alcohol, and infection can precipitate an attack. A first line drug used to treat gouty arthritis would be colchicine. **Uricosuric drugs** such as probenecid (Benemid®) increase elimination of uric acid and xanthine oxidase inhibitors such as allopurinol (Zyloprim®) interfere with uric acid synthesis.

MUSCULAR SYSTEM

The muscular system is a complex system of connecting and overlapping muscles that completely cover the body. There are cardiac muscles in the heart and smooth muscles in the arteries and digestive tract, but most muscles are skeletal muscles attached to the skeleton by tendons. These muscles are made up of long muscle fibers that expand and contract to push and pull bones and cause body movement.

gout a painful inflammatory condition in which excess uric acid accumulates in the joints.

rheumatoid arthritis a chronic and often progressive inflammatory condition with symptoms that include swelling, feelings of warmth, and joint pain.

Some Common Musculoskeletal Drugs

Type	Brand Name	Generic Name
Disease-modifying antirheumatic	Rheumatrex	methotrexate
Gold preparation	Solganal	aurothioglucose (suspended in oil)
Anti-gout	Colchine	colchicine
Anti-gout, uricosuric	Benemid	probenecid
Anti-gout, xanthine oxidase inhibitor	Zyloprim	allopurinol

Note: Drugs highlighted in green in the text and tables are parenteral drugs commonly found in hospitals and other institutional settings.

SKELETAL SYSTEM

The skeletal system works with the muscular system to provide precise and powerful movement. The system's 206 bones are called axial (brain and spinal column) or appendicular (arms, legs, and connecting bones). They are held together at joints by connective tissue called ligaments and cartilage. Joints range from rigid to those allowing full motion. The hinge joints of the knee, elbow and ankle allow motion along a single axis. The ball-and-socket joints of the hips and shoulders allow a much broader range of movement.

osteoarthritis a disorder characterized by weight-bearing bone deterioration, decreasing range of motion, pain, and deformity.

uricosuric drugs drugs used to treat gout that increase the elimination of uric acid.

Osteoarthritis and osteoporosis are marked by weight-bearing bone deterioration, decreasing range of motion, and increasing pain, deformity, and disability.

Water content changes in the bone cartilage weakens the bones, causes cartilage damage and prevents repair. Inflammation may occur. Deep aching and local pain is experienced but can initially be relieved by rest. However, as the disease progresses, pain becomes chronic. Deformity also occurs in the later stages and bony enlargements (osteophytes) develop on the fingers and toes. Post-menopausal women, osteoporotic males and those with Paget disease may suffer from osteoporosis, resulting in bone mass and density loss. Common osteoporotic agents include risedronate (Actonel®) and alendronate (Fosamax®).

Drug therapy, physical therapy, adaptive or assistive devices, patient education, and possibly surgery are part of a comprehensive treatment approach.

Drug therapy primarily consists of analgesics, NSAID's, and corticosteroids. Since the majority of patients are elderly, drug treatment is directed at pain relief and is traditionally more conservative than aggressive.

Muscle spasms are painful occurrences that can be infrequent, chronic, or acute, depending on their origin and the patient's underlying medical condition.

Trauma, overwork, or a disorder such as connective tissue irritation can cause painful muscle contractions and involuntary spasms. Severe spasticity is usually linked to central nervous system disorders. Traditionally, treatment of muscle spasms is directed at muscle relaxation, pain relief, ability to exercise the muscle, and prevention of motion loss. Centrally acting antispasmodics such as diazepam (Valium®) eliminate contracture and cramps without affecting normal muscle activity. The sedative action of agent carisoprodol (Soma®) helps relieve acute musculoskeletal pain while cyclobenzaprine (Flexeril®) decreases muscle tone and reduces spasm.

Some Common Musculoskeletal Drugs

Type	Brand Name	Generic Name
Osteoporotic	Actonel	risedronate
Osteoporotic	Fosamax	alendronate
Centrally acting antispasmodics	Valium	diazepam
Muscle relaxant	Soma	carisoprodol
Muscle relaxant	Flexeril	cyclobenzaprine

NEUROLOGICAL AGENTS

Since nerve cells do not contact other neurons and the muscles they affect directly, nerve impulses are communicated by chemical transmission.

These chemical mediators are neurotransmitters or neurohormones. They cross the synapses (the junctions between nerve cells) and allow transmission of impulses from one neuron to another. Two common peripheral nerve neurotransmitters are acetylcholine and norepinephrine.

Several common neurological disorders are affected by abnormalities in neurotransmitter release and/or response.

This includes the following disorders: Parkinson's Disease, Alzheimer's Disease, epilepsy, migraine headaches, multiple sclerosis, and attention deficit (hyperactivity) disorder.

The Nervous System

The nervous system is divided into two main subsystems: the central nervous system (CNS) and the peripheral nervous system. The central nervous system consists of the brain and spinal cord. The peripheral nervous system carries information throughout the body and links the body's systems together. It is made up of the somatic nervous system and the autonomic nervous system.

The somatic nervous system is associated with voluntary movements of the musculoskeletal system and sensations (heat, cold, pressure and pain). The autonomic nervous system is responsible for automatic movements (breathing, digestion, etc.).

The autonomic nervous system is divided into the sympathetic and parasympathetic systems. The sympathetic branch works with the adrenal

NERVOUS SYSTEM

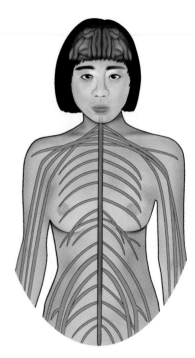

gland's medulla and regulates energy in times of stress such as danger, emotional tensions and severe illness. The parasympathetic branch influences bodily functions to slow down and conserve energy. The sympathetic and parasympathetic nervous systems effect a delicate balance and maintain homeostasis on a daily basis within the human body. Drugs referred to as mimics act upon these systems to affect this balance and force a reaction.

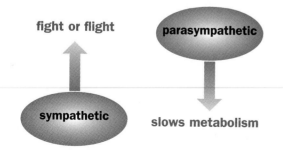

A Delicate Balance

The balance between the sympathetic and parasympathetic systems is illustrated in the "fight or flight" response. In the event of being threatened and frightened, the sympathetic system reacts to increase heart rate, deep breathing, and blood pressure (increases circulation of oxygen), dilate pupils (provides extra light for vision), increase liver glycogen breakdown (supplies glucose and oxygen to muscles for energy), and halt peristalsis. The parasympathetic system will restart digestive and peristaltic actions, constrict the pupils, slow the heart and respiratory rates, and lower blood pressure when the threat is removed.

DISORDERS

Parkinson's Disease

Parkinson's Disease is a progressive neuromuscular condition that usually affects patients above 50 years of age and is characterized by flat emotionless expression, bent posture, shuffling and unsteady gait, fine tremors, and difficulty chewing and swallowing. Early symptoms may include muscle aches, numbness, coldness, and loss of sensation or tingling. It is associated with low levels of the neurotransmitter dopamine in the brain and increased levels of acetylcholine. Brain tumors, arteriosclerosis, severe infectious processes, and excessive use of some antipsychotic drugs may also cause this disease.

Alzheimer's Disease

Alzheimer's, a progressive dementia often classified as a psychiatric disorder, has been linked to neurotransmitter abnormalities. It primarily affects the elderly. Loss of memory is often one of the first signs of this condition, with speech impairment, frustration, depression and decreased socialization soon occurring. These symptoms are generally followed by an inability to conduct the activities of daily living as well as a loss of spatial relationships. Ultimately, an inability to recognize familiar people and surroundings, wandering, combative aggression, and incontinence occur.

THERAPIES

Drug therapy will not stop the progress of this disease. Instead, an increased quality of life, decreased side effects, and minimization of disabilities are the goals of chemical treatment. Levodopa, carbidopa and levodopa together (Sinemet®), amantadine (Symmetrel®), and selegiline hydrochloride (Eldepryl®) are commonly prescribed antiparkinsonian drugs. In addition, dopamine agonists such as pergolide (Permax®) and bromocriptine (Parlodel®) are indicated when patients are experiencing a decrease in L-dopa's responsiveness. Anticholinergics are used for the treatment of tremors and decreased muscle tone.

Drug therapy can be divided into treatment for cognitive symptoms most closely associated with dementias and noncognitive symptoms such as depression. Tacrine (Cognex®) and donepezil (Aricept®) are examples of cognitive symptom agents while secondary amine tricyclic antidepressants such as nortriptyline (Pamelor®) and desipramine (Norpramin®) and SSRI's such as paroxetine (Paxil®) and sertraline (Zoloft®) are indicated for symptoms such as depression in the Alzheimer patient.

Some Common Neurological Drugs: Antiparkinsoniaon and Anti-Alzheimer

Type	Brand Name	Generic Name
Antiparkinsonian	Sinemet	carbidopa/levodopa
Antiparkinsonian	Eldepryl	selegiline hydrochloride
Antiparkinsonian	Symmetrel	amantadine
Antiparkinsonian/dopamine agonist	Permax	pergolide
Antiparkinsonian/dopamine agonist	Parlodel	bromocriptine
Antiparkinsonian/anticholinergic	Cogentin	benztropine
Cognitive symptom agent	Cognex	tacrine
Cognitive symptom agent	Aricept	donepezil
Antidepressant	Pamelor	nortriptyline
Antidepressant	Norpramin	desipramine
SSRI	Paxil	paroxetine
SSRI	Zoloft	sertraline

See Additional Common Drugs by Classification on pp 473–477 for more drugs in this class.

NEUROLOGICAL AGENTS (cont'd)

DISORDERS

THERAPIES

Epilepsy

Epilepsy is a neurologic disorder associated with neuron transmission instability and characterized by recurrent seizure activity. Though there are other causes for seizures (trauma, fever, stress, etc.), the excess excitability seen in seizures may be linked to an imbalance of dopamine and acetylcholine release coupled with factors such as improper pH balance or an inadequate supply of glucose, oxygen, potassium, calcium, or amino acids.

Common antiepileptic drugs include phenytoin (Dilantin®) and phenobarbital. Other drugs include valproic acid (Depakene®), divalproex sodium (Depakote®), and carbamazepine (Tegretol®). With anticonvulsant agents, the diagnosis needs to be conclusive and the most appropriate drug for the specific seizure type is chosen.

Migraine Headaches

There are two common theories on the causes of migraine headaches: the *vascular* and *nerve theories.* The vascular theory is that arterial vasoconstriction causes loss of oxygen and inflammation that stimulates sensory nerves in the head and results in possible auras and pain. An aura is an unusual sensation that can include hallucination. Stress, intense lights, colors, and sounds, and sleep deprivation are all considered stimulants of vasoconstriction. The nerve theory is that inflammation of nerve endings in the brain by inflammatory neurotransmitters (i.e., prostaglandins) causes pain.

Aspirin is considered the drug of choice (with caution used when treating children), and NSAID's are especially useful if the patient is female and menstruating. Other drug therapies include: sumatriptan (Imitrex®), and ibuprofen (Motrin®). Prophylactic treatment may include: beta-blockers, antidepressants, calcium channel blockers, corticosteroids and anticonvulsants.

Multiple Sclerosis

Multiple sclerosis is a disease in which the body's immune response attacks the person's central nervous system. In multiple sclerosis, nerve cells become demyelinated.

Treatment is aimed at improving function after an attack, preventing new attacks, and preventing disability. Immunomodulators (e.g., interferon beta-1-a and interferon beta-1-b) are used to reduce symptoms and slow the development of disability in patients with some forms of multiple sclerosis.

Attention Deficit (Hyperactivity) Disorder AD(H)D

Attention-deficit (hyperactivity) disorder or AD(H)D is a condition that can affect children and often continues into adulthood. Problems associated with ADHD include inattention, hyperactivity and impulsive behavior.

Examples of drugs to treat ADHD include methylphenidate (Concerta®, Methylin®, Ritalin®) and dextroamphetamine/amphetamine (Adderall®).

Some Common Neurological Drugs for Epilepsy, Migraine, Multiple Sclerosis, and AD(H)D

Type	Brand Name	Generic Name
Antiepileptic	Dilantin	phenytoin
Antiepileptic	Luminal	phenobarbital
Antiepileptic	Depakene	valproic acid
Antiepileptic	Depakote	divalproex sodium
Antiepileptic	Tegretol	carbamazepine
Antimigraine	Bayer Aspirin	aspirin
Antimigraine	Imitrex	sumatriptan
Antimigraine	Motrin	ibuprofen
Immunomodulator	Avonex	interferon beta-1a
Immunomodulator	Betaseron	interferon beta-1b
Immunomodulator	Copaxone	glatiramer acetate
Immunomodulator	Rebif	interferon beta-1a
AD(H)D	Concerta	methylphenidate
AD(H)D	Methylin	methylphenidate
AD(H)D	Ritalin	methylphenidate
AD(H)D	Adderall	dextroamphetamine/amphetamine

See Additional Common Drugs by Classification on pp 473–477 for more drugs in this class.

Rx safety you should know

- There are many important drug interactions with some seizure medications such as carbamazepine, phenytoin, and phenobarbital. Some drugs are contraindicated with some seizure medications. Alert your pharmacist when prompted about drug interactions.

- Divalproex sodium and valproic acid have been associated with birth defects if taken by women during pregnancy.

- Anticonvulsants should not be stopped abruptly when used as anticonvulsants.

- Many drugs used to treat AD(H)D are in DEA Schedule II and have a high potential for abuse. Because they are in DEA Schedule II, they have special requirements for inventory, labeling, and recordkeeping.

- Some drug interactions for selegiline are dangerous and therefore contraindicated. Alert the pharmacist when drug interactions with selegiline arise.

- Sumatriptan and related drugs have some serious drug interactions and are therefore contraindicated. Alert the pharmacist when drug interactions with sumatriptan or other related drugs for treating migraines arise.

OPHTHALMIC & OTIC AGENTS

Ophthalmic agents are used to treat various conditions or disorders of the eye.

Disorders include **glaucoma**, infection, pain, and inflammation, but agents may also be used for eye examinations and in preparation for surgery. Ophthalmic agents are generally applied topically as drops or ointments.

Due to the special requirements for ophthalmic formulations, there are often many ingredients in a product besides the active ingredient.

Preservatives, antioxidants, buffers, and wetting agents that control such factors as pH, sterility, and proper isotonic percentages are often included.

Glaucoma represents several disorders characterized by abnormally high pressure within the eye that leads to optic nerve damage and progressive loss of vision.

The onset of glaucoma can be a slow process that may not be apparent to the patient and may only be detected during an eye examination. Early detection is essential for successful treatment and prevention of vision loss.

Although infection and inflammation can increase *intraocular* pressure temporarily, the common cause of glaucoma is a structural defect in the eye.

This form is called primary glaucoma and is divided into two types: narrow- or closed-angle and wide- or open-angle. Narrow-angle glaucoma is corrected with surgery. Open-angle glaucoma can be successfully treated with antiglaucoma drugs such as cholinergic receptor agonists, acetylcholinesterase inhibitors, carbonic anhydrase inhibitors, beta-adrenergic receptor antagonists, and adrenergic receptor agonists.

THE EYE

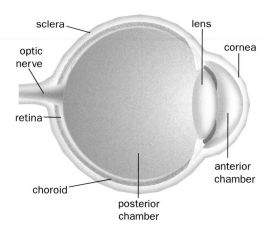

The eyeball has three layers:
- ➥ the outer layer contains the sclera (white part) and the cornea (clear);
- ➥ the middle vascular layer called the choroid contains the iris and pupil;
- ➥ the inner layer contains the retina, responsible for visual reception.

Both the anterior and posterior optic chambers are filled with a liquid called aqueous humor. The lens is located behind the iris. Ocular muscles control the movement of the eyeball and accommodate focusing. The thickness of the lens helps determine the distance at which one can see an object. Behind the lens, a jelly-like substance called the vitreous body helps maintain the shape of the eyeball.

Similar to a camera, the pupil allows light to enter. The lens focuses the light, and the retina receives the image. A complex chemical reaction within the retina processes the picture. The optic nerve then carries the image to the visual area of the brain.

Accessory structures to the eyeball include eyelids, ocular muscles, conjunctiva, eyelashes, and lacrimal glands.

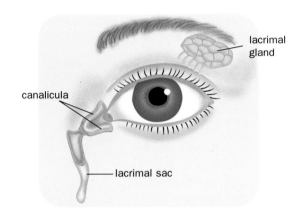

canalicula

lacrimal gland

lacrimal sac

Ophthalmic Administration

➡ Hands should always be washed prior to drug administration.

➡ If more than one agent is to be instilled, wait the suggested time (5 minutes between solutions, 10–15 minutes before ointments) between administrations.

➡ Do not rub eyes. Carefully instill, as per order, onto conjunctiva, one eye at a time.

➡ Do not touch the applicator to the eye at any time.

➡ Replace the applicator cap carefully and do not touch the top of the applicator.

➡ Be aware that temporary vision distortion may occur and encourage the patient accordingly.

➡ The physician should be notified if condition symptoms do not alleviate.

Note: The incidence of adverse reactions to ophthalmic agents is small. Systemic absorption may cause allergic response and steroidal side effects in some cases.

*C*onjunctivitis ("pink eye") is a common eye infection resulting from conjuctival irritation due to infectious organism or allergy.

Conjunctivitis infections are highly contagious. Symptoms are redness of the conjunctiva and pus-like crusty exudate that often leads to the eyelid closing. Antibiotics such as gentamicin, sodium sulfacetamide, and norfloxacin are indicated if the infection is bacterial. For viral infections such as herpes simplex and cytomegalovirus retinitis, vidarabine, and trifluridine are used. If the conjunctivitis is caused by an allergy, histamine blocking agents such as levocabastine, olopatadine, and emedastine may be ordered.

Inflammation of the eye may be treated with both NSAID's and corticosteriods.

Agents such as medrysone and prednisolone are common ophthalmic cortico-steroids while flurbiprofen and ketorolac are NSAID's available for ophthalmic application. Note: flurbiprofen and ketorolac are often used following cataract extraction surgery.

Other drugs include *mydriatics*, anesthetics, and lubricating agents.

Mydriatics are drugs that dilate the pupil and are commonly indicated prior to eye exams. When the pupil is dilated, more light is allowed in and visualization into the eye is enhanced. Phenylephrine is a popular example. For optic related pain, a topical anesthetic such as proparacaine may be prescribed. To provide lubrication to the eyes if abnormal drying is occurring, Lacrisert® is a prescription lubricating drug.

conjunctivitis inflammation of the conjunctiva (eyelid lining).

mydriatics drugs that dilate the pupil.

OPHTHALMIC & OTIC AGENTS (cont'd)

Antiglaucoma Agents

Cholinergic receptor agonists such as pilocarpine and acetylcholine were the first antiglaucoma drugs developed. Beta-adrenergic receptor antagonists are now used more commonly than the cholinergic receptor agonists as they are considered more effective and have fewer side effects. Examples of this type include: betaxolol, carteolol, metipranolol, and timolol.

Adrenergic receptor agonists such as atropine, and dipivefrin are used to lower intraocular pressure by increasing outflow of aqueous humor from the eye.

Some Common Ophthalmic Drugs

Type	Brand Name	Generic Name
Antibiotic	Garamycin	gentamicin
Antibiotic	Sodium Sulamyd	sodium sulfacetamide
Antibiotic	Chibroxin	norfloxacin
Antibiotic	Ciloxan	ciprofloxacin
Antiviral	Vira-a	vidarabine
Antiviral	Viroptic	trifluridine
Antihistamine	Livostin	levocabastine
Antihistamine	Patanol	olopatadine
Antihistamine	Emadine	emedastine
Ophthalmic cortico-steroids	HMS	medrysone
Ophthalmic cortico-steroids	Pred Forte	prednisolone
NSAID	Ocufen	flurbiprofen
NSAID	Acular	ketorolac
Mydriatic	Mydfrin	phenylephrine
Topical anesthetic	Alcaine	proparacaine
Ocular lubricant	Lacrisert	hydroxypropyl cellulose
Antiglaucoma	Betoptic	betaxolol
Antiglaucoma	Ocupress	carteolol
Antiglaucoma	Optipranolol	metipranolol
Antiglaucoma	Timoptic	timolol
Antiglaucoma	Isopto Atropine	atropine
Antiglaucoma	Propine	dipivefrin

See Additional Common Drugs by Classification on pp 473-477 for more drugs in this class.

℞ safety you should know
➡ Cortisporin® Otic Solution and Cortisporin® Otic Suspension are not the same: The active ingredients are identical but the vehicles are different and the solution is more acid than the suspension.

℞ Note: Drugs highlighted in green in the text and tables are parenteral drugs commonly found in hospitals and other institutional settings.

THE EAR

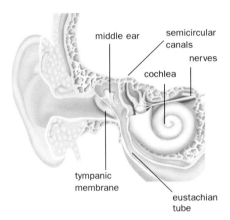

middle ear
semicircular canals
nerves
cochlea
tympanic membrane
eustachian tube

The ear has three main sections: the outer ear, the middle ear, and the inner ear.

The outer ear contains the external part of the ear as well as the part of the ear canal that leads up to the tympanic membrane. Cerumen (ear wax) is produced in the skin of the ear canal.

The middle ear contains the three ear bones or ossicles: the malleus, incus, and stapes. The middle ear also contains the Eustachian tube. The Eustachian tube functions to equalize pressure and allow mucus drainage.

The inner ear contains the cochlea which is the organ of hearing. The inner ear also contains three semi-circular canals and the vestibule which have function for balance.

Otic agents are used to treat conditions associated with the ear.

The most common conditions treated with otic products are associated with accumulation of ear wax and infections of the outer ear. The pH of most otic products is acidic. *Otic products can never be used in the eye because the acidity of otic products can damage the eye.* However, sometimes ophthalmic products are prescribed to treat infections of the ear.

Otic Administration

➡ Hands should always be washed prior to drug administration.

➡ The medicine should be warmed to body temperature by holding the bottle between the hands for a few minutes.

➡ The head should be placed so the affected ear is on top.

➡ The ear canal should be straightened

➡ For children younger than 3 years old: Hold ear lobe and pull down and back.

➡ For children 3 years and older: Hold upper part of ear and pull up and back.

➡ The dropper should not touch the ear; the drops should be placed onto the side of the ear canal (not dropped directly down the ear canal).

➡ The head should remain in place for 5 minutes or insert a cotton plug into the ear.

➡ The physician should be notified if condition symptoms do not alleviate.

Note: While the incidence of adverse reactions to otic agents is small, systemic absorption may cause allergic response and steroidal side effects.

Some Common Otic Drugs		
Type	**Brand Name**	**Generic Name**
Anti-infective	Cortisporin Otic Solution	neomycin, polymixin b, hydrocortisone
Anti-infective	Cortisporin Otic Suspension	neomycin, polymixin b, hydrocortisone
Ear wax softener	Cerumenex	triethanolamine polypeptide oleate-condensate
Ear wax softener	Debrox	carbamide peroxide
Anti-infective	VoSol HC	acetic acid, hydrocortisone
Anti-infective	Ciprodex	ciprofloxacin/dexamethasone

PSYCHOTROPIC AGENTS

Psychotropic agents are drugs that affect behavior, psychiatric state, and sleep.

They act on specialized areas of the brain to suppress or control the symptoms of common psychological disorders such as bipolar disorder, anxiety, depression, schizophrenia, and drug abuse. The primary drug types in this class are antidepressants, antipsychotics, and antianxiety agents. Other related psychotropic agents include sedatives and hypnotics.

THE BRAIN

The brain is an incredibly versatile and complex organ responsible for a vast number of the body's functions. To a great extent, the structures or areas of the brain are specialized by function. These specialized structures are shown below.

Cerebrum

➡ concerned mostly with learned behavior, thought, memory, sensation and voluntary motion. It is divided into lobes: Frontal, Occipital (back) Parietal (top) and Temporal (side).

Cerebellum

➡ controls balance and muscle coordination.

Medulla Oblongata (brain stem)

➡ controls processes that affect the heart, breathing, temperature control and circulation.

Pons

➡ bridges from the medulla oblongata to the cerebellum and also works on muscle coordination.

Thalamus

➡ above the Pons, receives sensations such as heat, cold, pressure and pain.

Hypothalamus

➡ below the Thalamus, controls blood sugar levels, body temperature, emotions, appetite and sleep.

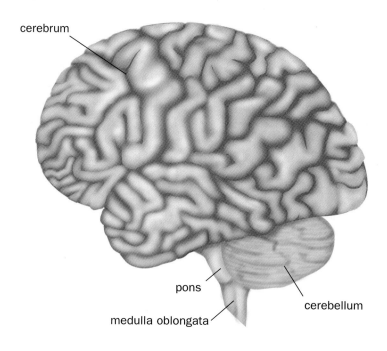

cerebrum

pons

cerebellum

medulla oblongata

Midbrain

➡ works to control blood pressure and the Pineal Gland secretes the hormone melatonin which effects the body's biological rhythms.

Limbic System

➡ an interconnecting network of brain cells inside the brain that affects behavior, emotions, sociosexual drives, motivation, learning, and memory storage and retrieval.

Sedatives and Hypnotics

Sedatives are drugs that are intended to relax and calm. They reduce restlessness and may produce mild drowsiness. Antianxiety medications that include benzodiazepines (e.g., diazepam and chlordiazepoxide) are included in this group.

Hypnotics are often referred to as "sleeping pills" and are designed to induce and, in some cases, prolong sleep. This group includes barbiturates such as secobarbital and pentobarbital. Nonbarbiturate sedative-hypnotics include chloral hydrate and meprobamate.

DISORDERS

Bipolar Disorder

Also known as Manic-Depression, this disorder is characterized by mood, energy, and behavior swings from periods of elation to episodes of depression. These swings are found to occur in a cyclical and recurring pattern. Theories of cause include chemical imbalance and neurotransmitter alterations in the brain. There is a high degree of family history associated with this disorder.

Schizophrenia

This is characterized by extreme and inappropriate behavior and dysfunctional daily routine. Hearing "voices," experiencing delusions, becoming agitated or hostile and perhaps a lack of response at all (flat affect) are examples of schizophrenic behavior. Theories of cause include: family history and chemical imbalances, especially norepinephrine and serotonin, noted in the limbic system.

THERAPIES

Although psychotherapy is included in the suggested treatment, antipsychotic drugs such as quetiapine (Seroquel®) and risperidon (Risperdal®) are commonly prescribed. Carbamazepine (Tegretol®), valproic acid (Depakene®) and clonazepam (Klonopin®) are often added to this therapy to treat seizure activity secondary to psychotropic agents.

Patients experiencing schizophrenia must undergo a complete medical and psychological examination. The drug therapy selected will result from the findings. Antipsychotic agents commonly used may include: chlorpromazine (Thorazine®) and trifluoperazine (Stelazine®).

Some Common Psychotropic Drugs: Antipsychotic and Antiseizure

Type	Brand Name	Generic Name
Antipsychotic/bipolar	Seroquel	quetiapine
Antipsychotic/bipolar	Risperdal	risperidon
Antipsychotic/schizophrenia	Thorazine	chlorpromazine
Antipsychotic/schizophrenia	Stelazine	trifluoperazine
Antiseizure	Tegretol	carbamazepine
Antiseizure	Depakene	valproic acid
Antiseizure	Klonopin	clonazepam

See Additional Common Drugs by Classification on pp 473–477 for more drugs in this class.

Some Common Psychotropic Drugs: Sedatives and Hypnotics

Type	Brand Name	Generic Name
Sedative/antianxiety	Valium	diazepam
Sedative/antianxiety	Librium	chlordiazepoxide
Hypnotic/barbiturate	Seconal	secobarbital
Hypnotic/barbiturate	Nembutal	pentobarbital
Hypnotic/nonbarbiturate	Noctec	chloral hydrate
Hypnotic/nonbarbiturate	Miltown	meprobamate

See Additional Common Drugs by Classification on pp 473–477 for more drugs in this class.

PSYCHOTROPIC AGENTS (cont'd)

DISORDERS

Anxiety

People experiencing anxiety may appear abnormally tired or energetic, withdrawn, tremorous, tense and restless, and may suffer from insomnia, phobias, and panic attacks. Theories of cause include a hypersensitive sympathetic nervous system, excessive serotonin release, and an inability to chemically receive the body's natural calming agents.

Depression

Depression is characterized by mood disturbances that may be mild (e.g., lack of interest or inability to experience joy) or severe (e.g., physical aggression or suicide attempts). Sleep disturbances, crying episodes, gastrointestinal upset and heart palpitations may occur. Theories of cause include: experience of trauma (real or perceived), loss, as well as poor neurotransmitter response of norepinephrine.

THERAPIES

In conjunction with psychotherapy and various relaxation techniques, the commonly prescribed drugs include antianxiety agents such as the benzodiazepines diazepam (Valium®), lorazepam (Ativan®), and alprazolam (Xanax®).

While psychotherapy and even shock therapy are often prescribed treatment, antidepressants such as amitriptyline (Elavil®) and sertraline (Zoloft®) are common drug suggestions. Others are escitalopram (Lexapro®), venlafaxine (Effexor®), and fluoxetine (Prozac®).

Some Common Psychotropic Drugs: Antianxiety

Type	Brand Name	Generic Name
Antianxiety	Valium	diazepam
Antianxiety	Librium	chlordiazepoxide
Antianxiety	Ativan	lorazepam
Antianxiety	Xanax	alprazolam

Some Common Psychotropic Drugs: Antidepressant

Type	Brand Name	Generic Name
Antidepressant	Elavil	amitriptyline
Antidepressant	Zoloft	sertraline
Antidepressant	Lexapro	escitalopram
Antidepressant	Effexor	venlafaxine
Antidepressant	Prozac	fluoxetine

See Additional Common Drugs by Classification on pp 473–477 for more drugs in this class.

DISORDERS

THERAPIES

Drug Dependency

Addiction to drugs and alcohol may occur for various reasons, including chronic usage without adequate physician supervision, chemical intolerance, error in personal judgement or purposeful abuse. Family history and social situation may be contributing factors.

Treatment for dependency often encompasses an on-site treatment program designed to identify and address the patient holistically. Adjunct drug therapy may or may not be included in this. For example, naltrexone (ReVia®) may be used to dissuade the alcoholic from drinking, desipramine (Norpramin®) curbs cocaine desire, and methadone is prescribed for narcotic detoxification.

Some Common Psychotropic Drugs for Treating Alcohol or Drug Dependency

Type	Brand Name	Generic Name
Treatment for alcoholism	Antabuse	disulfiram
Treatment for alcoholism	ReVia	naltrexone
Treatment for cocaine addiction	Norpramin	desipramine
Narcotic detoxification	Dolophine	methadone

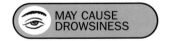

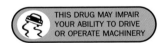

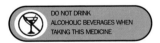

℞ **safety you should know**

➡ Psychotropic drugs, by their nature, often impair the central nervous system and can cause drowsiness. Technicians should consult with their pharmacists to see if auxiliary labels should be used to provide a reminder to the patient.

RESPIRATORY AGENTS

Balancing oxygen and carbon dioxide levels correctly is essential to health.

The cells of the body use oxygen for energy and produce carbon dioxide as waste. The respiratory system is responsible for exchanging oxygen from the air with carbon dioxide from the body. High carbon dioxide levels alert the medulla of the brain to signal inspiration (breathing in) to the diaphragm and intercostal muscles of the rib cage. It is their action that drives normal respiration. There are two phases of respiration: the mechanical phase which involves the diaphragm and the rib cage and allows air to enter the lungs, and the physiologic phase in which oxygen and carbon dioxide are exchanged between the lungs and the blood cells. Dysfunction can occur at any time during either phase.

Emotional stimuli as well as medical disorders may alter gas exchange and breathing patterns.

Abnormal breathing patterns can occur for a variety of reasons and include dyspnea (labored breathing), wheezing, hyperventilation, and apnea (absence of breathing). Common respiratory disorders include: asthma, emphysema, bronchitis, COPD, croup, pneumonia, and allergy (see below).

Drugs commonly indicated in the treatment of respiratory diseases and disorders include antihistamines, decongestants, antitussives, and bronchodilators.

These agents act in a variety of ways to clear the airways and restore normal respiration.

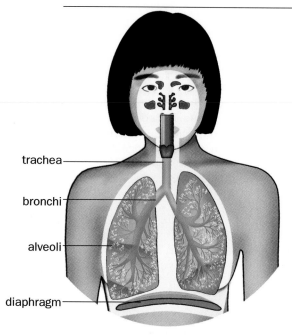

trachea

bronchi

alveoli

diaphragm

The trachea ("windpipe") connects the larynx or "voicebox" and the bronchi, the two airway branches that carry air to the lungs. The smaller bronchial tubes are called bronchioles, They carry the air to the alveoli (air sacs) of the lungs where gas exchange takes place.

Common Respiratory Disorders

➡ **Asthma**: chronic airway inflammation related to stimuli hyperresponsiveness, resulting in airflow obstruction with symptoms such as wheezing and potentially acute spasms and breathlessness.

➡ **Allergy**: allergic response to food, drugs, animals, insect bites, pollens, or dust.

➡ **Emphysema**: chronic airway obstruction due to lung hyperinflation and diminished oxygen intake, characterized by breathlessness and flushed color.

➡ **Croup** (bronchiolitis): an infection of the bronchioles occurring in young children and resulting in airway obstruction and labored breathing.

➡ **Bronchitis**: infection producing excess mucus in the bronchial tree that makes breathing difficult.

➡ **COPD** (chronic obstructive pulmonary disease): also termed COLD (lung) or COAD (airway) by some sources. Abnormal lung function that generally encompasses both emphysema and chronic bronchitis that is present at least for 3 months a year for 2 consecutive years.

➡ **Pneumonia**: infectious process of either bacterial or viral origin whereby fluid accumulates in the lungs causing inadequate or in severe cases, impossible, air exchange at the alveolar level.

CLASSES

Antihistamines

Antihistamines respond to the release of histamine or inflammation producing substance from white blood cells that occurs with injury or allergic reaction. Antihistamine agents replace histamine at the inflammation receptor sites to reduce inflammation, swelling, and irritation. Additional properties include: antipruritic (anti-itching), antiemetic, and sedative. Common antihistamines include hydroxyzine (Atarax®, Vistaril®), promethazine (Phenergan®) and loratadine (Claritin®).

Decongestants

Decongestants cause mucous membrane vasoconstriction, reduce nasal passage drainage, and relieve stuffiness. Pseudoephedrine (Sudafed®) is a common decongestant that is restricted by the Combat Methamphetamine Epidemic Act (CMEA) and must be kept behind the pharmacy counter (see Chapter 3 for more information about the CMEA). Phenylephrine (Sudafed PE®) is another common decongestant that is not restricted by the CMEA.

Antitussives

Antitussives treat both productive (with phlegm) and non-productive (without phlegm) coughs. They are available in both narcotic and non-narcotic preparations. Dextromethorphan is the most widely used antitussive agent. Hydrocodone and chlorpheniramine (Tussionex®) is a common antihistamine/antitussive combination drug. Codeine and hydrocodone are examples of popular narcotic antitussive agents that are used in combination with other respiratory agents to treat coughing.

Some Common Respiratory Drugs: Antihistamines, Decongestants, and Antitussives

Type	Brand Name	Generic Name
Antihistamine	Atarax/Vistaril	hydroxyzine
Antihistamine	Phenergan	promethazine
Antihistamine	Claritin	loratadine
Decongestant	Sudafed	pseudoephedrine
Decongestant	Sudafed PE	phenylephrine
Antitussive	Delsym	dextromethorphan
Antitussive (narcotic)/antihistamine	Tussionex	hydrocodone and chlorpheniramine

See Additional Common Drugs by Classification on pp 473–477 for more drugs in this class.

℞ **safety you should know**
➥ Narcotic antitussives and some antihistamines can cause severe drowsiness. Patients should use caution when taking medications that cause drowsiness.

RESPIRATORY AGENTS (cont'd)

CLASSES

Expectorants and Mucolytic Agents

Expectorants are used to treat chest congestion. Expectorants work by thinning the mucus that collects in the breathing passages. As the mucus becomes thinner, it is easier to cough up so the airways become more clear. An example of an expectorant is guaifenesin (Robitussin®). Mucolytic drugs that liquefy thickened bronchial mucus and assist in clearing airways are sometimes included in this category; acetylcysteine (Mucomyst®) is a common mucolytic agent.

Bronchodilators

Bronchodilators relieve bronchospasm (a narrowing of the bronchi, accompanied by wheezing and coughing, i.e., an "asthma attack," as seen in disorders such as asthma, emphysema and bronchitis). Sympathomimetics (e.g., Proventil HFA® and albuterol) dilate the bronchi. Xanthine derivatives such as theopylline (Theo-Dur®) directly relax the smooth muscle of the bronchi. Both categories increase the opening of the bronchi and allow more airflow to occur. Corticosteroids such as Beclomethasone (QVAR®) and anticholinergics such as ipratropium (Atrovent®) may be used to decrease respiratory airway inflammation and produce some bronchodilation.

Some Common Respiratory Drugs: Expectorants and Mucolytics		
Type	**Brand Name**	**Generic Name**
Expectorant	Robitussin	guaifenesin
Expectorant/antitussive (narcotic)	Robitussin AC	guaifenesin and codeine
Expectorant/antitussive (narcotic)	Vicodin Tuss	guaifenesin and hydrocodone
Mucolytic	Mucomyst	acetylcysteine

Some Common Respiratory Drugs: Bronchodilators		
Type	**Brand Name**	**Generic Name**
Bronchodilator/sympathomimetic	Proventil HFA	albuterol
Bronchodilator/xanthine derivative	Theo-Dur	theopylline
Bronchial corticosteroid	QVAR	beclomethasone
Anticholinergic	Atrovent	ipratropium

See Additional Common Drugs by Classification on pp 473–477 for more drugs in this class.

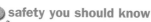
℞ safety you should know

➡ Inhalers should be cleaned regularly. If inhalers are not properly cleaned they may become blocked and may not spray medication. Cleaning is also important to prevent germs from growing on the devices. Manufacturers provide instructions for patients to clean their inhalers.

ADDITIONAL COMMON DRUGS BY CLASSIFICATION

Following are additional common drugs compiled from Drug Topic's 2008 Top 200 list that are not already included in the tables for each of the classification sections in this chapter. Drug Topics' web site is at http://drugtopics.modernmedicine.com/Pharmacy+Facts+&+Figures.

Class/Type	Brand Name	Generic Name
Analgesics		
Analgesic	Ultram ER	tramadol
NSAID	Celebrex	celecoxib
Opiate	Endocet	oxycodone and acetaminophen
Opiate	OxyContin	oxycodone
Anesthetics		
Local	Lidoderm	lidocaine transdermal
Ophthalmic	Alcaine	proparacaine
Anti-infectives		
Anti-infective	Avelox	moxifloxacin
Anti-infective	Floxin	ofloxacin
Anti-infective	Levaquin	levofloxacin
Anti-infective	Vibramycin	doxycycline hyclate
Antiviral	Tamiflu	oseltamivir
Antineoplastics		
Hormone	Arimidex	anastrozole
Hormone	Femara	letrozole
Radioactive isotope	Bexxar	tositumomab and iodine 131
Cardiovascular Agents		
Cardiovascular	Plavix	clopidogrel
Antiarrhythmic	Digitek	digoxin
Anticoagulant	Lovenox	enoxaparin
Anticoagulant	Jantoven	warfarin
Antihyperlipidemic	Crestor	rosuvastatin
Antihyperlipidemic	Lipitor	atorvastatin
Antihyperlipidemic	Lovaza	omega-3 fatty acid
Antihyperlipidemic	Niaspan	niacin
Antihyperlipidemic	Tricor	fenofibrate
Antihyperlipidemic	Zetia	ezetimibe
Antihypertensive	Atacand	candesartan
Antihypertensive	Avalide	irbesartan and hydrochlorothiazide
Antihypertensive	Avapro	irbesartan
Antihypertensive	Benicar	olmesartan
Antihypertensive	Benicar HCT	olmesartan and hydrochlorothiazide
Antihypertensive	Catapres-TTS	clonidine

ADDITIONAL COMMON DRUGS BY CLASSIFICATION

Class/Type	Brand Name	Generic Name
Antihypertensive	Coreg CR	carvedilol
Antihypertensive	Cozaar	losartan
Antihypertensive	Diovan	valsartan
Antihypertensive	Diovan HCT	hydrochlorothiazide and valsartan
Antihypertensive	Hyzaar	losartan and hydrochlorothiazide
Antihypertensive	Micardis	telmisartan
Antihypertensive	Micardis HCT	telmisartan and hydrochlorothiazide
Antihypertensive	Sular	nisoldipine
Antihypertensive	Toprol XL	metoprolol
Dermatologicals		
Dermatological	Aldara	imiquimod
Dermatological	Bactroban	mupirocin
Dermatological	BenzaClin	clindamycin and benzoyl peroxide
Dermatological	Differin	adapalene
Dermatological	Zovirax Topical	acyclovir
Gastrointestinal Agents		
Gastrointestinal	Asacol	mesalamine
Antacid/antiulcer	Aciphex	rabeprazole
Antacid/antiulcer	Nexium	esomeprazole
Antacid/antiulcer	Prevacid	lansoprazole
Antacid/antiulcer	Protonix	pantoprazole
Antidiarrheal	Polymaga Plain	attapulgite
Laxative	Halflytely Bowel Prep Kit	PEG-3350, sodium chloride, sodium bicarbonate and potassium chloride and bisacodyl
Laxative	Trilyte	PEG-3350, sodium chloride, sodium bicarbonate and potassium chloride
Hematological Agents		
Hematological/hematopoietic	Primacare One	prenatal multivitamins with folic acid
Hormones & Modifiers		
Thyroid	Cytomel	liothyronine
Thyroid	Levothroid	levothyroxine
Thyroid	Levoxyl	levothyroxine
Insulin	Humalog	insulin lispro
Insulin	Humulin 70/30	insulin (human recombinant)
Insulin	Lantus SoloSTAR	insulin glargine [rDNA origin]
Insulin	Levemir	insulin detemir (rDNA origin)
Insulin	NovoLog Mix 70/30	insulin aspart protamine and insulin aspart (rDNA origin)

Class/Type	Brand Name	Generic Name
Insulin	Novolin 70/30	human insulin isophane suspension and regular, human insulin injection (rDNA origin)
Oral antidiabetic	Actos	pioglitazone
Oral antidiabetic	Actoplus Met	metformin and pioglitazone
Oral antidiabetic	Avandamet	rosiglitazone and metformin
Oral antidiabetic	Avandia	rosiglitazone
Oral antidiabetic	Byetta	exenatide
Oral antidiabetic	Glipizide XL	glipizide
Oral antidiabetic	Janumet	metformin and sitagliptin
Oral antidiabetic	Januvia	sitagliptin
Androgen	AndroGel	testosterone
Phosphodiesterase inhibitor	Levitra	vardenafil
Contraceptive	Apri	desogestrel and ethinyl estradiol
Contraceptive	Aviane	levonorgestrel and ethinyl estradiol
Contraceptive	Cryselle	ethinyl estradiol and norgestrel
Contraceptive	Junel FE	norethindrone acetate, ethinyl estradiol and ferrous fumarate
Contraceptive	Kariva	desogestrel and ethinyl estradiol
Contraceptive	Levora	levonorgestrel and ethinyl estradiol
Contraceptive	Loestrin 24 Fe	ethinyl estradiol and norethindrone and iron
Contraceptive	Low-Ogestrel	ethinyl estradiol and norgestrel
Contraceptive	Necon 1/35	norethindrone and ethinyl estradiol
Contraceptive	NuvaRing	etonogestrel and ethinyl estradiol
Contraceptive	Ocella	drospirenone and ethinyl estradiol
Contraceptive	Ortho Evra	norelgestromin and ethinyl estradiol
Contraceptive	Ortho Tri Cyclen	norgestimate and ethinyl estradiol
Contraceptive	Sprintec	norgestimate and ethinyl estradiol
Contraceptive	Tri-Sprintec	norgestimate and ethinyl estradiol
Contraceptive	Trivora-28	levonorgestrel and ethinyl estradiol
Contraceptive	Yaz	drosperinone and ethinyl estradiol
Estrogen	Vivelle-DOT	estradiol
Progestin	Prometrium	progesterone
Estrogen and progestin	Prempro	conjugated estrogens and medroxyprogesterone
Other	CellCept	mycophenolate
Other	Propecia	finasteride

Musculoskeletal Agents

Class/Type	Brand Name	Generic Name
Muscle relaxant	Skelaxin	metaxalone
Osteoporitics	Evista	raloxifene

ADDITIONAL COMMON DRUGS BY CLASSIFICATION

Class/Type	Brand Name	Generic Name
Osteoporitics	Fosamax Plus D	alendronate sodium and cholecalciferol
Neurological Agents		
Neurological	Lyrica	pregabalin
Neurological	Topamax	topiramate
Anti-Alzheimer's	Namenda	memantine
Antiepileptic	Keppra	levetiracetam
Antiepileptic	Lamictal	lamotrigine
Antimigraine	Relpax	eletriptan
Antimigraine	Maxalt	rizatriptan
Antiparkinsonian	Mirapex	pramipexole
Antiparkinsonian	Requip	ropinirole
Ophthalmic Agents		
Ophthalmic/anti-infective	Tobradex	tobramycin and dexamethasone
Ophthalmic/anti-infective	Vigamox	moxifloxacin ophthalmic
Ophthalmic/anti-infective	Zymar	gatifloxacin
Antiglaucoma	Alphagan	brimonidine
Antiglaucoma	Alphagan P	brimonidine
Antiglaucoma	Azopt	brinzolamide
Antiglaucoma	Cosopt	dorzolamide and timolol
Antiglaucoma	Diamox	acetazolamide
Antiglaucoma	Iopidine	apraclonidine
Antiglaucoma	Lumigan	bimatoprost
Antiglaucoma	Neptazane	methazolamide
Antiglaucoma	Rescula	unoprostone
Antiglaucoma	Travatan	travoprost
Antiglaucoma	Travatan Z	travoprost
Antiglaucoma	Trusopt	dorzolamide
Antiglaucoma	Xalatan	latanoprost
Psychotropic Agents		
Psychotropic/neurologic/AD(H)D	Adderall XR	dextroamphetamine and amphetamine
Psychotropic	Budeprion XL	bupropion
Psychotropic/neurologic/AD(H)D	Concerta	methylphenidate
Psychotropic	Cymbalta	duloxetine
Psychotropic/neurologic/AD(H)D	Focalin XR	dexmethylphenidate
Psychotropic/neurologic/AD(H)D	Methylin	methylphenidate
Psychotropic	Provigil	modafinil
Psychotropic/neurologic/AD(H)D	Strattera	atomoxetine
Psychotropic/neurologic/AD(H)D	Vyvanse	lisdexamfetamine
Antidepressant	Budeprion SR	bupropion

Class/Type	Brand Name	Generic Name
Antidepressant	Paxil CR	paroxetine
Antidepressant	Wellbutrin XL	bupropion
Antipsychotic	Abilify	aripiprazole
Antipsychotic	Geodon Oral	ziprasidone
Antipsychotic	Risperdal	risperidone
Antipsychotic	Seroquel	quetiapine
Antipsychotic	Zyprexa	olanzapine
Drug dependency	Chantix	varenicline
Drug dependency	Suboxone	buprenorphine and naloxone
Hypnotic	Ambien CR	zolpidem
Hypnotic	Lunesta	eszopiclone
Respiratory Agents		
Respiratory	Advair Diskus	fluticasone and salmeterol
Respiratory	Allegra-D 12 Hour	fexofenadine and pseudoephedrine
Respiratory	Allegra-D 24	fexofenadine and pseudoephedrine
Respiratory	Asmanex	mometasone
Respiratory	Combivent	ipratropium and albuterol
Respiratory	C-Phen DM	chlorpheniramine, dextromethorphan and phenylephrine
Respiratory	Epipen	epinephrine
Respiratory	Flovent HFA	fluticasone
Respiratory	Nasacort AQ	triamcinolone
Respiratory	Nasonex	mometasone
Respiratory	Pulmicort Respules	budesonide
Respiratory	QVAR	beclomethasone
Respiratory	Rhinocort Aqua	budesonide
Respiratory	Singulair	montelukast
Respiratory	Spiriva	tiotropium
Respiratory	Symbicort	formoterol and budesonide
Respiratory	Veramyst	fluticasone
Antihistamine	Astelin	azelastine
Antihistamine	Benadryl	diphenhydramine
Antihistamine	Clarinex	desloratadine
Antihistamine	Xyzal	levocetirizine
Antihistamine	Zyrtec	cetirizine
Bronchodilator	ProAir HFA	albuterol
Bronchodilator	Ventolin HFA	albuterol
Bronchodilator	Xopenex	levalbuterol
Bronchodilator	Xopenex HFA	levalbuterol

REVIEW

KEY CONCEPTS

DRUG NAMES AND CLASSES

✔ A drug's name begins with a chemical name.

✔ Marketed drugs under patent protection have one nonproprietary or generic name and one proprietary or brand name.

✔ The United States Adopted Names Council (USAN) designates the official nonproprietary names for drugs.

CLASSIFICATION SCHEMES

✔ There are various systems for classifying drugs: by disorder, body system affected, type of receptor acted on, type of action, etc.

ANALGESICS

✔ Analgesic drugs create a state in which the pain from a painful medical condition is reduced or not felt.

✔ Common types of analgesics include salicylates, acetaminophen, non-steroidal anti-inflammatory, and opiate-type.

ANESTHETIC AGENTS

✔ Anesthetics cause an absence of sensation or pain.

✔ Anesthetics are classified as local or general.

✔ Local anesthetics block pain conduction without causing a loss of consciousness.

✔ General anesthetics are administered by inhalation or intravenously by an anesthesiologist and depress the central nervous system to the level of unconsciousness.

ANTI-INFECTIVES

✔ Anti-infectives treat disease produced by microorganisms such as bacteria, viruses, fungi, protozoa, and parasitic worms.

ANTINEOPLASTICS

✔ Antineoplastics inhibit new growth of cancer cells.

✔ Side effects caused by many antineoplastic agents are often uncomfortable and serious.

✔ Pharmacists and pharmacy technicians must be very careful with all calculations associated with drugs that are used to treat cancer.

CARDIOVASCULAR AGENTS

✔ Cardiovascular agents include antianginals, antiarrhythmics, antihypertensives, vasopressors, antihyperlipidemics, thrombolytics, and anticoagulants.

DERMATOLOGICALS

✔ The skin is the body's protective barrier and is the largest organ of the body.

✔ Dermatologicals are drugs used to treat diseases or conditions related to the skin.

ELECTROLYTIC AGENTS

✔ Electrolytes are water-soluble substances that are contained in our body fluids as salts.

✔ Electrolyte balance is important for healthy body function.

GASTROINTESTINAL & URINARY TRACT AGENTS

✔ Gastrointestinal agents are used to treat disorders of the stomach and/or intestines.

✔ Urinary agents are used to treat conditions affecting the flow of urine.

HEMATOLOGICAL AGENTS

✔ Each stage of the formation of blood clots can be affected by intrinsic clotting factors as well as drugs.

✔ Hematopoietics are drugs that treat various forms of anemias.

✔ Hemostatic drugs are used to treat or prevent excessive bleeding.

HORMONES & MODIFIERS

✔ Hormones are secreted by glands of the endocrine system.

✔ The pancreas secretes the hormones insulin and glucagon. Insulin and glucagon are involved in regulating serum glucose

IMMUNOBIOLOGIC AGENTS & VACCINES

✔ Immune globulins provide passive immunity.

✔ Vaccines provide active immunity.

✔ Immune globulins provide a shorter period of protection than vaccines.

MUSCULOSKELETAL AGENTS

✔ Musculoskeletal agents are used to treat rheumatoid arthritis, osteoarthritis, gout, osteoporosis, and muscle spasms.

NEUROLOGICAL AGENTS

✔ Several common disorders are affected by abnormalities in neurotransmitter release and/or response and include Parkinson's Disease, Alzheimer's Disease, epilepsy, migraine headaches, multiple sclerosis, and attention deficit (hyperactivity) disorder.

OPHTHALMIC & OTIC AGENTS

✔ Ophthalmic agents are used to treat conditions including glaucoma, eye infection, eye pain, and inflammation. Ophthalmic agents are also used for eye examinations and in preparation for surgery.

✔ Otic agents are used to treat conditions including accumulation of ear wax and infections of the outer ear.

PSYCHOTROPIC AGENTS

✔ Psychotropic agents are used to treat conditions such as bipolar disorder, anxiety, depression, schizophrenia, and drug abuse.

RESPIRATORY AGENTS

✔ Common respiratory disorders include asthma, allergy, emphysema, croup, bronchitis, chronic obstructive pulmonary disease, and pneumonia.

REVIEW

SELF TEST

MATCH THE TERMS: I   *the answer key begins on page 511*

1. analgesia ____

2. androgens ____

3. anemia ____

4. anion ____

6. anthelmintic ____

6. anti-pyretic ____

7. bactericidal ____

8. bacteriostatic ____

9. blocker ____

10. cation ____

11. chyme ____

12. clotting factors ____

13. conjunctivitis ____

14. corticosteroid ____

15. dermatological ____

16. diabetes mellitus ____

17. dissociation ____

18. electrolytes ____

19. endocrine system ____

20. estrogens ____

21. extracellular fluids ____

22. fibrin ____

23. fibrinogen ____

a. inflammation of the conjunctiva (eyelid lining).

b. another term for an antagonist drug, because antagonists block the action of neurotransmitters.

c. a state in which pain is not felt even though a painful condition exists.

d. reduces fever.

e. drug that destroys worms.

f. bacteria killing.

g. bacteria inhibiting.

h. a product used to treat a skin condition.

i. when a compound breaks down and separates into smaller components.

j. a substance that in solution forms ions that conduct an electrical current.

k. the fluid outside the body's individual cells found in plasma and tissue fluid.

l. the semi-liquid form of food as it enters the intestinal tract.

m. factors in the blood coagulation process.

n. Factor I.

o. the fiber that serves as the structure for clot formation.

p. a decrease in hemoglobin or red blood cells.

q. the system of hormone secreting glands.

r. male sex characteristic hormones.

s. female sex characteristic hormones that are involved in calcium and phosphorus conservation.

t. hormonal steroid substances produced by the cortex of the adrenal gland.

u. a condition in which the body does not produce enough insulin or is unable to use it efficiently.

v. a negatively charged ion.

w. a positively charged ion.

MATCH THE TERMS: II

the answer key begins on page 511

1. glaucoma ____

2. glucagon ____

3. gout ____

4. hematopoietics ____

5. hemostatic drugs ____

6. homeostasis ____

7. hormone ____

8. hyperthyroidism ____

9. hypothyroidism ____

10. insulin ____

11. ions ____

12. integumentary system ____

13. interstitial fluid ____

14. intracellular fluid ____

15. intraocular ____

16. Islands (or Islets) of Langerhans ____

17. lymphocyte ____

18. medullary paralysis ____

19. metastasis ____

20. mimetic ____

21. mydriatics ____

22. neoplasm ____

23. neurotransmitter ____

24. osteoarthritis ____

a. a chemical secretion that influences or controls an organ or organs in the body.

b. a type of white blood cell that releases antibodies that destroy disease cells.

c. a hormone that helps convert amino acids to glucose.

d. electrically charged particles.

e. disorders characterized by abnormally high pressure within the eye that leads to optic nerve damage and loss of vision.

f. the skin, hair, and nails.

g. a painful inflammatory condition in which excess uric acid accumulates in the joints.

h. a hormone that controls the body's use of glucose.

i. specialized cells of the pancreas that secrete insulin.

j. the state of equilibrium of the body.

k. drugs that dilate the pupil.

l. inside the eye.

m. drugs used to treat anemia.

n. cell fluid.

o. drugs that prevent excessive bleeding.

p. tissue fluid.

q. underproduction of thyroid hormone.

r. when cancer cells spread beyond their original site.

s. overproduction of thyroid hormone.

t. another term for an agonist, because agonists imitate or "mimic" the action of the neurotransmitter.

u. a new and abnormal tissue growth, often referring to cancer cells.

v. substances that carry the impulses from one neuron to another.

w. an overdose of anesthesia that paralyzes the respiratory and heart centers of the medulla, leading to death.

x. a disorder characterized by weight-bearing bone deterioration, decreasing range of motion, pain, and deformity.

REVIEW

MATCH THE TERMS: III   *the answer key begins on page 511*

1. peristalsis ____

2. progestins ____

3. protease inhibitor ____

4. remission ____

5. rheumatoid arthritis ____

6. serum glucose ____

7. surgical anesthesia ____

8. testosterone ____

9. topical hemostatics ____

10. uricosuric drugs ____

a. a chronic and often progressive inflammatory condition with symptoms that include swelling, feelings of warmth, and joint pain.

b. drugs used to treat gout that increase the elimination of uric acid.

c. the stage of anesthesia in which surgery can be safely conducted.

d. an antiviral used for HIV and Hepatitis C that blocks the enzyme responsible for viral replication.

e. a state in which cancer cells are inactive.

f. the wave-like motion of the intestines that moves food through them.

g. drugs used for minor bleeding when sutures are not appropriate.

h. blood sugar.

i. a female sex characteristic hormones that are involved in ovulation prevention.

j. the primary androgen.

CHOOSE THE BEST ANSWER   *the answer key begins on page 511*

1. Substances that carry impulses from one neuron to another are
   a. blockers.
   b. agonists.
   c. neurotransmitters.
   d. antagonists.

2. The _____ designates nonproprietary names for drugs.
   a. APhA
   b. ASH
   c. USAN
   d. pharmaceutical company

3. An example of a naturally occurring opiate drug is
   a. morphine.
   b. meperidine.
   c. ibuprofen.
   d. naproxen.

4. All of the following are anti-pyretic EXCEPT
   a. opiate-type analgesics.
   b. NSAIDs.
   c. acetaminophen.
   d. salicylates.

5. Which anesthetic is administered through an IV?
   a. propofol
   b. isoflurane
   c. sevoflurane
   d. desflurane

6. Which antibiotic contains sulfa?
   a. Sumycin®
   b. Bactrim DS®
   c. Ceclor®
   d. Geocillin®

7. _____ is an example of an antiviral drug.
   a. Zithromax®
   b. Flagyl®
   c. Valtrex®
   d. Vermox®

8. An example of an anthelmintic drug is
   a. Geocillin®.
   b. Vermox®.
   c. Zithromax®.
   d. Augmentin®.

9. A term for a state in which cancer cells are inactive is
   a. neoplasm.
   b. metastasis.
   c. lymphocyte.
   d. remission.

10. _____ is an example of an ACE inhibitor.
   a. Lasix®
   b. Vasotec®
   c. Cardizem®
   d. Norvasc®

11. _____ is an example of an antianginal drug.
   a. Heparin
   b. Pravastatin
   c. Warfarin
   d. Nitroglycerin

12. A term for non-malignant skin growths is
   a. keratoses.
   b. herpes simplex.
   c. psoriasis.
   d. eczema.

13. An isotonic solution of sodium chloride is
   a. Lactated Ringer's Solution™.
   b. D5LR.
   c. normal saline.
   d. Klor Con®.

14. An example of a histamine receptor antagonist is
   a. nizatidine.
   b. loperamide.
   c. furosemide.
   d. omeprazole.

15. An example of a stool softener is
   a. docusate sodium.
   b. loperamide.
   c. diphenoxylate plus atropine.
   d. pancrelipase.

16. Accidental overdose from _____ is a leading cause of fatal poisoning in children under the age of 6.
   a. cyanocobalamin
   b. aprotinin
   c. iron
   d. vitamin K

17. _____ is the main hormone that controls the body's use of glucose.
   a. Glucagon
   b. Insulin
   c. Epinephrine
   d. Cortisone

18. The generic name for Lantus® is
   a. lente.
   b. glyburide.
   c. glipizide.
   d. glargine.

19. Female sex characteristic hormones that are involved in ovulation prevention are
   a. progestins.
   b. estrogens.
   c. androgens.
   d. methylprednisolone.

20. A live attenuated influenza vaccine is
   a. Fluarix®.
   b. Fluvirin®.
   c. Flumist®.
   d. Fluzone®.

REVIEW

21. A disorder characterized by weight-bearing bone deterioration, decreasing range of motion, pain, and deformity is
    a. rheumatoid arthritis.
    b. osteoarthritis.
    c. gout.
    d. osteoporosis.

22. All of the following drugs are used to treat muscle spasms except
    a. cyclobenzaprine.
    b. carisoprodol.
    c. diazepam.
    d. alendronate.

23. A progressive dementia is
    a. Alzheimer's Disease.
    b. Parkinson's Disease.
    c. rheumatoid arthritis.
    d. osteoarthritis.

24. The following drugs are associated with migraine prophylactic treatment EXCEPT
    _____.
    a. beta blockers
    b. calcium channel blockers
    c. antidepressants
    d. diuretics

25. Which of the following statements is false?
    a. Otic products can never be used in the eye.
    b. Ophthalmic products can never be used in the ear.
    c. The most common conditions treated with otic products are associated with accumulation of ear wax and infections of the outer ear.
    d. The technique for administering ear drops is different for children under three years than for children older than three years old.

26. A disorder also known as Manic-Depression is
    a. schizophrenia.
    b. bipolar disorder.
    c. anxiety.
    d. ADHD.

27. A drug used to treat depression is
    a. Lexapro®.
    b. lithium.
    c. Ativan®.
    d. Seconal®.

28. An example of an expectorant is
    a. pseudoephedrine.
    b. dextromethorphan.
    c. guaifenesin.
    d. albuterol.

29. An example of a sympathomimetic agent used to dilate the bronchi in asthma
    a. albuterol.
    b. prednisone.
    c. Benadryl®.
    d. Claritin®.

30. An infection of the bronchioles that occurs in young children is
    a. COPD.
    b. asthma.
    c. emphysema.
    d. croup.

APPENDICES

LOOK-ALIKE / SOUND-ALIKE

It is important to recognize that a number of drugs have similar sounding or looking names, but very different properties.

Besides similarity, one of the primary problems with accuracy in drug name identification is that prescriptions are still largely written by hand. However, it is also true that there are many ways drug names may be miscommunicated (by mispronunciation, typos, etc.). Therefore, the identification of a drug should be verified as many ways as possible.

Accuracy in handling and using drugs is essential.

Confusing one drug with another can lead to terrible, sometimes fatal consequences. It is critical to make certain that you have the name correct when involved in any aspect of the prescription process. At right is a list of drugs that can be mistaken for one another either by their sound or how they appear when written. There are many others, but this should illustrate the need for accuracy in drug names.

IDENTIFYING DRUG NAMES

At right is a list of drug names that might be easily misread, mispronounced, or otherwise mistaken for each other. Note that this is only a sample and that there are many other drugs with similar looking or sounding names.

Identifying Forms

Frequent handling of a drug will help you to remember its physical characteristics (size, shape, color, markings, etc.), and this can be a valuable skill in the safe handling of drugs. It should be noted, however, that the most important step in identifying drugs is identifying the correct name. All drug information from the manufacturer to the prescriber, pharmacist, and ultimately the user is based upon communicating the correct name of the drug.

Acetazolamide	Acetohexamide	Hydralazine	Hydroxyzine
Alfentanil	Fentanyl, Sufentanil	Hydrochlorothiazide	Hydroflumethiazide
Amitriptyline	Aminophylline	Hydrocortisone	Hydrocodone
Atenolol	Albuterol	Kanamycin	Garamycin®, Gentamicin
Azathioprine	Azatadine		
Baclofen	Bactroban®, Beclovent®	Lisinopril	Fosinopril
Bupropion	Buspirone	Magnesium Sulfate	Manganese Sulfate
Calcitonin	Calcitriol	Methicillin	Mezlocillin
Captopril	Capitrol	Metolazone	Metaxalone
Cefamandole	Cefmetazole	Metoprolol	Metaproterenol
Cefonicid	Cefobid®	Nifedipine	Nicardipine
Cefotaxime	Ceftizoxime	Oxymorphone	Oxymetholone
Cefoxitin	Cefotaxime	Pancuronium	Pipecuronium
Ceftizoxime	Ceftazidime	Pentobarbital	Phenobarbital
Cephalexin	Cephalothin	Phenytoin	Mephenytoin
Chlorpropamide	Chlorpromazine	Pramoxine	Pralidoxime
Clomiphene	Clomipramine	Prazosin	Prednisone
Clonazepam	Clofazimine	Prednisone	Prednisolone
Clorazepate	Clofibrate	Primidone	Prednisone
Clotrimazole	Co-trimoxazole	Proparacaine	Propoxyphene
Cyclosporine	Cycloserine	Quazepam	Oxazepam
Dapsone	Daypro®	Reserpine	Risperidone
Dexamethasone	Desoximetasone	Ribavirin	Riboflavin
Digoxin	Digitoxin	Ritodrine	Ranitidine
Diphenhydramine	Dimenhydrinate	Sucralfate	Salsalate
Dopamine	Dobutamine	Sulfadiazine	Sulfasalazine
Doxazosin	Doxorubicin	Sulfamethizole	Sulfamethoxazole
Doxepin	Doxapram, Doxidan®	Terbutaline	Tolbutamide
Dronabinol	Droperidol	Terconazole	Tioconazole
Dyclonine	Dicyclomine	Testoderm®	Estraderm®
Encainide	Flecainide	Thyrar®	Thyrolar®
Enflurane	Isoflurane	Thyrolar®	Theolair®
Etidronate	Etretinate	Timolol	Atenolol
Flunisolide	Fluocinonide	Tolazamide	Tolbutamide
Glyburide	Glipizide	Torsemide	Furosemide
Guanadrel	Gonadorelin	Tretinoin	Trientine
Guanethidine	Guanidine	Triamterene	Trimipramine
Guanfacine	Guaifenesin, Guanidine	Vincristine	Vinblastine
Halcinonide	Halcion®	Zofran®	Zoloft®

TOP 200 BRAND NAME DRUGS

Following is a list of the Top 200 Brand Name Drugs cross-referenced with corresponding generic drug names and the classifications used in this text. Rankings are based on Drug Topic's 2008 Top 200 list (available at http://drugtopics.modernmedicine.com/Pharmacy+Facts+&+Figures).

	Brand Name	Generic Name	Classification
1.	Lipitor	atorvastatin	Cardiovascular, Antihyperlipidemic
2.	Nexium	esomeprazole	Gastrointestinal, Antacid/Antiulcer
3.	Lexapro	escitalopram	Psychotropic, Antidepressant
4.	Singulair	montelukast	Respiratory
5.	Plavix	clopidogrel	Cardiovascular
6.	Synthroid	levothyroxine	Hormones and Modifiers, Thyroid
7.	Prevacid	lansoprazole	Gastrointestinal, Antacid/Antiulcer
8.	Advair Diskus	fluticasone and salmeterol	Respiratory
9.	Effexor XR	venlafaxine	Psychotropic, Antidepressant
10.	Diovan	valsartan	Cardiovascular, Antihypertensive*
11.	Crestor	rosuvastatin	Cardiovascular, Antihyperlipidemic
12.	Vytorin	ezetimibe and simvastatin	Cardiovascular, Antihyperlipidemic
13.	Cymbalta	duloxetine	Psychotropic
14.	ProAir HFA	albuterol	Respiratory, Bronchodilator
15.	Klor-Con	potassium chloride	Electrolyte
16.	Diovan HCT	hydrochlorothiazide and valsartan	Cardiovascular, Antihypertensive*
17.	Levaquin	levofloxacin	Anti-infective
18.	Actos	pioglitazone	Hormones and Modifiers, Oral antidiabetic
19.	Flomax	tamsulosin	Urinary
20.	Seroquel	quetiapine	Psychotropic, Antipsychotic
21.	Zetia	ezetimibe	Cardiovascular, Antihyperlipidemic
22.	Tricor	fenofibrate	Cardiovascular, Antihyperlipidemic
23.	Celebrex	celecoxib	Analgesic, NSAID
24.	Nasonex	mometasone	Respiratory
25.	Premarin Tablets	conjugated estrogens	Hormones and Modifiers, Estrogen
26.	Lantus	insulin glargine	Hormones and Modifiers, Insulin
27.	Viagra	sildenafil	Hormones and Modifiers, Phosphodiesterase inhibitor
28.	Yaz	drosperinone and ethinyl estradiol	Hormones and Modifiers, Contraceptive
29.	Lyrica	pregabalin	Neurological
30.	Adderall XR	dextroamphetamine and amphetamine	Psychotropic/Neurologic/AD(H)D
31.	Valtrex	valacyclovir	Anti-infective, Antiviral

*An asterisk next to a drug's classification indicates there are additional common uses for that drug.

Brand Name	Generic Name	Classification
32. Cozaar	losartan	Cardiovascular, Antihypertensive*
33. Topamax	topiramate	Neurological
34. Concerta	methylphenidate	Psychotropic/Neurologic/AD(H)D
35. Levoxyl	levothyroxine	Hormones and Modifiers, Thyroid
36. Actonel	risedronate	Musculoskeletal, Osteoporitic
37. Ambien CR	zolpidem	Psychotropic, Hypnotic
38. Spiriva	tiotropium	Respiratory
39. Benicar	olmesartan	Cardiovascular, Antihypertensive*
40. Xalatan	latanoprost	Ophthalmic, Antiglaucoma
41. Benicar HCT	olmesartan and hydrochlorothiazide	Cardiovascular, Antihypertensive*
42. Aricept	donepezil	Neurological, Anti-Alzheimer's
43. Ortho Tri Cyclen	norgestimate and ethinyl estradiol	Hormones and Modifiers, Contraceptive
44. Hyzaar	losartan and hydrochlorothiazide	Cardiovascular, Antihypertensive*
45. Tri-Sprintec	norgestimate and ethinyl estradiol	Hormones and Modifiers, Contraceptive
46. Cialis	tadalafil	Hormones and Modifiers, Phosphodiesterase inhibitor
47. OxyContin	oxycodone	Analgesic, Opiate
48. Aciphex	rabeprazole	Gastrointestinal, Antacid/Antiulcer
49. Lunesta	eszopiclone	Psychotropic, Hypnotic
50. Lamictal	lamotrigine	Neurological, Antiepileptic*
51. Detrol LA	tolterodine	Urinary
52. Chantix	varenicline	Psychotropic, Drug dependency
53. Avapro	irbesartan	Cardiovascular, Antihypertensive*
54. Proventil HFA	albuterol	Respiratory, Bronchodilator
55. Abilify	aripiprazole	Psychotropic, Antipsychotic
56. Yasmin 28	drospirenone and ethinyl estradiol	Hormones and Modifiers, Contraceptive
57. Budeprion XL	bupropion	Psychotropic
58. Niaspan	niacin	Cardiovascular, Antihyperlipidemic
59. Combivent	ipratropium and albuterol	Respiratory
60. Januvia	sitagliptin	Hormones and Modifiers, Oral antidiabetic
61. Boniva	ibandronate	Musculoskeletal, Osteoporitic
62. Trinessa	norgestimate and ethinyl estradiol	Hormones and Modifiers, Contraceptive
63. NuvaRing	etonogestrel and ethinyl estradiol	Hormones and Modifiers, Contraceptive
64. Risperdal	risperidone	Psychotropic, Antipsychotic
65. Polymagma Plain	attapulgite	Gastrointestinal, Antidiarrheal

TOP 200
BRAND NAME DRUGS

	Brand Name	Generic Name	Classification
66.	Flovent HFA	fluticasone	Respiratory
67.	Imitrex Oral	sumatriptan	Neurological, Antimigraine
68.	Evista	raloxifene	Musculoskeletal, Osteoporitic
69.	Avelox	moxifloxacin	Anti-infective
70.	Depakote ER	divalproex sodium	Neurological
71.	Protonix	pantoprazole	Gastrointestinal, Antacid/Antiulcer
72.	Avalide	irbesartan and hydrochlorothiazide	Cardiovascular, Antihypertensive*
73.	Lidoderm	lidocaine transdermal	Anesthetic, Local
74.	Zyprexa	olanzapine	Psychotropic, Antipsychotic
75.	Namenda	memantine	Neurological, Anti-Alzheimer's
76.	Tussionex	hydrocodone and chlorpheniramine	Respiratory
77.	Thyroid, Armour	desiccated thyroid	Hormones & Modifiers, Thyroid
78.	Humalog	insulin lispro	Hormones and Modifiers, Insulin
79.	Vigamox	moxifloxacin ophthalmic	Ophthalmic
80.	Tamiflu	oseltamivir	Anti-infective, Antiviral
81.	Budeprion SR	bupropion	Psychotropic, Antidepressant
82.	Suboxone	buprenorphine and naloxone	Psychotropic, Drug dependency
83.	Lanoxin	digoxin	Cardiovascular, Antiarrhythmic
84.	Loestrin 24 Fe	ethinyl estradiol and norethindrone and iron	Hormones and Modifiers, Contraceptive
85.	Avodart	dutasteride	Urinary
86.	Coumadin	warfarin	Cardiovascular, Anticoagulant
87.	Wellbutrin XL	bupropion	Psychotropic, Antidepressant
88.	Endocet	oxycodone and acetaminophen	Analgesic, Opiate
89.	Skelaxin	metaxalone	Musculoskeletal, Muscle relaxant
90.	Nasacort AQ	triamcinolone	Respiratory
91.	Keppra	levetiracetam	Neurological, Antiepileptic
92.	Allegra-D 12 Hour	fexofenadine and pseudoephedrine	Respiratory
93.	Strattera	atomoxetine	Psychotropic
94.	Lovaza	omega-3 fatty acid	Cardiovascular, Antihyperlipidemic
95.	Avandia	rosiglitazone	Hormones and Modifiers, Oral antidiabetic
96.	Ocella	drospirenone and ethinyl estradiol	Hormones and Modifiers, Contraceptive
97.	Vyvanse	lisdexamfetamine	Psychotropic
98.	Toprol XL	metoprolol	Cardiovascular, Antihypertensive*
99.	Levitra	vardenafil	Hormones and Modifiers, Phosphodiesterase inhibitor

Brand Name	Generic Name	Classification
100. Astelin	azelastine	Respiratory, Antihistamine
101. Vivelle-DOT	estradiol	Hormones and Modifiers, Estrogen
102. Glipizide XL	glipizide	Hormones and Modifiers, Oral antidiabetic
103. Xopenex HFA	levalbuterol	Respiratory, Bronchodilator
104. Aviane	levonorgestrel and ethinyl estradiol	Hormones and Modifiers, Contraceptive
105. Fosamax	alendronate	Musculoskeletal, Osteoporitic
106. Kariva	desogestrel and ethinyl estradiol	Hormones and Modifiers, Contraceptive
107. Byetta	exenatide	Hormones and Modifiers
108. Mirapex	pramipexole	Neurological, Antiparkinsonian
109. Prempro	conjugated estrogens and medroxyprogesterone	Hormones and Modifiers
110. Low-Ogestrel	ethinyl estradiol and norgestrel	Hormones and Modifiers, Contraceptive
111. Patanol	olopatadine	Ophthalmic
112. Lumigan	bimatoprost	Ophthalmic, Antiglaucoma
113. Provigil	modafinil	Psychotropic
114. Pulmicort Respules	budesonide	Respiratory
115. Altace	ramipril	Cardiovascular, Antihypertensive*
116. Necon 1/35	norethindrone and ethinyl estradiol	Hormones and Modifiers, Contraceptive
117. Micardis	telmisartan	Cardiovascular, Antihypertensive*
118. Depakote	divalproex sodium	Neurological
119. Fosamax Plus D	alendronate sodium and cholecalciferol	Musculoskeletal, Osteoporitic
120. Alphagan P	brimonidine	Ophthalmic, Antiglaucoma
121. Geodon Oral	ziprasidone	Psychotropic, Antipsychotic
122. Micardis HCT	telmisartan and hydrochlorothiazide	Cardiovascular, Antihypertensive*
123. Vesicare	solifenacin	Urinary
124. Focalin XR	dexmethylphenidate	Psychotropic/Neurologic/AD(H)D
125. Digitek	digoxin	Cardiovascular, Antiarrhythmic
126. Sprintec	norgestimate and ethinyl estradiol	Hormones and Modifiers, Contraceptive
127. Xopenex	levalbuterol	Respiratory, Bronchodilator
128. Tobradex	tobramycin and dexamethasone	Ophthalmic
129. Humulin N	insulin (human recombinant)	Hormones and Modifiers, Insulin
130. Clarinex	desloratadine	Respiratory, Antihistamine
131. Ciprodex Otic	ciprofloxacin and dexamethasone	Otic
132. Coreg CR	carvedilol	Cardiovascular, Antihypertensive*
133. Apri	desogestrel and ethinyl estradiol	Hormones and Modifiers, Contraceptive
134. Atacand	candesartan	Cardiovascular, Antihypertensive*

TOP 200 BRAND NAME DRUGS

Brand Name	Generic Name	Classification
135. Levothroid	levothyroxine	Hormones and Modifiers, Thyroid
136. Restasis	cyclosporine	Ophthalmic
137. Ventolin HFA	albuterol	Respiratory, Bronchodilator
138. Rhinocort Aqua	budesonide	Respiratory
139. Prometrium	progesterone	Hormones and Modifiers, Progestin
140. Trivora-28	levonorgestrel and ethinyl estradiol	Hormones and Modifiers, Contraceptive
141. Xyzal	levocetirizine	Respiratory, Antihistamine
142. Ortho Evra	norelgestromin and ethinyl estradiol	Hormones and Modifiers, Contraceptive
143. Cosopt	dorzolamide and timolol	Ophthalmic, Antiglaucoma
144. Arimidex	anastrozole	Antineoplastic, Hormone
145. Veramyst	fluticasone	Respiratory
146. Requip	ropinirole	Neurological, Antiparkinsonian
147 Humulin 70/30	insulin (human recombinant)	Hormones and Modifiers, Insulin
148. BenzaClin	clindamycin and benzoyl peroxide	Dermatological
149. Differin	adapalene	Dermatological
150. Methylin	methylphenidate	Psychotropic/Neurologic/AD(H)D
151. Asacol	mesalamine	Gastrointestinal
152. Dilantin	phenytoin	Neurological, Anti-epileptic
153. Zymar	gatifloxacin	Ophthalmic
154. Vagifem	estrogen	Hormones and Modifiers, Estrogen
155. AndroGel	testosterone	Hormones and Modifiers, Androgen
156. Ethedent	sodium fluoride	Dental
157. Lantus SoloSTAR	insulin glargine [rDNA origin]	Hormones and Modifiers, Insulin
158. Fluvirin	influenza vaccine, inactivated	Immunobiologic, Vaccine
159. Premarin Vaginal	conjugated estrogens	Hormones and Modifiers, Estrogen
160. Actoplus Met	metformin and pioglitazone	Hormones and Modifiers, Oral antidiabetic
161. Propecia	finasteride	Hormones and Modifiers
162. NovoLog Mix 70/30	insulin aspart protamine and insulin aspart (rDNA origin)	Hormones and Modifiers, Insulin
163. Asmanex	mometasone	Respiratory
164. Levora	levonorgestrel and ethinyl estradiol	Hormones and Modifiers, Contraceptive
165. Uroxatral	alfuzosin	Urinary
166. Allegra-D 24	fexofenadine and pseudoephedrine	Respiratory
167. Epipen	epinephrine	Respiratory
168. Zyrtec	cetirizine	Respiratory, Antihistamine
169. Enablex	darifenacin	Urinary

Brand Name	Generic Name	Classification
170. Levemir	insulin detemir (rDNAorigin)	Hormones and Modifiers, Insulin
171. Fluzone	influenza vaccine, inactivated	Immunobiologic, Vaccine
172. Relpax	eletriptan	Neurological, Antimigraine
173. Symbicort	formoterol and budesonide	Respiratory
174. Janumet	metformin and sitagliptin	Hormones and Modifiers, Oral antidiabetic
175. Pataday	olopatadine	Ophthalmic
176. Travatan	travoprost	Ophthalmic, Antiglaucoma
177. Halflytely Bowel Prep Kit	PEG-3350, sodium chloride, sodium bicarbonate and potassium chloride for oral solution and bisacodyl	Gastrointestinal, Laxative
178. Travatan Z	travoprost	Ophthalmic, Antiglaucoma
179. Primacare One	prenatal multivitamins with folic acid	Hematological
180. Bactroban	mupirocin	Dermatological
181. C-Phen DM	chlorpheniramine, dextromethorphan and phenylephrine	Respiratory
182. Trilyte	PEG-3350, sodium chloride, sodium bicarbonate and potassium chloride	Gastrointestinal, Laxative
183. Welchol	colesevelam	Cardiovascular, Antihyperlipidemic
184. Lovenox	enoxaparin	Cardiovascular, Anticoagulant
185. Junel FE	norethindrone acetate, ethinyl estradiol and ferrous fumarate	Hormones and Modifiers, Contraceptive
186. Novolin 70/30	human insulin isophane suspension and regular, human insulin injection (rDNA origin)	Hormones and Modifiers, Insulin
187. Sular	nisoldipine	Cardiovascular, Antihypertensive*
188. Ultram ER	tramadol	Analgesic
189. Zovirax Topical	acyclovir	Dermatological
190. Catapres-TTS	clonidine	Cardiovascular, Antihypertensive*
191. Avandamet	rosiglitazone and metformin	Hormones & Modifiers, Oral antidiabetic
192. Maxalt	rizatriptan	Neurological, Anti-migraine
193. Jantoven	warfarin	Cardiovascular, Anticoagulant
194. Paxil CR	paroxetine	Psychotropic, Antidepressant
195. Femara	letrozole	Antineoplastic, Hormone
196. Aldara	imiquimod	Dermatological
197. Cytomel	liothyronine	Hormones & Modifiers, Thyroid
198. Cryselle	ethinyl estradiol and norgestrel	Hormones & Modifiers, Contraceptive
199. CellCept	mycophenolate	Hormones & Modifiers
200. QVAR	beclomethasone	Respiratory

TOP 200 GENERIC DRUGS

Following is a list of the Top 200 Generic Drugs cross-referenced with corresponding brand name(s) and the classifications used in this text. Rankings are based on Drug Topic's 2008 Top 200 Generic Drugs by Prescriptions list (available at http://drugtopics.modernmedicine.com/Pharmacy+Facts+&+Figures).

	Generic Name	Brand Name	Classification
1.	Hydrocodone/APAP	Vicodin	Analgesic, Opiate
2.	Lisinopril	Zestril, Prinivil	Cardiovascular, Antihypertensive*
3.	Simvastatin	Zocor	Cardiovascular, Antihyperlipidemic
4.	Levothyroxine	Synthroid	Hormones & Modifiers, Thyroid
5.	Amoxicillin	Trimox	Anti-infective
6.	Azithromycin	Zithromax	Anti-infective
7.	Hydrochlorothiazide	Hydrodiuril	Cardiovascular, Antihypertensive*
8.	Alprazolam	Xanax	Psychotropic
9.	Atenolol	Tenormin	Cardiovascular, Antihypertensive*
10.	Metformin	Glucophage	Hormones & Modifiers, Oral antidiabetic
11.	Metoprolol Succinate	Toprol	Cardiovascular, Antihypertensive*
12.	Furosemide Oral	Lasix	Cardiovascular, Antihypertensive*
13.	Metoprolol Tartrate	Lopressor	Cardiovascular, Antihypertensive*
14.	Sertraline	Zoloft	Psychotropic, Antidepressant
15.	Omeprazole	Prilosec	Gastrointestinal, Antacid/Antiulcer
16.	Zolpidem Tartrate	Ambien	Psychotropic, Hypnotic
17.	Oxycodone w/APAP	Percocet	Analgesic, Opiate
18.	Ibuprofen	Motrin	Analgesic, NSAID
19.	Prednisone Oral	Deltasone	Hormones & Modifiers, Adrenal corticosteroid
20.	Fluoxetine	Prozac	Psychotropic, Antidepressant
21.	Warfarin	Coumadin	Cardiovascular, Anticoagulant
22.	Cephalexin	Keflex	Anti-infective
23.	Lorazepam	Ativan	Psychotropic
24.	Clonazepam	Klonopin	Psychotropic
25.	Citalopram HBr	Celexa	Psychotropic, Antidepressant
26.	Tramadol	Ultram	Analgesic
27.	Gabapentin	Neurontin	Neurological, Anti-epileptic
28.	Ciprofloxacin HCl	Cipro	Anti-infective
29.	Propoxyphene-N/APAP	Darvocet N-100	Analgesic, Opiate
30.	Lisinopril/HCTZ	Prinizide, Zestoretic	Cardiovascular, Antihypertensive*
31.	Triamterene w/HCTZ	Dyazide, Maxzide	Cardiovascular, Antihypertensive*

*An asterisk next to a drug's classification indicates there are additional common uses for that drug.

	Generic Name	Brand Name	Classification
32.	Amoxicillin/Potassium Clavulanate	Augmentin	Anti-infective
33.	Cyclobenzaprine	Flexeril	Musculoskeletal, Muscle relaxant
34.	Trazodone HCl	Desyrel	Psychotropic, Antidepressant
35.	Fexofenadine	Allegra	Respiratory, Antihistamine
36.	Fluticasone Nasal	Flonase	Respiratory
37.	Paroxetine	Paxil	Psychotropic, Antidepressant
38.	Lovastatin	Mevacor	Cardiovascular, Antihyperlipidemic
39.	Trimethoprim/Sulfamethoxazole	Bactrim, Septra	Anti-infective
40.	Albuterol Aerosol	Ventolin, Proventil, AccuNeb, Vospire, ProAir	Respiratory, Bronchodilator
41.	Diazepam	Valium	Psychotropic
42.	Pravastatin	Pravachol	Cardiovascular, Antihyperlipidemic
43.	Acetaminophen w/Codeine	Tylenol w/Codeine	Analgesic, Opiate
44.	Alendronate	Fosamax	Musculoskeletal, Osteoporitic
45.	Amitriptyline	Elavil	Psychotropic, Antidepressant
46.	Naproxen	Naprosyn	Analgesic, NSAID
47.	Fluconazole	Diflucan	Anti-infective, Antifungal
48.	Enalapril	Vasotec	Cardiovascular, Antihypertensive*
49.	Carvedilol	Coreg	Cardiovascular
50.	Ranitidine HCl	Zantac	Gastrointestinal, Antacid/Antiulcer
51.	Doxycycline	Vibramycin	Anti-infective
52.	Carisoprodol	Soma	Musculoskeletal, Muscle relaxant
53.	Allopurinol	Zyloprim	Musculoskeletal, Antigout
54.	Methylprednisolone	Medrol	Hormones & Modifiers, Adrenal corticosteroid
55.	Meloxicam	Mobic	Analgesic, NSAID
56.	Amlodipine Besylate/Benazepril	Lotrel	Cardiovascular, Antihypertensive*
57.	Potassium Chloride	K-Dur, K-Lor, K-Tab, Kaon CL, Klorvess, Slow-K, Ten-K, Klotrix, K-Lyte CL	Electrolyte
58.	Clonidine	Catapres	Cardiovascular, Antihypertensive*
59.	Promethazine	Phenergan	Respiratory, Antihistamine
60.	Isosorbide Mononitrate	Imdur, Ismo, Monoket	Cardiovascular
61.	Folic Acid	Folvite	Hematological, Hematopoietic
62.	Spironolactone	Aldactone	Cardiovascular, Antihypertensive*
63.	Glimepiride	Amaryl	Hormones & Modifiers, Oral antidiabetic
64.	Pantoprazole	Protonix	Gastrointestinal, Antacid/Antiulcer

TOP 200 GENERIC DRUGS

Generic Name	Brand Name	Classification
65. Glyburide	Micronase, Diabeta, Glynase Prestab	Hormones & Modifiers, Oral antidiabetic
66. Verapamil SR	Calan SR, Isoptin SR	Cardiovascular, Antihypertensive*
67. Albuterol Nebulizer Solution	Proventil, Ventolin	Respiratory, Bronchodilator
68. Cefdinir	Omnicef	Anti-infective
69. Temazepam	Restoril	Psychotropic, Hypnotic
70. Triamcinolone Acetenoide Topical	Kenalog, Aristocort	Dermatological
71. Penicillin VK	Pen Vee K	Anti-infective
72. Oxycodone	Oxycontin	Analgesic, Opiate
73. Metformin HCl ER	Glucophage XR	Hormones & Modifiers, Oral antidiabetic
74. Benazepril	Lotensin	Cardiovascular, Antihypertensive*
75. Glipizide	Glucotrol	Hormones & Modifiers, Oral antidiabetic
76. Clindamycin	Cleocin	Anti-infective
77. Ramipril	Altace	Cardiovascular, Antihypertensive*
78. Metronidazole	Flagyl	Anti-infective
79. Digoxin	Lanoxin, Digitek	Cardiovascular, Antiarrhythmic
80. Metoclopramide	Reglan	Gastrointestinal
81. Estradiol Oral	Estrace	Hormones and Modifiers, Estrogen
82. Hydroxyzine HCl	Atarax	Respiratory, Antihistamine
83. Amphetamine Salt Combination	Adderall	Psychotropic/Neurologic/AD(H)D
84. Diclofenac Sodium SR	Voltaren SR	Analgesic, NSAID
85. Gemfibrozil	Lopid	Cardiovascular, Antihyperlipidemic
86. Propranolol	Inderal	Cardiovascular, Antihypertensive*
87. Vitamin D	Vitamin D	Vitamin
88. Quinapril	Accupril	Cardiovascular, Antihypertensive*
89. Promethazine/Codeine	Phenergan with Codeine	Respiratory
90. Doxazosin	Cardura	Cardiovascular, Antihypertensive*
91. Mirtazapine	Remeron	Psychotropic, Antidepressant
92. Glipizide ER	Glucotrol XL	Hormones & Modifiers, Oral antidiabetic
93. Phentermine	Adipex-P, Fastin, Obenix, Oby-Trim	Gastrointestinal
94. Acyclovir	Zovirax	Anti-infective, Antiviral
95. Meclizine HCl	Antivert	Gastrointestinal, Antiemetic
96. Potassium Chloride ER	Klor-Con	Electrolyte
97. Nitrofurantoin Monohydrate Micronized	Macrobid	Anti-infective
98. Sulfamethoxazole/Trimethoprim	Bactrim, Septra	Anti-infective

Generic Name	Brand Name	Classification
99. Fentanyl Transdermal	Duragesic	Analgesic, Opiate
100. Buspirone HCl	Buspar	Psychotropic
101. Diltiazem	Cardizem	Cardiovascular, Antihypertensive*
102. Nifedipine ER	Adalat CC	Cardiovascular, Antihypertensive*
103. Glyburide/Metformin HCl	Glucovance	Hormones & Modifiers, Oral antidiabetic
104. Methotrexate	Rheumatrex, Trexall	Antineoplastic, Antimetabolite
105. Cheratussin AC	Robitussin AC	Respiratory
106. Clotrimazole/Betamethasone	Lotrisone	Dermatological
107. Mupirocin	Bactroban	Dermatological
108. Benzonatate	Tessalon	Respiratory, Antitussive
109. Methadone HCl (Non-Injectable)	Dolophine	Analgesic, Opiate
110. Butalbital/APAP/Caffeine	Fioricet, Esgic	Analgesic
111. Polyethylene Glycol	MiraLAX	Gastrointestinal, Laxative
112. Diltiazem CD	Cardizem CD	Cardiovascular, Antihypertensive*
113. Bisoprolol/HCTZ	Ziac	Cardiovascular, Antihypertensive*
114. Minocycline	Minocin	Anti-infective
115. Terazosin	Hytrin	Cardiovascular, Antihypertensive*
116. Nabumetone	Relafen	Analgesic, NSAID
117. Famotidine	Pepcid	Gastrointestinal, Antacid/Antiulcer
118. Tizanidine HCl	Zanaflex	Musculoskeletal, Muscle relaxant
119. Ferrous Sulfate	Feosol	Hematological, Hematopoietic
120. Methocarbamol	Robaxin	Musculoskeletal, Muscle relaxant
121. Finasteride	Proscar	Urinary
122. Phenytoin Sodium	Dilantin	Neurological, Anti-epileptic
123. Insulin Aspart	NovoLog	Hormones & Modifiers, Antidiabetic
124. Clobetasol	Temovate	Dermatological
125. Chlorhexidine Gluconate	Peridex, Periochip, Perichlor, Periogard	Dental
126. Clarithromycin	Biaxin	Anti-infective
127. Dicyclomine HCl	Bentyl	Gastrointestinal
128. Phenazopyridine HCl	Pyridium	Urinary
129. Colchicine	Colchicine	Musculoskeletal, Antigout
130. Atenolol/Chlorthalidone	Tenoretic	Cardiovascular, Antihypertensive*
131. Felodipine ER	Plendil	Cardiovascular, Antihypertensive*
132. Bupropion XL	Wellbutrin XL	Psychotropic, Antidepressant
133. Bupropion SR	Wellbutrin SR	Psychotropic, Antidepressant

TOP 200 GENERIC DRUGS

Generic Name	Brand Name	Classification
134. Hydroxychloroquine	Plaquenil	Anti-infective, Antimalarial
135. Aspirin Enteric-Coated	Ecotrin	Analgesic
136. Baclofen	Lioresal	Musculoskeletal, Muscle relaxant
137. Tramadol HCl/APAP	Ultracet	Analgesic
138. Ketoconazole Topical	Nizoral	Dermatological
139. Nortriptyline	Pamelor, Aventyl	Psychotropic, Antidepressant
140. Risperidone	Risperdal	Psychotropic, Antipsychotic
141. Cefuroxime	Ceftin	Anti-infective
142. Nystatin Topical	Mycostatin	Dermatological
143. Prednisolone Sd. Phs. Oral	Orapred, Pediapred, Prelone	Hormones & Modifiers, Adrenal corticosteroid
144. Nitroquick	Nitrostat	Cardiovascular, Antianginal
145. Hydroxyzine Pamoate	Vistaril	Respiratory, Antihistamine
146. Etodolac	Lodine	Analgesic, NSAID
147. Benztropine	Cogentin	Neurological
148. Nitroglycerin	Nitro-Bid	Cardiovascular, Antianginal
149. Phenobarbital	Luminal	Neurological, Anti-epileptic
150. Nystatin Systemic	Mycostatin	Anti-infective, Antifungal
151. Morphine Sulfate ER	MS Contin	Analgesic, Opiate
152. Fluocinonide	Lidex	Dermatological
153. Hydrocortisone Topical	Hytone	Dermatological
154. Oxybutynin Chloride	Ditropan	Urinary
155. Lamotrigine	Lamictal	Neurological, Anti-epileptic
156. Labetalol	Normodyne, Trandate	Cardiovascular, Antihypertensive*
157. Hydralazine	Apresoline	Cardiovascular, Antihypertensive*
158. Nitrofurantoin Macrocrystals	Macrodantin	Anti-infective
159. Amiodarone	Cordarone, Pacerone	Cardiovascular, Antiarrhythmic
160. Indomethacin	Indocin	Analgesic, NSAID
161. Carbidopa/Levodopa	Sinemet	Neurological, Antiparkinsonian
162. Clindamycin Topical	Cleocin T	Dermatological
163. Ondansetron	Zofran	Gastrointestinal, Antiemetic
164. Lithium Carbonate	Eskalith	Psychotropic
165. Fosinopril Sodium	Monopril	Cardiovascular, Antihypertensive*
166. Medroxyprogesterone	Provera	Hormones and Modifiers, Progestin
167. Hydrocodone/Ibuprofen	Vicoprofen	Analgesic, Opiate, NSAID
168. Ropinirole HCl	Requip	Neurological, Antiparkinsonian

Generic Name	Brand Name	Classification
169. Terbinafine HCl	Lamisil	Anti-infective, Antifungal
170. Bupropion ER	Zyban	Psychotropic, Drug dependency
171. Promethazine DM	Phen-Tuss DM, Phenergan w/Dextromethorphan	Respiratory, Antitussive, Antihistamine
172. Diltiazem SR	Cardizem SR	Cardiovascular, Antihypertensive*
173. Carbamazepine	Tegretol	Neurological, Anti-epileptic
174. Benazepril/HCTZ	Lotensin HCT	Cardiovascular, Antihypertensive*
175. Oxcarbazepine	Trileptal	Neurological, Anti-epileptic
176. Prednisone Intensol	Intensol	Hormones & Modifiers, Adrenal corticosteroid
177. Tetracycline	Sumycin	Anti-infective
178. Doxepin	Sinequan, Adapin	Psychotropic, Antidepressant
179. Dexamethasone	Decadron	Hormones & Modifiers, Adrenal corticosteroid
180. Prochlorperazine Maleate	Compazine	Gastrointestinal, Antiemetic
181. Venlafaxine	Effexor	Psychotropic, Antidepressant
182. Nystatin/Triamcinolone	Myco-Triacet II, Mycolog II	Dermatological
183. Mometasone Topical	Elocon	Dermatological
184. Oxybutynin ER	Ditropan XL	Urinary
185. Cyanocobalamin	Cobal, Cyanoject, Cyomin, Vibal	Hematological, Hematopoietic
186. Sotalol	Betapace	Cardiovascular, Antiarrhythmic
187. Erythromycin Ophthalmic	Ilotycin	Ophthalmic
188. Piroxicam	Feldene	Analgesic, NSAID
189. Oxycodone HCl ER	Oxycontin	Analgesic, Opiate
190. Hyoscyamine	Anaspaz, Cystospaz, Donnamar, Levsin	Gastrointestinal, Antispasmodic
191. Torsemide	Demadex	Cardiovascular, Antihypertensive*
192. Naproxen Sodium	Anaprox	Analgesic, NSAID
193. Nadolol	Corgard	Cardiovascular, Antihypertensive*
194. Hydromorphone HCl	Dilaudid	Analgesic, Opiate
195. Bumetanide	Bumex	Cardiovascular, Antihypertensive*
196. Methylphenidate	Concerta, Ritalin	Psychotropic/Neurologic/AD(H)D
197. Nifedical XL	Procardia XL	Cardiovascular, Antihypertensive*
198. Microgestin Fe 1/20	Loestrin Fe 1/20	Hormones and Modifiers, Contraceptive
199. Prednisolone Acetate Ophthalmic	Pred Mild, Pred Forte	Ophthalmic
200. Diphenoxylate w/Atropine	Lomotil	Gastrointestinal, Antidiarrheal

COMMONLY REFRIGERATED DRUGS

Many products must be stored at refrigerated temperatures to ensure stability. Following is a list of commonly refrigerated drugs. As per the manufacturer's product information, some products need to be refrigerated immediately upon receipt from the manufacturer. Others may be stored at room temperature but will require refrigeration once reconstituted or when a diluent is added. A few drugs are stored in the refrigerator at the pharmacy but can be kept at room temperature when in use by the patient. For reconstituted products, the manufacturer will provide information as to how long the product is stable once reconstituted.

Brand Name & Dosage Form	Generic Name
ActHib vials	haemophilus b conjugate vaccine (tetanus toxoid conjugate)
Actimmune vials	interferon gamma-1b
Adacel vials	tetanus toxoid, reduced diphtheria toxoid, acellular pertussis vaccine adsorbed (Tdap) vaccine
Alcaine ophthalmic solution	proparacaine
Amoxil suspension	amoxicillin
Anectine vials	succinylcholine chloride
Aspirin Uniserts suppositories	aspirin
Atgam vials	lymphocyte immune globulin
Augmentin suspension	amoxicillin/clavulanic acid
Avonex syringes	interferon beta-1a
Azasite ophthalmic solution	azithromycin
BACiiM vials	bacitracin
Benzamycin gel	erythromycin/benzoyl peroxide
Bicillin syringes	penicillin G benzathine
Cardizem vials	diltiazem hydrochloride
Caverject vials	alprostadil
Ceftin suspension	cefuroxime axetil
Cefzil suspension	cefprozil
Cerebyx vials	fosphenytoin sodium
Cipro suspension	ciprofloxacin
Combipatch transdermal patch	estradiol/norethindrone
Copaxone	glatiramer acetate
DDAVP vials	desmopressin
Digibind vials	digoxin immune Fab
Enbrel syringes	etanercept
Engerix-B vials	hepatitis B vaccine
Epogen vials	epoetin alfa
Genotropin cartridges	somatropin
Havrix vials, syringes	hepatitis A vaccine
Hemabate vial	carboprost tromethamine
Humalog vials, pens	insulin lispro

Brand Name & Dosage Form	Generic Name
Humira syringes	adalimumab
Humulin R vials	regular insulin
Infergen vials	interferon alfacon-1
Kaletra solution, capsules	lopinavir/ritonavir
Lactinex tablets	Lactobacillus acidophilus/bulgaricus
Lantus vials, pens	insulin glargine
Leukeran tablets	chlorambucil
Meruvax vials	rubella virus vaccine live
Methergine vials	methylergonovine maleate
Miacalcin nasal spray	calcitonin salmon
MMR II vials	measles, mumps, rubella virus vaccine live
Mycostatin pastilles	nystatin
Neupogen vials, syringes	filgrastim
Nimbex vials	cisatracurium besylate
Norditropin cartridges	somatropin
Norvir soft gels	ritonavir
Neulasta syringe	pegfilgrastim
Neurontin suspension	gabapentin
Pavulon	pancuronium bromide
Phenergan suppositories	promethazine
Pneumovax 23 vaccine	pneumococcal vaccine polyvalent
Premarin Secule® vials	conjugated estrogens
RabAvert vial	rabies vaccine
Rapamune solution	sirolimus
Rebetron	ribavirin/interferon alfa-2b
Regranex gel	becaplermin
Risperdal Consta kits	risperidone
Sandostatin vials	octreotide acetate
Suprax suspension	cefixime
Survanta vials	beractant
Tamiflu suspension	oseltamivir phosphate
Thyrolar tablets	liotrix
Tracrium vials	atracurium besylate
Veetids suspension	penicillin V
VePesid capsules	etoposide
Vibramycin suspension	doxycycline
Viroptic ophthalmic solution	trifluridine
Xalatan ophthalmic solution	latanoprost
Zemuron vials	rocuronium bromide
Zithromax suspension	azithromycin

GLOSSARY

absorption the movement of the drug from the dosage formulation to the blood.

abstracting services services that summarize information from various primary sources for quick reference.

active transport the movement of drugs from an area of lower concentration to an area of higher concentration; cellular energy is required.

acute condition a sudden condition requiring immediate treatment.

acute viral hepatitis a virus-caused systemic infection that causes inflammation of the liver.

additive a drug that is added to a parenteral solution.

additive effects the summation in effect when two drugs with similar pharmacological actions are taken.

admixture the resulting solution when a drug is added to a parenteral solution.

adverse drug reaction an unintended side affect of a medication that is negative or in some way injurious to a patient's health.

agonists drugs that activate receptors to accelerate or slow normal cell function.

alimentary tract the organs from the mouth to the anus. The GI tract is a portion of the alimentary tract.

aliquot a portion of a mixture.

alveolar sacs (alveoli) the small sacs of specialized tissue that transfer oxygen out of inspired air into the blood and carbon dioxide out of the blood and into the air for expiration.

ampules sealed glass containers with an elongated neck that must be snapped off.

analgesia a state in which pain is not felt even though a painful condition exists.

anaphylactic shock a potentially fatal hypersensitivity reaction producing severe respiratory distress and cardiovascular collapse.

androgens male sex hormones.

anemia a deficiency of red blood cells in blood.

anhydrous without water molecules.

antagonists drugs that bind with receptors but do not activate them. They block receptor action by preventing other drugs or substances from activating them.

anthelmintics drugs that destroys worms.

antibiotic a substance which harms or kills microorganisms like bacteria and fungi.

antibiotic therapy a common home infusion service used for treating AIDS-related and other infections.

antidote a drug that antagonizes the toxic effect of another drug.

antihyperlipidemics drugs that lower cholesterol and triglyceride levels.

anti-pyretic reduces fever.

antitoxin a substance that acts against a toxin in the body; also, a vaccine containing antitoxins, used to fight disease.

antitussive a drug that acts against a cough.

aqueous water based.

arrest knob the knob on a balance that prevents any movement of the balance pans.

arrhythmia an abnormal heart rhythm.

aseptic techniques methods that maintain the sterile condition of products.

automated dispensing system a system in which medications are dispensed from an automated unit at the point of use upon confirmation of an order communicated by computer from a central system.

automated filling machines automated machines that fill and label pill bottles with correct quantities of ordered drugs.

auxiliary labels labels regarding specific warnings, foods or medications to avoid, potential side effects, etc.

bactericidal kills bacteria.

bacteriostatic retards bacteria growth

batching preparation of large quantities of unit-dose oral solutions/suspensions or small volume parenterals for future use.

bevel an angled surface at the tip of a needle.

beyond-use date a date assigned to a compounded prescription telling the patient when the formulation should no longer be taken.

bioavailability the relative amount of an administered dose that reaches the general circulation and the rate at which this occurs.

biocompatibility not irritating; does not promote infection or abscess.

bioequivalency the comparison of bioavailability between two dosage forms.

biopharmaceutics the study of the factors associated with drug products and physiological processes, and the resulting systemic concentrations of the drugs.

blocker another term for an antagonist drug, because antagonists block the action of neurotransmitters.

body surface area a measure used for dosage that is calculated from the height and weight of a person and measured in square meters.

bronchodilators a medication that decongests the bronchial tubes.

browser a software program that allows users to view Web sites on the World Wide Web.

buccal inside the cheek.

buffer system ingredients in a formulation designed to control the pH.

bulk compounding log a record of medications that are compounded in the pharmacy for non-specific patients. Information must include a list of all the ingredients, amounts used, manufacturer, lot numbers and expiration dates of each specific ingredient.

calcium channel blockers drugs that lower blood pressure by relaxing blood vessels.

calibrate to set, mark, or check the graduations of a measuring device.

carcinogenicity the ability of a substance to cause cancer.

cardiac cycle the contraction and relaxation of the heart that pumps blood through the cardiovascular system.

central pharmacy the main in-patient pharmacy in a hospital that has pharmacy satellites. It is the place where most of the hospital's medications are prepared and stored.

certification a legal proof or document that an individual meets certain objective standards, usually provided by a neutral professional organization.

Chapter <795> regulations from USP/NF pertaining to the nonsterile compounding of formulations.

Chapter <797> regulations from USP/NF pertaining to the sterile compounding of formulations.

chronic condition a continuing condition that requires ongoing treatment for a prolonged period.

chyme the semi-liquid form of food as it enters the intestinal tract.

cirrhosis a chronic and potentially fatal liver disease causing loss of function and increased resistance to blood flow through the liver.

clean room area designed for the preparation of sterile products.

closed formulary a limited list of approved medications.

clotting factors factors in the blood coagulation process.

CMS-1500 (formerly HCFA 1500) form the standard form used by health care providers, such as physicians, to bill for services. It can be used to bill for disease state management services.

CMS-10114 form the standard form used by health care providers to apply for a National Provider Identifier (NPI).

co-insurance an agreement for cost-sharing between the insurer and the insured.

co-pay the portion of the price of medication that the patient is required to pay.

code cart a locked cart of medications designed for emergency use only.

colloids particles up to a hundred times smaller than that those in suspensions that are, however, likewise suspended in a solution.

Combat Methamphetamine Epidemic Act (CMEA) Federal law that sets daily and monthly limits on OTC sale of pseudoephedrine and ephedrine.

combining vowel a vowel used to connect the prefix, root word, or suffix parts of a term.

competent being qualified and capable.

complexation when molecules of different chemicals attach to each other.

compliance doing what is required.

compounded sterile preparation (CSP) a compounded sterile parenteral dosage form that will be parenterally administered.

compounding record a record of what actually happened when the formulation was compounded.

compression molding a method of making suppositories in which the ingredients are compressed in a mold.

concentration the strength of a solution as measured by the weight-to-volume or volume-to-volume of the substance being measured.

confidentiality the requirement of health care providers to keep all patient information private among the patient, the patient's insurer, and the providers directly involved in the patient's care.

conjunctiva the eyelid lining.

conjunctivitis inflammation of the conjunctiva (eyelid lining).

consultant pharmacist develops and maintains an individual pharmaceutical plan for each long-term care patient.

contraceptive device or formulation designed to prevent pregnancy.

controlled substance mark the mark (CII-CV) which indicates the control category of a drug with a potential for abuse.

controlled substances five groups of drugs identified by the 1970 Controlled Substances Act (CSA) as having the potential for abuse and whose distribution is therefore strictly controlled by five control schedules set forth in the CSA.

conversions the change of one unit of measure into another so that both amounts are equal.

coring when a needle damages the rubber closure of a parenteral container causing fragments of the closure to fall into the container and contaminate its contents.

cornea the transparent outer part of the eye.

corticosteroid hormonal steroid substances produced by the cortex of the adrenal gland.

counting tray a tray designed for counting pills.

GLOSSARY

Current Procedural Terminology Codes (CPT Codes) identifiers used for billing pharmacist-provided MTM Services.

data information that is entered into and stored in a computer system.

database a collection of information structured so that specific information within it can easily be retrieved and used.

DEA number required on all controlled drug prescriptions; identifies the prescriber.

deductible a set amount that must be paid by the patient for each benefit period before the insurer will cover additional expenses.

denominator the bottom or right number in a fraction which is divided into the numerator to give the fraction's value.

depot the area in the muscle where a formulation is injected during an intramuscular injection.

depth filter a filter that can filter solutions being drawn into or expelled from a syringe, but not both ways in the same procedure.

dermatological a product used to treat a skin condition.

diabetes mellitus a condition in which the body does not produce enough insulin or is unable to use it efficiently.

dialysis movement of particles in a solution through permeable membranes.

diastolic phase the blood pressure after the heart has completed a pumping stroke.

diastolic pressure the minimum blood pressure when the heart relaxes; the second number in a blood pressure reading.

diluent a solvent that dissolves a freeze-dried powder or dilutes a solution.

disintegration the breaking apart of a tablet into smaller pieces.

dispense as written (DAW) mechanism by which a prescriber may indicate that the brand product, not the equivalent generic, must be dispensed.

displacement a drug bound to a plasma protein is removed when another drug of greater binding potential binds to the same protein.

disposition a term sometimes used to refer to all of the ADME processes together.

dissociation when a compound breaks down and separates into smaller components.

dissolution when the smaller pieces of a disintegrated tablet dissolve in solution.

distributive pharmacist makes sure long-term care patients receive the correct medications ordered.

diuretics drugs that increase the elimination of salts and water through urination.

drip rounds a process in which the pharmacy technician goes to specific nursing units to find out what IV drips will be needed later that day.

drug-diet interactions when elements of ingested nutrients interact with a drug and this affects the disposition of the drug.

drug recall voluntary or involuntary removal of a drug product by the manufacturer; usually pertaining to a particular shipment or lot number.

DSL a digital subscriber line that provides digital data transmission over the wires of a local phone network.

dual co-pay co-pays that have two prices: one for generic and one for brand medications.

dual marketing status of medications like Plan B® that are classified as both prescription and OTC drugs.

duration of action the time drug concentration is above the minimum effective concentration (MEC).

edema swelling from abnormal retention of fluid.

electrocardiogram (EKG or ECG) a graph of the heart's rhythms.

electrolytes a substance that in solution forms ions that conduct an electrical current.

electronic medical record (EMR) or electronic health record (EHR) a computerized patient medical record.

elimination the processes of metabolism and excretion.

embolism, embolus a clot that has traveled in the bloodstream to a point where it obstructs flow.

emergency drug procurement to quickly obtain a medication not currently in stock in the pharmacy in situations where the drug is urgently needed.

emulsifier a stabilizing agent in emulsions.

emulsions mixture of two liquids that do not mix with each other; one liquid is spread through the other by mixing and using an emulsifier for stability.

endocrine system a system of glands that secrete hormones into the bloodstream.

enteral a route of administration to any organ in the alimentary tract (ie., from the mouth to the anus).

enterohepatic cycling the transfer of drugs and their metabolites from the liver to the bile in the gall bladder, and then into the intestine, and then back into circulation.

enzyme a complex protein that catalyzes chemical reactions.

enzyme induction the increase in hepatic enzyme activity that results in greater metabolism of drugs.

enzyme inhibition the decrease in hepatic enzyme activity that results in reduced metabolism of drugs.

epidural a sterile, preservative-free medication administered into a patient's epidural space (located near the spinal cord and backbone).

equivalent weight a drug's molecular weight divided by its valence; a common measure of electrolyte concentration.

estrogens female sex characteristic hormones that are involved in calcium and phosphorus conservation.

eustachian tube the tube that connects the middle ear to the throat.

exempt narcotics medications with habit-forming ingredients that can be dispensed by a pharmacist without a prescription to persons at least 18 years of age.

extemporaneous compounding the on-demand preparation of a drug product according to a physician's prescription, formula, or recipe.

extracellular fluid the fluid outside the body's individual cells found in plasma and tissue fluid.

fibrin the fiber that serves as the structure for clot formation.

fibrinogen Factor I.

final filter a filter that filters solution immediately before it enters a patient's vein.

finger cots protective coverings for fingers.

first-pass metabolism the substantial degradation of an orally administered drug caused by enzyme metabolism in the liver before the drug reaches the systemic circulation.

Flashball flexible rubber tubing near the needle adapter on an administration set; used to determine if the needle is properly placed in the veins.

flexor movement an expansion or outward movement by muscles.

flocculating agent electrolytes used in the preparation of suspensions.

flow rate the rate (in ml/hour or ml/minute) at which solution is administered to the patient.

Food and Drug Administration (FDA) a national regulatory body in the United States that oversees the approval, manufacture, and distribution of drugs, for the safety of the public.

formulary a list of stocked drugs that have been selected based on therapeutic factors as well as cost or a list of drugs covered by a third party plan.

formulation record formulas and procedures (i.e., recipes) for what should happen when a formulation is compounded.

fusion molding a suppository preparation method in which the active ingredients are dispersed or dissolved in a melted suppository base.

gastric emptying time the time a drug will stay in the stomach before it is emptied into the small intestine.

gauge a measurement with needles: the higher the gauge, the smaller the lumen.

geometric dilution a technique for mixing two powders of unequal quantity.

glaucoma disorders characterized by abnormally high pressure within the eye that leads to optic nerve damage and loss of vision.

glomerular filtration the blood filtering process of the nephron.

glucagon a hormone that helps convert amino acids to glucose.

gout a painful inflammatory condition in which excess uric acid accumulates in the joints.

Health Insurance Portability and Accountability Act (HIPAA) a federal act that, among other things, protects the privacy of individuals and the sharing of protected health information.

hematopoietics drugs used to treat anemia.

hemorrhoid painful swollen veins in the anal/rectal area, generally caused by strained bowel movements from hard stools.

hemostatic drugs drugs that prevent excessive bleeding.

HEPA filter a high efficiency particulate air filter.

heparin lock an injection device which uses heparin to keep blood from clotting in the device.

HMOs a network of providers for which costs are covered inside but not outside of the network.

home care agencies home nursing care businesses that provide a range of health care services, including infusion.

homeostasis the state of equilibrium of the body.

horizontal flow hood a laminar flow hood where the air crosses the work area in a horizontal direction.

hormones chemicals produced by the body that regulate body functions and processes.

hub the part of the needle that attaches to the syringe.

human genome the complete set of genetic material contained in a human cell.

hydrates absorbs water.

hydrophilic capable of associating with or absorbing water.

hydrophilic emulsifier a stabilizing agent for water-based dispersion mediums.

hydrophobic water repelling; cannot associate with water.

hypersensitivity an abnormal sensitivity generally resulting in an allergic reaction.

hyperthyroidism a condition in which thyroid hormone secretions are above normal, often referred to as an overactive thyroid.

hypertonic when a solution has a greater osmolarity than that of blood.

GLOSSARY

hypothyroidism a condition in which thyroid hormone secretions are below normal, often referred to as an underactive thyroid.

hypotonic when a solution has a lesser osmolarity than that of blood.

idiosyncrasy an unexpected reaction the first time a drug is taken, generally due to genetic causes.

immiscible cannot be mixed.

infusion the gradual intravenous injection of a volume of fluid into a patient.

injectability the ease of flow when a suspension is injected into a patient.

injunction a court order preventing a specific action, such as the distribution of a potentially dangerous drug.

in-patient pharmacy pharmacy located in a hospital or inpatient facility which services only those patients in the hospital/facility and ancillary areas.

inspiration breathing in.

insulin a hormone that controls the body's use of glucose.

integumentary system the body covering, i.e., skin, hair, and nails.

Internet Service Provider (ISP) a company that provides access to the Internet.

interpersonal skills skills involving relationships between people.

interstitial fluid tissue fluid.

intracellular fluid cell fluid.

intraocular inside the eye.

intrauterine device (IUD) an intrauterine contraceptive device that is placed in the uterus for a prolonged period of time.

intravenous piggyback (IVPB) a small volume parenteral that will be added into or "piggybacked" into a large volume parenteral (LVP).

inventory to make an accounting of items on hand; also, with people, to assess characteristics, skills, qualities, etc.

ions molecular particles that carry electric charges.

irrigation solution large volume splash solutions used during surgical or urologic procedures to bathe and moisten body tissues.

Islands (or Islets) of Langerhans specialized cells of the pancreas that secrete insulin.

isotonic when a solution has an osmolarity equivalent to that of blood.

lacrimal canalicula the tear ducts.

lacrimal gland the gland that produces tears for the eye.

laminar flow continuous movement at a uniform rate in one direction.

least common denominator smallest possible denominator for an equivalent fraction so that two fractions can be added or subtracted and have the same denominator.

legend drug any drug which requires a prescription and either of these "legends" on the label: "Caution: Federal law prohibits dispensing without a prescription," or "Rx only."

levigation triturating a powder drug with a solvent in which it is insoluble to reduce its particle size.

liability legal responsibility for costs or damages arising from misconduct or negligence.

lipoidal fat like substance.

lipophilic emulsifier a stabilizing agent for oil-based dispersion mediums.

local effect when drug activity is at the site of administration.

look-alikes drug names that have similar appearance, particularly when written.

lumen the hollow center of a needle.

lymphocytes a type of white blood cells that helps the body defend itself against bacteria and diseased cells.

lyophilized freeze-dried.

maintenance medication a medication that is required on an ongoing basis for a chronic condition.

mark-up the difference between the retailer's sale price and their purchase price.

materia medica generally pharmacology, but also refers to the drugs in use (from the Latin materia, matter, and medica, medical).

Material Safety Data Sheets (MSDS) OSHA required notices for hazardous substances that provide hazard, handling, clean-up, and first aid information.

maximum allowable cost (MAC) the maximum price per tablet (or other dispensing unit) an insurer or PBM will pay for a given product.

Medicaid a federal-state program, administered by the states, providing health care for the needy.

Medicare a federal program providing health care to people with certain disabilities over age 65; it includes basic hospital insurance, voluntary medical insurance, and voluntary prescription drug insurance.

medication administration record (MAR) a form that tracks the medications administered to a patient in institutional settings.

medication order the form used to prescribe medications for patients in institutional settings.

Medication Therapy Management Services (MTMS) services provided to some Medicare beneficiaries who are enrolled in Medicare Part D and who are taking multiple medications or have certain diseases.

medullary paralysis an overdose of anesthesia that paralyzes the respiratory and heart centers of the medulla, leading to death.

membrane filter a filter that attaches to a syringe and filters solution through a membrane as the solution is expelled from the syringe.

meniscus the curved surface of a column of liquid.

metabolite the substance resulting from the body's transformation of an administered drug.

metastasis when cancer cells spread beyond their original site.

milliequivalent (mEq) a unit of measure for electrolytes in a solution.

mimetic another term for an agonist, because agonists imitate or "mimic" the action of the neurotransmitter.

minimum effective concentration (MEC) the blood concentration needed for a drug to produce a response.

minimum toxic concentration (MTC) the upper limit of the therapeutic window. Drug concentrations above the MTC increase the risk of undesired effects.

miscible capable of being mixed together.

modem computer hardware that enables a computer to communicate through telephone lines.

molecular weight the sum of the atomic weights of a molecule.

mucilage a wet, slimy liquid formed as an initial step in the wet gum method.

mydriatics drugs that dilate the pupil.

myocardium heart muscle.

nasal cavity the cavity behind the nose and above the roof of the mouth that filters air and moves mucous and inhaled contaminants outward and away from the lungs.

nasal inhaler a device which contains a drug that is vaporized by inhalation.

nasal mucosa the cellular lining of the nose.

National Drug Code (NDC) number the number assigned by the manufacturer of a drug. The first five digits indicate the manufacturer. The next four indicate the medication, its strength, and dosage form. The last two indicate the package size.

National Provider Identifier a unique, national, ten-digit, health care provider identification number, required for all HIPAA regulated claims submissions.

necrosis increase in cell death.

negligence failing to do something that should or must be done.

neoplasm a new and abnormal tissue growth, often referring to cancer cells.

nephron the functional unit of the kidneys.

nephrotoxicity the ability of a substance to harm the kidneys.

neuron the functional unit of the nervous system.

neurotransmitter chemicals released by nerves that interact with receptors to cause an effect.

nomogram a chart showing relationships between measurements.

non-formulary drugs not on the formulary which the physician can order; a physician may have to fill out a form stating why that particular drug is needed.

numerator the top or left number in a fraction that indicates a portion of the denominator to be used.

obstructive jaundice an obstruction of the bile excretion process.

off-label indication a use of a medication for an indication not approved by the FDA.

oil-in-water emulsion an emulsion in which oil is dispersed through a water base.

Omnibus Budget Reconciliation Act of 1990 (OBRA '90) a federal act that is generally credited for states mandating pharmacist counseling on all new prescriptions.

online adjudication the resolution of prescription coverage through the communication of the pharmacy computer with the third party computer.

onset of action the time MEC is reached and the response occurs.

open formulary a system that allows the pharmacy to purchase any medication that is prescribed

ophthalmic related to the eye.

"Orange Book" the common name for the FDA's *Approved Drugs Products with Therapeutic Equivalence.*

osmosis the action in which a drug in a higher concentration solution passes through a permeable membrane to a lower concentration solution.

osmotic pressure a characteristic of a solution determined by the number of dissolved particles in it.

osseous tissue the rigid portion of the bone tissue.

osteoarthritis a disorder characterized by weight-bearing bone deterioration, decreasing range of motion, pain, and deformity.

outpatient pharmacy a pharmacy attached to a hospital servicing patients who have left the hospital or who are visiting doctors in a hospital outpatient clinic.

over-the-counter (OTC) drugs medications that do not require a prescription but may be filled with a prescription. Some insurance companies cover prescriptions for OTC drugs.

panacea a cure-all (from the Greek panakeia, same meaning).

GLOSSARY

par amount of drug product that should be kept on the pharmacy shelf. Each drug product may have a different par value. Par levels may also be assigned to drug products in automated dispensing cabinets.

parenteral a route of administration to any organ outside of the alimentary tract (e.g., ophthalmic, dermal).

passive diffusion the movement of drugs from an area of higher concentration to lower concentration.

patient assistance programs manufacturer sponsored prescription drug programs for the needy.

pediatric having to do with the treatment of children.

percutaneous absorption the absorption of drugs through the skin, often for a systemic effect.

peristalsis the wave like motion of the intestines that moves food through them.

peritoneal dialysis solution a solution placed in and emptied from the peritoneal cavity to remove toxic substances.

perpetual inventory a system that maintains a continuous record of every item in inventory so that it always shows the stock on hand.

personal inventory to assess one's personal characteristics, skills, qualities, etc.

pH the pH scale measures the acidity or the opposite (alkalinity) of a substance. 7 is the neutral midpoint of the scale, values below which represent increasing acidity, and above which represent increasing alkalinity.

pharmaceutical of or about drugs; also, a drug product.

pharmaceutical alternative drug products that contain the same active ingredient, but not necessarily in the same salt form, amount, or dosage form.

pharmaceutical equivalent drug products that contain identical amounts of the same active ingredient in the same dosage form.

pharmacogenetics a new field of study which defines the hereditary basis of individual differences in absorption, distribution, metabolism, and excretion (the ADME processes).

pharmacognosy derived from the Greek words "pharmakon" or drug and "gnosis" or knowledge; the study of physical, chemical, biochemical and biological properties of drugs as well as the search for new drugs from natural sources.

pharmacology the study of drugs—their properties, uses, application, and effects (from the Greek pharmakon: drug, and logos: word or thought).

pharmacopeia an authoritative listing of drugs and issues related to their use.

pharmacy benefit managers companies that administer drug benefit programs.

pharmacy satellite a branch of the in-patient pharmacy responsible for preparing, dispensing, and monitoring medication for specific patient areas.

piggybacks small volume solutions added to an LVP.

placebo an inactive substance given in place of a medication.

pneumatic tube a system which shuttles objects through a tube using compressed air as the force; commonly used in hospitals for delivery of medication.

point of sale system (POS) an inventory system in which the item is deducted from inventory as it is sold or dispensed.

positional notation the position of the number carries a mathematical significance or value.

POSs a network of providers where the patient's primary care physician must be a member and costs outside the network may be partially reimbursed.

potentiation when one drug with no inherent activity of its own increases the activity of another drug that produces an effect.

PPOs a network of providers where costs outside the network may be partially reimbursed and the patient's primary care physician need not be a member.

prefix a modifying component of a term located before the other components of the term.

prescription a written order from a practitioner for the preparation and administration of a medicine or device.

prescription drug benefit cards cards that contain third party billing information for prescription drug purchases.

Prescription Drug Plans (PDPs) third party programs for Medicare Part D.

primary emulsion the initial emulsion to which ingredients are added to create the final product.

primary literature original reports of clinical and other types of research projects and studies.

PRN order an order for medication to be administered only on an as needed basis.

product labeling important associated information that is not on the label of a drug product itself.

professionals individuals who receive extensive and advanced levels of education before being allowed to practice, such as physicians and pharmacists.

progestins a female sex characteristic hormones that are involved in ovulation prevention.

protease inhibitor an antiviral used for HIV and Hepatitis C that blocks the enzyme responsible for viral replication.

protein binding the attachment of a drug molecule to a plasma or tissue protein, effectively making the drug inactive, but also keeping it within the body.

protocols specific guidelines for practice.

punch method a method for filling capsules by repeatedly pushing or "punching" the capsule into an amount of drug powder.

purchase order number the number assigned to each order for identification.

pyrogens chemicals produced by microorganisms that can cause pyretic (fever) reactions in patients.

qs ad the quantity needed to make a prescribed amount.

ready-to-mix a specially designed minibag where a drug is put into the SVP just prior to administration.

recall the action taken to remove a drug from the market and have it returned to the manufacturer.

receptor the cellular material at the site of action that interacts with the drug.

reconstitute addition of water or other diluent to commercially made drug bottles or vials in order to make a solution or suspension from a pre-made powder form of the drug. This may include oral or parenteral products.

remission a state in which cancer cells are inactive.

reorder points minimum and maximum stock levels which determine when a reorder is placed / for how much.

restricted distribution medications having limited availability due to cost, manufacturing problems, or safety concerns. Typically pharmacies must ensure enrollment before obtaining the restricted drug.

retina the inner lining of the eye that translates light into nerve impulses.

rheumatoid arthritis a disease in which the body's immune system attacks joint tissue.

root word the base component of a term which gives a word its meaning and which may be modified by other components.

safety caps a child-resistant cap.

Schedule II drugs drugs that have a high potential for abuse or addiction but that also have safe and accepted medical uses; they require special handling.

scope of practice what individuals may and may not do in their jobs.

search engine software that searches the Web for information related to criteria entered by the user.

secondary literature general reference works based upon primary literature sources.

selective (action) the characteristic of a drug that makes its action specific to certain receptors and the tissues they affect.

sensitivity the amount of weight that will move the balance pointer one division mark on the marker plate.

serum glucose blood sugar.

shaft the stem of the needle that provides the overall length of the needle.

sharps needles, jagged glass or metal objects, or any items that might puncture or cut the skin.

shelf stickers stickers with bar codes that can be scanned for inventory identification.

short stability medication that will expire soon after preparation (i.e., within 1-6 hours after preparation).

signa the directions for use on the prescription that must be printed on the prescription label.

signature log a book in which patients sign for the prescriptions they receive, for legal and insurance purposes.

site of action the location where an administered drug produces an effect.

Slip-Tip®, Luer-Lok®, eccentric, oral different types of syringe tips.

solution a clear liquid made up of one or more substances dissolved in a solvent.

solvent a liquid that dissolves another substance in it.

sonication exposure to high frequency sound waves.

spatulation mixing powders with a spatula.

stability the chemical and physical integrity of the dosage form, and when appropriate, its ability to withstand microbiological contaminations.

standing order a standard medication order for patients to receive medication at scheduled intervals.

STAT order an order for medication to be administered immediately.

sterile a sterile condition is one which is free of all microorganisms, both harmful and harmless.

stratum corneum the outermost cell layer of the epidermis.

sublingual under the tongue.

suffix a modifying component of a term located after the other components of the term.

surgical anesthesia the stage of anesthesia in which surgery can be safely conducted.

suspensions formulations in which the drug does not completely dissolve in the liquid.

synergism when two drugs with similar pharmacological actions produce greater effects than the sum of the individual effects.

synthetic with chemicals, combining simpler chemicals into more complex compounds, creating a new chemical not found in nature as a result.

syringeability the ease with which a suspension can be drawn from a container into a syringe.

systemic effect when a drug is introduced into the circulatory system and carried to the site of activity.

systolic phase the blood pressure as the heart is pumping blood into the cardiovascular system.

systolic pressure the maximum blood pressure when the heart contracts; the first number in a blood pressure reading.

technicians individuals who are given a basic level of training designed to help them perform specific tasks.

teratogenecity the ability of a substance to cause abnormal fetal development when given to a pregnant woman.

tertiary literature condensed works based on primary literature, such as textbooks, monographs, etc.

testosterone the primary androgen.

therapeutic equivalent pharmaceutical equivalents that produce the same effects in patients.

therapeutic window a drug's blood concentration range between its minimum effective concentration and minimum toxic concentration.

thickening agent an ingredient used in the preparation of suspensions to increase the viscosity of the liquid.

thrombus a blood clot.

tier categories of medications that are covered by third party plans.

topical hemostatics drugs used for minor bleeding when sutures are not appropriate.

total nutrient admixture (TNA) solution a TPN solution that contains intravenous fat emulsion.

total parenteral nutrition (TPN) solution complex solutions with two base solutions (amino acids and dextrose) and additional micronutrients.

trade journals journals published commercially for pharmacists but not produced by the profession; they tend to contain large amounts of advertising material.

transaction window counter area designated for taking prescriptions and dispensing them.

transcorneal transport drug transfer into the eye.

trituration the process of grinding powders to reduce particle size.

turnover the rate at which inventory is used, generally expressed in number of days.

tympanic membrane the membrane that transmits sound waves to the inner ear.

uniform resource locator (URL) a Web address.

unit-dose packaging a package containing the amount of a drug required for one dose.

unit price the price of a unit of medication (such as an ounce of liquid cold remedy).

universal claim form a standard claim form accepted by many insurers.

uricosuric drugs drugs used to treat gout that increase the elimination of uric acid.

usual and customary (U&C or UCR) usual and customary—the maximum amount of payment for a given prescription, determined by the insurer to be a usual and customary (and reasonable) price.

valence the number of positive or negative charges on an ion.

variable an unknown value in a mathematical equation.

vasodilators drugs that relax and expand the blood vessels.

vertical flow hood a laminar flow hood where the air crosses the work area in a vertical direction.

viscosity the thickness of a liquid.

volumetric measures volume.

water-in-oil emulsion an emulsion in which water is dispersed through an oil base.

water soluble the property of a substance being able to dissolve in water.

waters of hydration water molecules that attach to drug molecules.

wheal a raised blister-like area on the skin caused by an intradermal injection.

workers' compensation an employer compensation program for employees accidentally injured on the job.

World Wide Web (WWW) a collection of electronic documents at Internet addresses called Web sites.

ANSWER KEY

Chapter 1
Match the Terms
1. h
2. g
3. l
4. i
5. j
6. f
7. d
8. c
9. k
10. e
11. b
12. a

Multiple Choice
1. c
2. b
3. b
4. b
5. a
6. b
7. d
8. c
9. c
10. a
11. d
12. c
13. a
14. c
15. a
16. a
17. b
18. c
19. d
20. c
21. d
22. c
23. a
24. c
25. b
26. d
27. d
28. c

Chapter 2
Match the Terms
1. e
2. d
3. c
4. h
5. b

6. g
7. a
8. f

Multiple Choice
1. d
2. b
3. c
4. c
5. d
6. b
7. b
8. d
9. b
10. a
11. c
12. d
13. d
14. a
15. a
16. a
17. a
18. d
19. b
20. b
21. b
22. a
23. d
24. c
25. c
26. d
27. c

Chapter 3
Match the Terms
1. *p*
2. *j*
3. *s*
4. *h*
5. *o*
6. *f*
7. *a*
8. *q*
9. *b*
10. *e*
11. *i*
12. *c*
13. *l*
14. *m*
15. *k*
16. *d*
17. *r*

18. *g*
19. *n*

Multiple Choice
1. a
2. b
3. c
4. d
5. b
6. b
7. c
8. b
9. c
10. d
11. b
12. d
13. a
14. c
15. a
16. d
17. b
18. c
19. c
20. b
21. a
22. a
23. b
24. a
25. c
26. a
27. d

Chapter 4
Match the Terms I
1. d
2. g
3. p
4. n
5. w
6. a
7. h
8. o
9. y
10. f
11. j
12. v
13. r
14. k
15. q
16. m
17. x
18. b

19. u
20. e
21. l
22. i
23. c
24. s
25. t

Match the Terms II
1. a
2. c
3. e
4. d
5. h
6. f
7. g
8. i
9. b

Match the Terms III
1. b
2. e
3. c
4. d
5. j
6. k
7. h
8. a
9. f
10. g
11. i
12. l

Multiple Choice
1. a
2. b
3. b
4. c
5. b
6. a
7. c
8. c
9. d
10. d
11. a
12. b
13. d
14. c
15. c
16. d
17. c
18. a

19. b
20. d
21. c
22. b
23. b
24. c

Chapter 5
Match the Terms I
1. g
2. d
3. i
4. f
5. c
6. b
7. a
8. h
9. e

Match the Terms II
1. h
2. b
3. d
4. k
5. i
6. a
7. n
8. f
9. e
10. l
11. m
12. g
13. j
14. c

Multiple Choice
1. c
2. c
3. d
4. b
5. a
6. c
7. d
8. d
9. a
10. d
11. c
12. b
13. b
14. b
15. b
16. b

ANSWER KEY

17. a
18. a
19. d
20. b
21. c
22. a
23. c
24. d

Chapter 6

p. 105
1. XVIII
2. LXIV
3. LXXII
4. CXXVI
5. C
6. VII
7. XXVIII
8. 33
9. 110
10. 1,100
11. 1.5
12. 19
13. 24
14. 14 capsules
15. 9 drops
16. 48 tablets
17. 21 tablets

p. 107
1. 0.33
2. 0.5
3. 0.25
4. 0.3
5. 0.1
6. 5/1
7. 3/2
8. 5/2
9. 9/2
10. 15/1

p. 108
1. 2/4 = 1/2
2. 8/8 = 1
3. 1/5
4. 4/8 = 1/2
5. 5/5 = 1
6. 4/8 = 1/2
7. 9/20
8. 7/15
9. 7/16
10. 3/8

p. 109
1. 1/16
2. 3/24 = 1/8
3. 2/9
4. 15/64
5. 2/3
6. 4/12 = 1/3
7. 10/5 = 2
8. 24/24 = 1

p. 110
1. 1.3
2. 7.4
3. 4.34
4. 23.798
5. 72.31
6. 4.6926
7. 276.096
8. 359.3404
9. 230.4465
10. 5288.5529

p. 111
1. -0.16
2. 8.63
3. 14.29
4. 0.9726
5. 71.965
6. 14.592
7. 251.1229
8. 20.6699
9. 459.8842
10. 368.32

p. 112
1. 0.35
2. 0.32
3. 0.09
4. 0.15
5. 22.2
6. 0.159
7. 0.144
8. 0.0264
9. 581.0248
10. 382.6764

p. 117
1. mcg
2. l or L
3. ml or mL
4. g (gm)
5. mg
6. kg
7. 1,000

8. 1,000
9. 129.6
10. 1,000
11. 0.001
12. 0.001

p. 117
1. 7,000
2. 3,200
3. 0.0648
4. 30
5. 300
6. 7,000
7. 437.5
8. 1.1
9. 2
10. 1
11. 32
12. 0.25

p. 127
1. 2 ml
2. 8 ml
3. 75 ml
4. 2.08 ml/mn
5. 4.8 mL

p. 129
1. 60%
2. 80%
3. 12%
4. .5
5. .125
6. .99
7. 35 g
8. 52.5 g
9. 14 g
10. 50 ml
11. 70 ml
12. 20 ml
13. 0.12%

p. 134
1. 73.5 ml Amin. 8.5%
2. 37.5 ml dext 50%
3. 2 ml KCl
4. 0.45 ml Ca Gl.
5. 5 ml Ped MVI
6. 131.55 mL sterile water is needed

p. 144
1. $45.76
2. $18.40
3. $11.50
4. $328.38
5. $27.05

p. 145
1. $8.54
2. $17.49
3. $37.24
4. $94.90
5. $122.09
6. $8.09
7. $16.64
8. $35.37
9. $8.91
10. $162.50

p. 147
1. gross $24.46 net $18.46
2. gross $17.18 net $11.18
3. gross $19.90 net $13.90
4. gross $29.31 net $23.31
5. gross $23.63 net $17.63
6. gross $31.39 net $25.39
7. gross $54.06 net $48.06
8. gross $6.71 net $0.71
9. gross $25.59 net $19.59
10. gross $22.63 net $16.63

Self-Test
Match the Terms
1. *l*
2. *g*
3. *d*
4. *b*
5. *f*
6. *o*
7. *j*
8. *m*
9. *c*
10. *a*
11. *i*

12. *h*
13. *n*
14. *k*
15. *e*

Self-Test *Multiple Choice*
1. b
2. c
3. c
4. d
5. d
6. a
7. b
8. b
9. b
10. c
11. b
12. c
13. a
14. b
15. c
16. b
17. b
18. d
19. b
20. c
21. c
22. a
23. c
24. c
25. a
26. c
27. c
28. b
29. b

Self-Test *Conversion Exercise*
1. 5,000 mg
2. 10,000 g
3. 0.3 L
4. 0.6 g
5. 0.12 mg
6. 224.4 lb
7. 2,200 g
8. 0.473 L
9. 65.9 kg
10. 10,000 mg

Self-Test *Problems*
1. 7.8°C
2. 2 mL
3. 2.5 ml

4. 143 ml Dext
    70% and 357
    ml sterile water

Chapter 7
Match the Terms I
1. p
2. d
3. l
4. f
5. b
6. k
7. o
8. s
9. j
10. h
11. w
12. x
13. c
14. g
15. a
16. i
17. q
18. r
19. n
20. m
21. e
22. t
23. u
24. v

Match the Terms II
1. m
2. c
3. b
4. g
5. a
6. k
7. e
8. h
9. f
10. j
11. d
12. l
13. i

Multiple Choice
1. b
2. d
3. c
4. c
5. d
6. c

7. b
8. b
9. a
10. d
11. a
12. d
13. d
14. c
15. c
16. a
17. b
18. d
19. d
20. b
21. b
22. c
23. c
24. b
25. a
26. c
27. a
28. a
29. c

Chapter 8
Match the Terms I
1. m
2. i
3. a
4. n
5. h
6. f
7. j
8. o
9. p
10. g
11. d
12. q
13. b
14. r
15. k
16. e
17. c
18. l

Match the Terms II
1. y
2. n
3. e
4. d
5. b
6. k
7. c

8. l
9. p
10. f
11. q
12. u
13. i
14. r
15. j
16. t
17. a
18. x
19. o
20. s
21. m
22. h
23. g
24. w
25. z
26. v

Multiple Choice
1. b
2. c
3. d
4. c
5. d
6. d
7. c
8. d
9. c
10. b
11. d
12. b
13. c
14. c
15. d
16. d
17. b
18. b
19. d
20. a
21. d

Chapter 9
Match the Terms I
1. h
2. b
3. c
4. i
5. a
6. d
7. g
8. k

9. j
10. m
11. e
12. f
13. l

Match the Terms II
1. a
2. r
3. q
4. p
5. s
6. d
7. c
8. b
9. l
10. m
11. o
12. f
13. i
14. h
15. e
16. j
17. n
18. g
19. k

Multiple Choice
1. b
2. b
3. b
4. d
5. d
6. d
7. c
8. d
9. d
10. a
11. a
12. a
13. a
14. b
15. d
16. b
17. a
18. b
19. c
20. d
21. a
22. c

Chapter 10
Match the Terms I
1. r
2. q
3. s
4. t
5. e
6. d
7. c
8. p
9. o
10. n
11. m
12. l
13. k
14. b
15. j
16. a
17. i
18. h
19. g
20. f
21. u

Match the Terms II
1. j
2. f
3. i
4. k
5. g
6. c
7. n
8. l
9. a
10. b
11. d
12. e
13. m
14. h

Multiple Choice
1. a
2. c
3. d
4. c
5. d
6. d
7. c
8. c
9. c
10. a
11. b
12. b

ANSWER KEY

13. d
14. a
15. c
16. c
17. b
18. c
19. b
20. a
21. b
22. b
23. d
24. c

Chapter 11
Match the Terms
1. j
2. f
3. p
4. c
5. h
6. e
7. i
8. a
9. r
10. k
11. t
12. s
13. b
14. m
15. n
16. d
17. l
18. o
19. q
20. g

Multiple Choice
1. b
2. d
3. a
4. c
5. a
6. c
7. c
8. b
9. b
10. c
11. d
12. b
13. a
14. c
15. a

16. a
17. c
18. d
19. a
20. a
21. a
22. c
23. c
24. a
25. d

Chapter 12
Match the Terms
1. d
2. n
3. j
4. e
5. h
6. m
7. p
8. l
9. f
10. a
11. i
12. k
13. c
14. b
15. o
16. g

Multiple Choice
1. b
2. c
3. a
4. c
5. b
6. b
7. b
8. c
9. c
10. c
11. d
12. b
13. b
14. a
15. a
16. b
17. c
18. c
19. a
20. b
21. d

22. b
23. a
24. b
25. c

Chapter 13
Match the Terms
1. m
2. b
3. f
4. n
5. k
6. g
7. a
8. j
9. d
10. h
11. e
12. l
13. c
14. i

Multiple Choice
1. b
2. a
3. a
4. b
5. b
6. d
7. c
8. c
9. a
10. a
11. a
12. b
13. c
14. c
15. d
16. c
17. b
18. a
19. d
20. c
21. d
22. a
23. a
24. a
25. c
26. b
27. d
28. b

Chapter 14
Match the Terms I
1. i
2. n
3. e
4. b
5. m
6. g
7. f
8. o
9. h
10. c
11. d
12. j
13. k
14. l
15. a

Match the Terms II
1. d
2. a
3. f
4. g
5. e
6. i
7. j
8. c
9. b
10. h

Multiple Choice
1. a
2. a
3. c
4. b
5. d
6. a
7. b
8. b
9. b
10. a
11. b
12. a
13. a
14. d
15. d
16. b
17. c
18. a
19. a
20. c
21. c

22. d
23. d

Chapter 15
Match the Terms
1. j
2. f
3. e
4. a
5. h
6. c
7. i
8. g
9. b
10. d

Multiple Choice
1. d
2. a
3. a
4. d
5. c
6. b
7. b
8. b
9. d
10. a
11. d
12. b
13. d
14. d
15. a
16. a
17. c
18. a
19. d
20. a
21. a
22. d
23. c
24. c
25. d
26. c
27. a
28. c
29. b

Chapter 16
Match the Terms I
1. d
2. h
3. i

4. g
5. b
6. k
7. q
8. n
9. c
10. l
11. a
12. p
13. j
14. m
15. e
16. f
17. o
18. r

Match the Terms II
1. m
2. g
3. b
4. d
5. e
6. f
7. h
8. a
9. i
10. j
11. k
12. c
13. l

Multiple Choice
1. c
2. d
3. c
4. a
5. d
6. a
7. d
8. d
9. c
10. d
11. d
12. d
13. b
14. d
15. d
16. c
17. b
18. b
19. a
20. b

21. d
22. c
23. b

Chapter 17
Match the Terms
1. d
2. e
3. h
4. a
5. b
6. g
7. f
8. c

Multiple Choice
1. a
2. a
3. c
4. a
5. b
6. b
7. c
8. d
9. a
10. a
11. d
12. a
13. c
14. b
15. b
16. d
17. c
18. a
19. c
20. a

Chapter 18
Match the Terms I
1. c
2. r
3. p
4. v
5. e
6. d
7. f
8. g
9. b
10. w
11. l
12. m
13. a

14. t
15. h
16. u
17. i
18. j
19. q
20. s
21. k
22. o
23. n

Match the Terms II
1. e
2. c
3. g
4. m
5. o
6. j
7. a
8. s
9. q
10. h
11. d
12. f
13. p
14. n
15. l
16. i
17. b
18. w
19. r
20. t
21. k
22. u
23. v
24. x

Match the Terms III
1. f
2. i
3. d
4. e
5. a
6. h
7. c
8. j
9. g
10. b

Multiple Choice
1. c
2. c

3. a
4. a
5. a
6. b
7. c
8. b
9. d
10. b
11. d
12. a
13. c
14. a
15. a
16. c
17. b
18. d
19. a
20. c
21. b
22. d
23. a
24. d
25. b
26. b
27. a
28. c
29. a
30. d